Into Teachers' Hands:
Creating Classroom Success

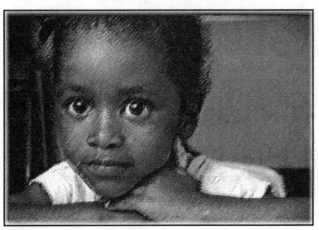

Contents:

ISSUES

MULTIYEAR EDUCATION

EARLY CHILDHOOD

UPPER ELEMENTARY

ASSESSMENT

FOR FURTHER THOUGHT

RESOURCES/ BIBLIOGRAPHY

Into Teachers' Hands: Creating Classroom Success.
SDE Sourcebook. © Copyright 1998 by The Society For Developmental Education.
All rights reserved. Printed in the United States of America.
Published by The Society For Developmental Education, Ten Sharon Road, PO Box 577, Peterborough, New Hampshire 03458.
Phone 1-800-924-9621
FAX 1-800-337-9929
e-mail: sde.csb@socdeved.com
website: www.socdeved.com

ELEVENTH EDITION Gift 4/00

President: Jay LaRoche
Executive Director: Jim Grant
Program Director: Irv Richardson
Publishing Manager: Lorraine Walker
Editor: Meredith Reed
Assistant Editor: Aldene Fredenburg
Cover and Book Design: Susan Dunholter
Production Coordinator: Christine Landry

ISBN 1-884548-22-9

Can EDUCATION Reduce Social Inequity?

There is a crisis of equity in U.S. schools. Once thought of as the most equalizing institution in our society, public schools play as much of a role in magnifying differences between children from wealthy and impoverished backgrounds and between children of different ethnic backgrounds as they do in overcoming these differences.

The equity gap relates both to the opportunities children are provided and to the outcomes they achieve. Regarding opportunities, children from lower-class homes start off at a disadvantage, with less access to prenatal and early health care, quality day care as infants, quality early childhood programs, and other supports that most children from middle-class homes take for granted. The school system often compounds these inequities. In most states, the amount of money spent on education is strongly influenced by local property values. As a result, children who live in low-wealth inner cities or rural areas are likely to receive much less in per-pupil funding than are children in wealthy suburbs. In most states, the difference in per-pupil funding between the highest-spending districts (95th percentile) and the lowest-spending (5th percentile) is a ratio of from 1.5:1 to 2:1.

For example, in 1990, high-spending districts in Pennsylvania spent $7,058 per pupil, compared to $3,794 for low-spending districts. The difference was $5,457 to $3,910 in Florida, $4,557 to $2,803 in Missouri, and $6,078 to $3,879 in Oregon (Riddle and White 1993). A difference of even $1,000, a typical difference between an inner city and its surrounding suburbs, translates into $25,000 per class per year for a class of 25 students, or a half-million dollars for a typical elementary school of 500 children. Of course, even equal dollars would not be equal in impact; schools serving many children in poverty also have to cope with higher needs for special education services, security guards, and other services not needed in wealthier jurisdictions.

This degree of inequity is unique in the industrialized world. All major trading partners of the United States at least *equalize* funding for all children, but in most cases they provide *additional* funding for poor or minority children. In the Netherlands, for example, a funding formula provides 25 percent more funding for each lower-class Dutch child in a school and 90 percent more funding for each minority child. European observers of our schools are aghast to discover that our system does exactly the opposite.

In outcomes, American students vary substantially according to social class and ethnicity. For example, on the 1994 National Assessment of Educational Progress (NAEP) (Campbell et al. 1996), 71 percent of white 4th graders scored at or above the *basic* level in reading. Only 31 percent of African-American and 36 percent of Latino students scored that well. These differences correspond closely with differences in social class. Among 4th graders whose parents graduated from college, 70 percent were reading at or above the basic level. This drops to 54 percent for children of high school graduates and 32 percent for children of high school dropouts. Among children whose homes had magazines, newspapers, encyclopedias, and at least 25 books, about 70 percent scored at or above basic; among those without these resources, fewer than half scored this well. Differences in mathematics, writing, and science are similar. Further, performance differences increase as students get older.

In some ways, the equity gap has been diminishing. Since the first NAEP assessments in 1971, the difference between African-American and white students in NAEP reading and other measures has been cut in half. Differences in Scholastic Assessment Test (SAT) scores have also been dropping. Dropout rates for African-American students have diminished substantially over the past 20 years, although those for Latino students remain very high.

Most of the gains made by minority students, however, took place during the 1970s, when major improvements in the education of African-American students were taking place in the South. Since 1980, the gap has slightly increased, with a particularly disturbing drop in the reading performance of African-American and Latino 4th graders in 1994.

The Equity Gap Is Unacceptable and Unnecessary

The differences in academic performance among children from different social class and ethnic backgrounds are

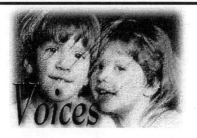

Voices

Regardless of race or ethnicity, poor children are much more likely than nonpoor children to suffer developmental delay and damage, to drop out of high school, and to give birth during the teen years.

— *Ruby Payne, Ph.D.,* quoted in Miranda, 1991

From *Poverty: A Framework for Understanding and Working With Students and Adults From Poverty,* by Ruby K. Payne, Ph.D. Baytown, TX: RFT Publishing, 1995.

unacceptably large, and they are not diminishing rapidly enough. These differences underlie many of the most polarizing issues in the United States, from affirmative action to immigration policies. Their consequences are getting progressively worse, as the income gap between well-educated and poorly educated workers is increasing. We cannot have a just or peaceful society if major segments of it see little hope for their children.

There will always be achievement differences, on average, among groups of students. No one realistically expects that the children of high school dropouts and those of college graduates will ever perform at exactly the same levels. Yet these gaps are far greater than they need to be. In particular, differences among ethnic groups are unacceptably high and completely unnecessary. Some portion of these differences results from socioeconomic differences among different ethnic groups, over which the schools have no control. Nevertheless, schools can have a powerful impact on the educational success of all children and can greatly increase the achievement of disadvantaged and minority children. As educators, we cannot wait for U.S. society to solve its problems of racism and economic inequity. We can and must take action now to prepare all children to achieve their full potential.

How Can We Reduce the Equity Gap?

The only way to decrease the equity gap in academic performance is to greatly increase the achievement and school success of disadvantaged and minority students. If we could place a high floor under the achievement of all children, regardless of social background, we would substantially reduce inequalities. Imagine, for example, that we could ensure that every American 4th grader were reading at or above the basic level on NAEP, as President Clinton has proposed. This would be enormously

beneficial for millions of white, middle-class students, of course, but it would have a far more dramatic effect on disadvantaged and minority children, as a group. Imagine how different U.S. schools and society would be if every child entering 5th grade had 5th grade reading and math skills.

No single policy or program can ensure the school success of every child, but a combination of approaches can. Research in education is increasingly identifying the kinds of approaches we could use if we decided as a society to

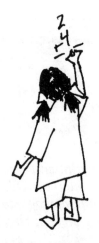

end the poor academic performance of so many of our children.

1. Begin to think of all children as being at promise. The first requirement for a policy designed to ensure the school success of all children is to change the mindset of educators and policymakers. As my colleague Wade Boykin (1996) puts it, we need to move away from seeing children as being *at risk* toward seeing them as being *at promise.* We identify and build on cultural and personal strengths, and accept nothing less than outstanding performance. Rather than thinking in terms of remediation or compensation,

we insist on high-quality instruction sensitive to students' needs from the beginning of their time in school and respond immediately and intensively if children start to fall behind.

2. Start early. As a rule, children enter preschool or kindergarten highly motivated, bright-eyed and bushy-tailed, fully confident in their abilities to learn. Schools can build on this energy and enthusiasm and thereby ensure children a good start in elementary school. Research on Head Start and other programs for 3- and 4-year-olds finds consistent and powerful impacts of high-quality early childhood programs on the cognitive performance of young children (McKey et al. 1985; Berrueta-Clement et al. 1984). Researchers debate long-term effects of preschool experiences; clearly, no one-year or two-year program will ensure the success of every child (see Karweit 1994). But there is no question that quality early childhood programs can

> We cannot have a just or peaceful society if major segments of it see little hope for their children.

greatly enhance children's preparation for elementary school; it's just up to the school to take advantage of this preparation.

One extraordinary study shows how much early intervention can contribute to the success of children who are placed at risk. The Abecedarian Project provided the children of low-income African-American parents in North Carolina with intensive services from infancy to age 8. The project included high-quality infant care, preschool, kindergarten, and school-age programs; support to parents; and other services. In comparison to matched controls, the children in the Abecedarian Project scored substantially higher on measures of IQ, reading, and mathematics, at ages 8, 12, and 15. By age 15, Abecedarian children were half as likely to have been assigned to special education or to have been retained (Campbell and Ramey 1995).

The Abecedarian Project is too expensive under current conditions to replicate widely, but it clearly establishes the principle that nothing is inevitable about the failure of so many at-risk children.

These results and those from other early intervention programs that continue into the early elementary grades (Karweit 1994) demonstrate that we can make a substantial difference in the school success of children placed at risk if we stop the process of falling behind before it begins.

3. Overdetermine success—work on many fronts at once. Children who are placed at risk by their life circumstances can fail for many reasons. Effective schooling, therefore, anticipates all the ways children might fail and then plans how each will be prevented or quickly and effectively dealt with. Wade Boykin (1996) calls this "over-determining success"— being *overprepared* to ensure the success of every child.

An example of over-determining success is our own Success for All program (Slavin et al. 1996). It provides elementary schools, mostly high-poverty schoolwide Title I schools, with an array of programs and services intended to ensure that children begin with success in preschool and then remain successful throughout the elementary grades. The program emphasizes research-based materials and instructional approaches from prekindergarten

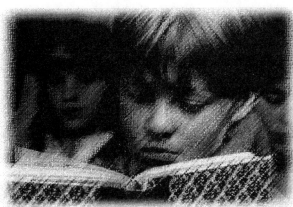

to 6th grade, with extensive professional development, follow-up, and assessment to be sure that all students are on track. If children begin to fall behind in reading, teachers or para-professionals may give them one-to-one tutoring until the children are able to progress on their own with their classmates. A family support program engages parents in their children's learning and solves such nonacademic problems as truancy, behavior problems, or the need for eyeglasses.

Research on Success for All in 12 school districts in the United States has shown consistent positive effects of the program. On average, Success for All children read almost three months

ahead of matched controls at the end of 1st grade, and more than a full year ahead at the end of 5th grade. That difference is maintained into middle school (Slavin et al. 1996). In nearly every study, the students who gain the most are those who are most at risk: low achievers, special education students, and speakers of languages other than English (a Spanish bilingual version of the program has been particularly successful). Special education referrals are typically cut in half or, in one study, cut to a quarter of what they had been before (Smith et al. 1994).

One study of Success for All found that the program eliminated an achievement gap between African-American and white students. This study (Ross et al. 1997) compared integrated Success for All and control schools in Ft. Wayne, Indiana. At pretest, African-American and white students showed large differences on reading scores. At post-test, these differences remained in the control schools, but in the Success for All schools they had essentially disappeared, because African-American students made substantial gains.

Other programs also demonstrate that if we want to place a high floor under the achievement of all children, we can do it. One widely known example is Reading Recovery, which provides one-to-one tutoring to 1st graders who are falling behind in reading. Studies of Reading Recovery find consistent positive effects of the program on student reading achievement (Lyons et al. 1993).

Reading Recovery and Success for All are expensive, of course, but large numbers of schools have shifted resources to fund them. As of fall 1997, Success for All is in 750 schools, and Reading Recovery is in more than 6,000. But consider: What does "expensive" mean? Imagine that all high-poverty schools received the funding typical in suburban schools. Every school could afford Success for All, Reading Recovery, high-quality preschool programs, and much more.

At present, schools and districts fund these programs primarily through Title I; but high-poverty, underfunded schools face very difficult choices in the use of these funds. All high-poverty schools should be able to provide effective programs for their students, even if these programs are costly.

Are We Willing to Do What It Takes?

The research on the Abecedarian Project, Success for All, Reading Recovery, and other programs demonstrates that if we, as a society, decided to substantially reduce the equity gap, we could do so. We could decrease the gap between middle-class and disadvantaged children—not by taking away from the middle class but by building a high floor under the achievement level of all children, of all backgrounds. Simply by giving high-poverty schools the resources typical of suburban schools, and focusing these new

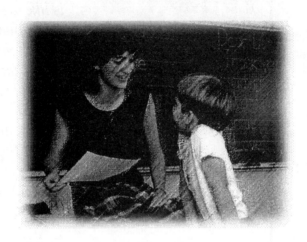

We can make a substantial difference in the school success of children placed at risk if we stop the process of falling behind before it begins.

resources on proven, replicable programs and practices, we could make profound changes in the achievement gaps that so bedevil our educational system and our society.

Certainly we need more research and more development to understand how to transform large numbers of schools and to solve remaining tough problems. But we already know enough to take action. So many children are suffering, and we know how to help them. How can we justify doing less? ■

References

Berrueta-Clement, J.R., L.J. Schweinhart, W.S. Barnett, A.S. Epstein, and D.P. Weikart. (1984). *Changed Lives*. Ypsilanti, Mich.: High/Scope.

Boykin, A.W. (April 10, 1996). "A Talent Development Approach to School Reform." Paper presented at the annual meeting of the American Educational Research Association, New York.

Campbell, F.A., and C.T. Ramey. (1995). "Cognitive and School Outcomes for High-risk African-American Students at Middle Adolescence: Positive Effects of Early Intervention." *American Educa-tional Research Journal* 32: 743–772.

Campbell, J.R., P.L. Donahue, C.M. Reese, and G.W. Phillips. (1996). *NAEP 1994 Reading Report Card for the Nation and the States*. Washington, D.C.: National Center for Education Statistics, U.S. Department of Education.

Karweit, N.L. (1994). "Can Preschool Alone Prevent Early Reading Failure?" In *Preventing Early School Failure*, edited by R.E. Slavin, N.L. Karweit, and B.A. Wasik. Boston: Allyn and Bacon.

Lyons, C.A., G.S. Pinnell, and D.E. DeFord. (1993). *Partners in Learning: Teachers and Children in Reading Recovery*. New York: Teachers College Press.

McKey, R., L. Condelli, H. Ganson, B. Barrett, C. McConkey, and M. Plantz. (1985). *The Impact of Head Start on Children, Families, and Communities*. Washington, D.C.: CSR, Inc.

Riddle, W., and L. White. (1993). *Variations in Expenditures per Pupil among Local Educational Agencies Within the States*. Washington, D.C.: Congressional Research Service.

Ross, S.M., L.J. Smith, and J.P. Casey. (1997). "Preventing Early School Failure: Impacts of Success for All on Standardized Test Outcomes, Minority Group Performance, and School Effectiveness." *Journal of Education for Students Placed at Risk* 2, 1: 29–53.

Slavin, R.E., N.A. Madden, L.J. Dolan, and B.A. Wasik. (1996). *Every Child, Every School: Success for All*. Thousand Oaks, Calif.: Corwin.

Smith, L.J., S.M. Ross, and J.P. Casey. (1994). *Special Education Analyses for Success for All in Four Cities*. Memphis. Tenn.: University of Memphis, Center for Research in Educational Policy.

Robert E. Slavin is Codirector of the Center for Research on the Education of Students Placed At Risk (CRESPAR), 3505 N. Charles St., Baltimore, MD 21218-2498 (e-mail: rslavin@inet.ed.gov). Web site (http://scov.csos.jhu.edu/crespar/CReSPaR.html).

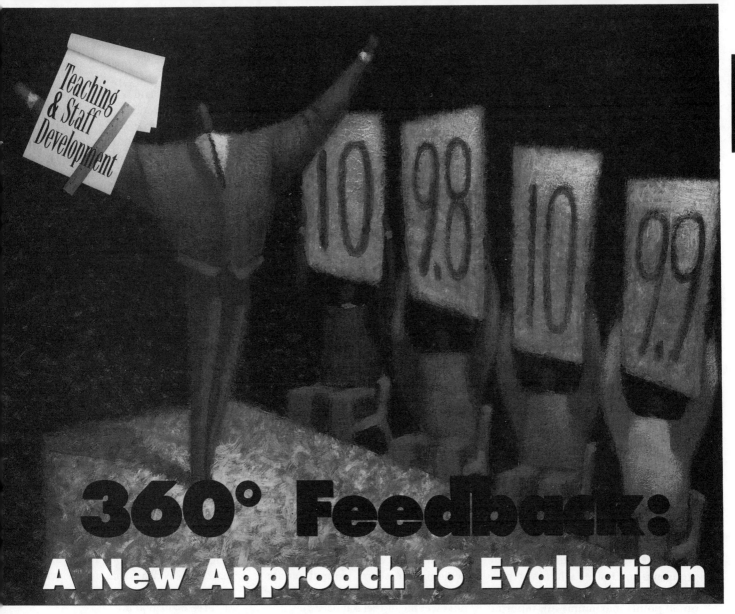

360° Feedback:
A New Approach to Evaluation

*You can learn a lot about a teacher when you get input
from students, parents, and other teachers.*

RICHARD P. MANATT AND MARI KEMIS

There is nothing more difficult to plan, more doubtful of success, nor more dangerous to manage than the creation of a new system. For the initiator has the enmity of all who would profit by the preservation of the old system, and merely lukewarm defenders in those who would gain by the new one.

Niccolo Machiavelli, 1513

Despite Machiavelli's dour prediction, some school districts have begun to create new systems that are more promising than the old. One of the most important of these reforms involves teacher evaluation. The old system, still widely practiced, calls for a single evaluator—usually the principal—to pass judgment on a teacher's ability. This places an enormous responsibility on principals who may not possess the necessary skills or experience.

Teacher evaluation was a major concern back in 1964, when professors and research specialists at the Iowa State University College of Education launched a long-term effort to measure and improve not only how teachers teach, but how administrators lead, and how students learn. By 1978, this research effort became the School Improvement Model (SIM).

SIM uses a total systems approach to measure and report teacher performance. It is an approach that focuses on student achievement and emphasizes validity, reliability, and discrimination.

• *Validity* means that the criteria and results—measured behaviors that result in effective learning—are truthful.

• *Reliability* means that the results remain consistent with different evaluators over different periods of time.

Richard P. Manatt is director of the School Improvement Model at Iowa State University in Ames.

Mari Kemis is senior research associate at the Research Institute for Studies in Education at Iowa State University.

"360° Feedback: A New Approach to Evaluation," by Richard C. Manatt and Mari Kemis. *Principal,* Volume 77, Number 1, September 1997, pp. 24, 26-27. Reprinted with permission.

- *Discrimination* means the ability to distinguish high performance from average performance from marginal performance.

Developing a Performance Evaluation

The heart of SIM's total systems approach to teacher evaluation is its 360° feedback from anyone who has had contact with the teacher, including the principal, other teachers, parents, and students. A similar approach is used to evaluate principals (*see box*).

Student feedback is an important component of the evaluation system. SIM has developed student feedback instruments for grades K-2, 3-5, 6-8, and 9-12 that rate teacher preparation, instructional delivery, and student interest (Omotani and Manatt 1993; Weber and Manatt 1993). These student ratings also can be used to show differences among teachers in the quality of instruction, and can be compared with national norms established by SIM's ratings of 500 teachers by more than 21,000 students.

SIM's reporting of student feedback consists of four components. First, a summary report provides aggregated total scores for each of the four grade groupings and for the school system as a whole. Second, total scores (based on 80 points maximum) are reported for each teacher. Third, mean scores and frequency distributions are reported for each of 20 items, by grade level and teacher. Fourth, mean scores and frequency distributions are reported by teacher for each class section surveyed.

Putting the System to Work

Lincoln County School District 1 is a small district in southwestern Wyoming that for the last six years has been a showcase for SIM's total systems approach to evaluation. It began when Superintendent Ron Maughan became concerned about the district's lack of consistency in determining which teachers would be advanced to tenure at the end of the state-mandated three years of probation.

"All too often," he said, "some marginal candidates worked really hard in their third year of probation, and then fell back into a marginal level of performance

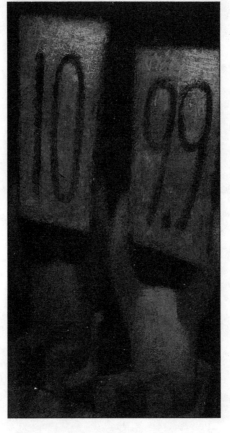

after tenure was granted." The district's Stanford Eight achievement tests and frequent observation by principals didn't seem to be effective.

Maughan turned to the SIM center for a better evaluation system. "We wanted to use a three-track approach that would have different evaluation standards for beginning teachers, tenured teachers, and those few teachers who cannot or will not meet the district standards."

Working with a planning committee comprised of teachers, parents, students,

"PRINCIPALS...

ARE ADVISED TO

START WITH

FEEDBACK

FROM TEACHERS

TO THEMSELVES."

administrators, and board members, SIM personnel introduced the concept of 360° feedback to evaluate both teachers and principals. By using surveys of students and parents for teachers, and teachers and parents for principals, SIM was able to supply data to supplement and strengthen both principals' ratings of teachers and the superintendent's ratings of principals.

By the time Terry Ebert became superintendent in 1996, all of the system's components were operational, including pre-test and post-test assessment of all students in all subjects at the elementary school level. Ebert marvels at how much easier it is to work in a district where multiple data sets provide rich information on the performance of students, teachers, and principals. "Educators in this district don't realize how lucky they are," Ebert says.

How a Principal Uses Feedback

Lyn Hendry, an experienced principal with thorough training in clinical supervision, recently completed her first year as principal of Kemmerer Elementary School and Burgoon Primary School in Lincoln County District 1. She reports that 360° feedback has made her job much easier as she works with teachers in all three evaluation tracks.

By consulting available feedback reports, Hendry was able to quickly assess the climate and achievement levels in her two buildings. Teachers' feedback from the previous year provided the new principal with their expectations for school administration as well as indicators of the teachers' cohesiveness, morale, and goal orientation.

Hendry also could examine student achievement gains for the past year by student, classroom, and building, using data based on district-specific curricula and learner outcomes, as measured by criterion-referenced tests.

Single-page reports for every teacher contained the teacher's self-rating on each of 20 questions, the ratings by the previous principal, and the mean ratings of the teacher's class. Hendry believes that such concise information enabled her to quickly orient herself to her new students and faculty, and to appreciate their accomplishments, concerns, and needs. She was able to pinpoint strengths across classrooms as well as problem areas.

Looking Ahead

Some or all components of 360° feedback are now in place in public school districts in five states, and longitudinal studies in two districts have demonstrated dramatic improvements in student achievement and equity.

Extensive research is now under way, using Lincoln County District No. 1's data, to explore the relationships of all elements of SIM's total systems approach: achievement test gains; students' characteristics; principals' ratings of teachers; teachers' ratings of principals; school climate; and subjects taught.

Principals seeking to use 360° feedback are advised to start with feedback from teachers to themselves. The three rating scales of SIM's School Improvement Inventory (SII) can give the principal insights into what teachers expect from the principal, as well as their perceptions of the quality of the principal's performance and school climate.

The next step is to offer teachers an opportunity to obtain student and parent feedback. It's wise to give both teachers and principals feedback on an "eyes only" basis for the first year. After that, feedback data should be shared with the appropriate evaluators.

Machiavelli warned those who introduce a new system to expect resistance, and this is certainly true for 360° feedback. But while many administrators seem to have a great fear of feedback, the linking of evaluation with national standards has caused a number of them to re-examine this approach.

Few of us would play a round of golf without asking "What's par for this course?" and runners always ask, "How'd I do this time?" as they cross the finish line. Principals will find 360° feedback a valuable tool as they seek to improve quality in their continuing quest for excellence. □

REFERENCES

Omotani, L. and Manatt, R. "Student Ratings Belong in Total Teacher Performance Evaluation Systems." *People and Education,* 1:3 (1993): 266-283.

Weber, B. and Manatt, R. "Elementary Students' Ratings of Teacher Performance: Issues of Bias, Reliability, and Discrimination Power." *People and Education,* 1:3 (1993): 284-302.

FOR MORE INFORMATION

To learn more about 360° feedback, contact the School Improvement Model Office at Iowa State University, 1-515-294-5521, or e-mail rmanatt@iastate.edu.

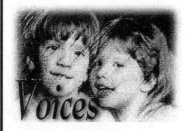

*P*eople forget how fast you did a job — but they remember how well you did it.

— *Howard W. Newton*

From *Teacher's Inspirations: Motivational Quotes for You and Your Students* © 1990, Great Quotations, Inc.

Thinking About Standards

By Nel Noddings

The current emphasis on national standards is distracting us from larger social problems that must be addressed, Ms. Noddings cautions.

REASONABLE, well-intentioned people often disagree about the wisdom and usefulness of national standards as a strategy for education reform. None of us would argue in favor of low standards or no standards, but some of us fear that the concept of standards has not been analyzed carefully enough to warrant establishing national standards, that proponents of such standards have not fully considered the possibility of undesirable consequences, and that many closely associated issues, consideration of which might counsel a different role for government, have largely been ignored.

What Is a Standard?

Even staunch supporters of national standards admit that there is considerable confusion about the idea of a standard.[1] Some see a standard as a flag of sorts — something to rally around. Others see it as a goal to be reached, and still others see it as a description of various proficiency levels. In this last sense, a standard is a norm for quality control. Perhaps the clearest statement comes from Diane Ravitch, who describes three interrelated categories of standards: content (or curriculum) standards, performance standards, and opportunity-to-learn standards.

Content standards describe "what teachers are supposed to teach and students are expected to learn."[2] Immediately, a matter that concerns many thoughtful educators arises. This innocent-sounding statement moves us too hastily past an important educational debate. Must students learn everything that teachers teach, or should the curriculum be rich in opportunities for the cooperative construction of learning objectives? Many of us who regard ourselves as good teachers provide much more than we expect students to learn, and we are often pleased and surprised when they learn things we hadn't anticipated. Of course, there are some things that we think all students should know as a result of taking a particular course, but specifying exactly which things is a task requiring considerable thought, and the list we construct for *all* students will properly be much shorter than lists we create or eventually report for each student; we recognize that students have varying interests and capabilities. My main point here is that a simple statement that equates what teachers should teach with what students are expected to learn cuts short what should be a rich and com-

NEL NODDINGS is Lee L. Jacks Professor of Child Education, School of Education, Stanford University, Stanford, Calif., and a professor of philosophy and education, Teachers College, Columbia University, New York, N.Y.

Reprinted with permission of Phi Delta Kappan (Vol. 79, Pages 184-186, November 1997).

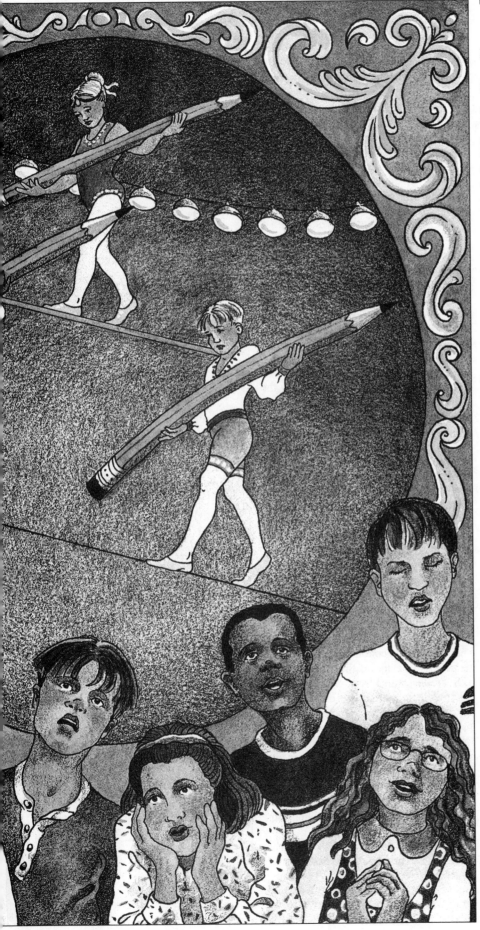

plex educational debate.

"Performance standards define degrees of mastery or levels of attainment."[3] We are familiar with performance standards from sports, from the commercial world of various instruments and appliances, and from licensing tests. Advocates of performance standards for schoolchildren neglect the fact that the performance standards for athletes and professionals are established for those who *choose* to take part in competitions or to enter certain fields. They require a voluntary commitment. K-12 education, by contrast, is compulsory. Students will use their educations for very different purposes; they are not voluntarily entering a particular field of endeavor. This is not to say that there are no skills that should be universally possessed at some level of proficiency, but it is not clear which ones should be specified, and whatever is specified for *all* is likely to be pathetically puny in contrast to what could be suggested if relevant differences in talents, plans, affiliations, and interests were taken into account. Any set of standards rich enough for a particular student will contain items unnecessary for many, and any set designed realistically for all will, paradoxically, be inadequate for anyone considered individually. I'll return to this problem in the next section, where I'll discuss some undesirable outcomes that may well emerge from the standards movement.

Opportunity-to-learn (OTL) standards "define the availability of programs, staff, and other resources that schools, districts, and states provide so that students are able to meet challenging content and performance standards."[4] How should these standards be determined? If all high school students in a given district are required to take algebra, for example, do they thereby have an "opportunity to learn" algebra? In particular, if students are not adequately prepared for algebra, if they see no reason to study it, if their teacher is not fully competent, if they are crowded into an unpleasant room, if they have to share outdated textbooks, can the *requirement* be regarded as an opportunity to learn? And if poor districts and states are to be held to the same OTL standards as wealthier ones (as poor students are to be held to the same performance standards as wealthier students), who will provide the necessary resources?

It is disheartening that so many adults are willing to prescribe standards that children must meet and yet are so unwilling to dedicate themselves and their resources to meet standards for school delivery. Most advocates of national standards admit that OTL standards in some form are needed, but the political debate has almost faded away. (See, however, the recent New Jersey Supreme Court decision.) At present, fear of federal mandates and interference has all but eliminated meaningful OTL standards at the national level. Children are expected to meet high standards for learning, but it is not clear how poor children and their teachers will meet this expectation. Perhaps the new slogan will be "Just do it!"

Who Will Benefit?
Who Will Be Harmed?

Well-intentioned advocates of national standards often argue that such standards will ensure students in poor districts of an education equal to that of wealthier students. All students will be expected to meet the standards. It is surely right to urge educators to believe in the innate capabilities of poor children. But when we know that the educational status of parents is the single strongest predictor of how children will do in school, it seems ludicrous to suppose that merely stating that "all children will perform task T at level P" will actually accomplish much. Clearly, some children have resources (both inside and outside schools) that make their success more likely.

Many of us fear that national standards may create the illusion that everyone now has a fair chance and that any resulting differences in outcomes — with regard to jobs or further education — are the fault of those who didn't try hard enough. Some people will be squeezed out in a system governed mainly by standards. Thus we have to ask who will benefit from national standards.

A couple of historical cases might prove helpful here. In the early part of this century, the Flexner Report resulted in sweeping changes in medical education. Many medical schools, unable to meet the new standards, had to close. Black schools and black people who needed physicians suffered under the new standards. It could be argued that, in the long run, the entire public benefited from higher standards for the training of physicians and that the temporary suffering of a few was more than offset by the eventual benefit to all. This claim is debatable on several levels, but let us suppose that the changes were intended to benefit all patients and that they accomplished this — lives were saved, pain reduced, more vigorous health maintained. Most of us would say, then, that a good thing was done.

Now consider the dramatic changes effected in college and university departments of literature in the 1920s.[5] In this case, changes were deliberately designed to raise the status of English departments. It was argued that instructors in English departments should look more like those in physics departments — that is, display roughly similar credentials. Sometimes it was explicitly stated that there were too many women in English departments and that their presence reduced the status of the discipline. Standards had to be raised. The result was a drastic reduction not only in female faculty members but in the number of women writers in the canon. Who benefited? Male scholars with the appropriate credentials clearly did so. It would not be easy to argue that students in general benefited from this move or that the general public received some demonstrable good.

Many more such examples could be given. Someone almost always bears a considerable cost when standards are raised or changed. I am not going to argue that the current standards movement is an effort to exclude some groups. But I think we must ask who will benefit and who will be harmed, whether the foreseeable harms are outweighed by the long-term benefits, and whether the immediate harms can be reduced. The benefits most often claimed are for the nation and its ability to compete in a world economy. But there is little persuasive evidence that workers in the U.S. are less capable or productive than other workers. Further, we can't argue, as we did in the 1960s and 1970s, that we need more mathematicians and physicists; we do not. If it is the nation that will benefit, we have to provide convincing evidence that the nation needs something that the schools could, but are now failing to, accomplish. We then have to show how this failing can be corrected by national standards.

Will the children benefit? It is often argued that all children need a "world-class" education to compete in today's economy. But if everyone were to meet new high standards, some would still have to do work that is ill paid today.[6] Even a high-

It seems ludicrous to suppose that merely stating that "all children will perform task T at Level P" will accomplish much.

tech society needs to have food grown, transported, packaged, and sold. It needs maintenance people, servers, cleaners, bus drivers, animal groomers, retail salespersons, clerks, construction workers, plumbers, and a host of other workers. Will we pay more for the same job simply because the workers are better educated? I raise this question because I believe that the current emphasis on national standards is distracting us from larger social problems that must be addressed. Education by itself is not the solution to poverty. Thus it is not clear that national standards will serve all our children.

We might argue that we are aiming at benefits beyond the material. I would be delighted to hear such an argument — that education is rightly aimed at enhancing life in personal, social, recreational, spiritual, moral, and aesthetic domains. Is the standards movement aimed at producing better citizens, more loving and effective parents, persons with greater moral sensitivities, individuals with enhanced social graces and healthy psyches? Wonderful! But now we need an argument that explains just how national standards will promote these benefits. My guess is that all such aims will be deliberately culled from an approved list of national standards because many of our citizens fear the state's intervention in "private" life.

Some advocates of national standards agree with my view of educational aims, and they are as disheartened as I am by the flagging commitment of those in political power to do anything substantial to promote real benefits for children. But others respond that schools are designed only to provide academic instruction, that the kinds of goals I've suggested must be pursued outside of schools, and that national standards are properly aimed at the academic goals for which schools are constituted. Then, of course, we have come full circle. We are once again at a point where we must ask substantial educational questions. How can we begin to decide whether children will benefit if we rush to national standards without considering what aims are defensible for contemporary education?

One group that will clearly benefit from the movement is a subset of professional educators who will work on the project. Some will benefit from the sort of "middle-class welfare" associated with grants, lectures, conferences, consultations, and other activities. I include myself in this group, even though I oppose the movement. Some general good can emerge from these projects, but self-interest will be evident everywhere. Mathematics educators will enthusiastically push math; art educators will push art; social studies educators will translate their own expertise into goals and standards for "all children" that few well-educated adults can meet. Because we know that professional self-interest is already at work, we have an obligation to slow the process, deepen our analysis, and urge a less parochial stance. What questions should we be asking, and how can we avoid the predictable competition among subject-matter experts?

Before leaving the question of harms and benefits, I want to examine a case that, on the surface at least, is less problematic than most others. My purpose is to show how complex the issues are. Suppose we decide to establish standards for a first course in algebra. Surely we cannot expect the same level of performance from all students. Even such a staunch advocate of national standards as Albert Shanker warned educators about this problem. Either our standards will be pitifully low, he said, or many children will fail. To avoid these unacceptable consequences, Shanker advised that we adopt more than one set of standards.[7]

We might, for example, adopt a scheme comparable to that of the National Assessment of Educational Progress; we could evaluate students as failing, basic, proficient, or advanced. Such a plan has the great merit of freeing educators to be honest about what students achieve. At present, we all know that many students are enrolled in "algebra" classes that hardly deserve the name. Students who complete these classes are often chagrined to learn that they must enroll in remedial classes at college. There are days, then, when I think it would be a good idea (at least a token of honesty) to enact such standards.

However, the issue is complicated. Lots of students will not be able to achieve even the basic level, and a reasonable question arises whether all children should be *forced* to take algebra. Here again, we have to retreat at least temporarily from a campaign for standards to a thoughtful discussion of what students really need and whether coercing them ("for their own good") is compatible with preparation for democratic life. In addition to the harm experienced by children who fail (at something they did not choose to do), what will be suf-fered by those who score at the "basic" level? In an age of diminishing commitment to affirmative action, many youngsters who would formerly have qualified on paper (they "took" algebra) will now be weak candidates. How do we feel about this? I confess to being torn. On the one hand, I do not think we should deceive students by letting them suppose they have learned algebra when they have not. On the other hand, if they are *compelled* to take it, when some other form of mathematics might better serve their interests and talents, then I hate to see them penalized for our narrow choices and insistence that "everyone can do it."

I taught high school mathematics for 12 years. It is simply not true that "everyone can do it." Many hard-working, cooperative children have a very hard time with mathematics. I'd like to see a thorough discussion of these matters before committing ourselves to national standards, and I'd like to see respectable — even exciting — alternatives to algebra. If we respect and love our children, there is no reason why courses once regarded as not college preparatory cannot be challenging and useful. Forcing everyone to take algebra in the name of equality is, ultimately, disrespectful and self-defeating.

Neglected Issues

The underlying idea of standards seems to be that we need to be clear about what we are trying to accomplish in schools. There are other ideas that add to the enthusiasm — for example, the simple-minded notion that the U.S. should have a national curriculum because other nations, some of which post high test scores, have centrally controlled education systems. These copycat enthusiasts ignore the fact that the evidence linking central control and educational achievement is scanty. Some centrally controlled systems show up well on tests; others do not. But the belief that a statement of standards will improve education by making the tasks of schooling clear and cogent is, perhaps, the dominant one.

If this is so, thoughtful educators should be led to ask how well such ideas have served us in the past. In the 1970s, for example, the big fad was behavioral objectives, and many school districts invested huge amounts of professional time in rewriting their curricula in terms of these carefully stated objectives. We were supposed to say exactly what students would do (content standards?), to what level of proficiency (performance standards?), and under what conditions (opportunity-to-learn standards?). The objectives movement, despite its vigor and the number of person-hours devoted to it, produced little demonstrable improvement. Indeed, some of us would argue that it reduced the quality of education by making it unnecessary for students to construct their own learning objectives, to learn how to make distinctions between important and less important material, and in general to take responsibility for organizing the material offered.

When objectives didn't "work," policy makers turned to "competencies." Many of us then asked the question I am asking now: How do competencies (or standards) differ from objectives? And if there is no significant difference, why should we waste valuable professional time formulating competencies or standards? Why not put our energies into tasks that are more promising?

During the decade of behavioral objectives, many teachers raised a question that we should take seriously now. They said, in effect: "Look, we've always known that kids are supposed to be able to add fractions with denominators up to 12 in fifth grade. That's not the question. The question is, How do we get them to do it?" Now *there's* a substantial task.

Why don't children learn what we think they should learn? Are our methods faulty? Are we teaching the wrong things? What *are* kids interested in? How can those interests be steered toward the material we deem important? Can schools impart knowledge without the cooperation of parents? These and many other questions point us toward the identification of deep problems that will not yield to the quick fix of stating goals, objectives, competencies, or standards.

Indeed, almost all schools have long had formal statements of goals; many also have detailed expositions of curriculum content. If the careful statement of goals hasn't worked at the local level, why should we suppose it will work at the national level? Of course, there are schools whose staffs seem to have given up and are serving their students badly. They must be reformed. But we don't need a set of national goals to tell us that something is badly wrong with these schools, and national goals will not solve these obvious

problems, because they simply skip over them.

Much more — volumes more — could be said about educational issues that need deep analysis and wide discussion, but I will close with a brief look at how we might approach the topic of standards in a democratic society.[8]

The Role of Standards In Democratic Education

We have long believed that democratic government requires at least the consent, if not the vigorous participation, of the governed. In consonance with this belief, John Dewey insisted on "the importance of the participation of the learner in the formation of the purposes which direct his activities in the learning process."[9] If we are serious about raising standards, we have to help students understand what standards are and how they are related to the students' own purposes. Talking about standards with both teachers and students is not a waste of time. It is a prelude to establishing and meeting any meaningful standards.

To return to my earlier example, how might we discuss algebra standards with our pupils? I would explain frankly to them that there are certain things they must be able to do in order for me to certify to the school that they have learned algebra. I would be honest in confessing that this "basic" level would not be enough for them to tackle further academic mathematics without great difficulty. In reaching this level, they and I would satisfy a contractual requirement laid on us by various credentialing bodies. We would do an honest job at a level compatible with purposes understood by all of us. Then I would describe what has to be done (or what the best professional minds at this time believe must be done) to prepare adequately for further academic mathematics. Again, there would be considerable open conversation about possibilities, purposes, tradeoffs, and commitments. Finally, I would describe an enhanced course with no fixed limits. If you really love mathematics, I would say, there is no clear limit to what we might do together this year, but in the tentative syllabus I'll share with you, you can get a sense of the possibilities.

In this continuing conversation, it should be clear to students that all honest student choices are respected by the teacher. A stu-

dent planning a career in art or journalism, for example, might well want to work toward only basic proficiency in algebra. He or she will thereby satisfy a somewhat arbitrary school requirement. Such students should understand, because the teacher takes the time to advise them conscientiously, that if they change their minds later, they will need further preparation. The conversation is characterized at every point by a cooperative commitment to making well-informed choices. This approach avoids both the coercion so popular today and an irresponsible attitude of laissez-faire. All forms of coercion should be at least questionable in a democracy, and the coercion even of children should be thoroughly examined and justified. At the other extreme, abandoning children to their own ill-considered passions and whims is equally reprehensible. Teaching, at its best, requires familiarity with individual students and their needs. It requires conversation and the cooperative construction of standards.

The discussion of my approach to standards in first-year algebra might lead readers to suppose that I would endorse national standards "done right." I don't think so. The discussion and ensuing standard-setting is best done locally. Professional groups at the national level, such as the National Council of Teachers of Mathematics, can certainly provide invaluable guidance, but local educators have to decide what the sequence of study will be and why. Ideally, they should work closely with community colleges, local four-year institutions, trade schools, and businesses to establish standards that will enable students to make well-informed decisions. Genuine school/business partnerships, for example, would include such cooperative standard-setting, and businesses would provide work/study experiences for young people planning to enter the work world directly from high school. "Partnerships" in which businesses give money or computers and then sit on the sidelines complaining about the school's failures are not genuine partnerships. Setting standards is a sophisticated process both within disciplines and within wage-earning communities.

Throughout this process, in every subject, teachers should continue to ask: Why am I requiring this? Do students understand the mutual commitments we are making? Are the standards defensible? A conversation of this sort might be promoted at the national level, but the actual establishment of standards at the national level might well defeat the whole purpose. If standards are to have meaning, the people who must meet them should be involved in their construction.

It has always been anathema to democratic life for authority to impose its dictates on unwilling subjects. To be sure, children are, by definition, not ready to make adult choices. But they can make some choices, and John Dewey argued that they must be helped to make *well-informed* choices at every stage of development if they are to become competent citizens in a democratic society. What responsibilities do adults — educators, policy makers, parents, citizens — have in aiding this process?

Mortimer Adler and others who advocate a uniform curriculum for all children have suggested that, unless they are coerced into taking certain subjects, some students will downgrade their own education.[10] But if we take our own responsibilities as adults seriously, this should not be possible. Instead of assuming (with little or no evidence to back our contention) that physics is automatically superior to photography,[11] we should pledge ourselves to high standards in every course we offer. The educational questions I raised earlier and a host of others should be directed at *every course* that is offered in our schools.

It should not be possible for students to downgrade their education by choosing among the courses responsible educators offer. A school should be ashamed to offer "good" courses and "bad" courses.

It should also be clear that standards apply to adults and not just children. It is ridiculous and irresponsible to set standards for children that well-educated adults cannot meet. An editorial in *Rethinking Schools* quite rightly mocked Wisconsin Gov. Tommy Thompson's proposal for a fourth-grade standard that states, "Show a basic understanding of the role played by religion and civic values in the history of Wisconsin and the nation, and describe how that role is similar to, or different from, that role in an ancient civilization and a feudal society in Europe or China."[12] The preposterous nature of this standard should underscore my point that standard setting is a complex process requiring sustained debate and sophisticated knowledge.

However, criticism of this one standard should not be taken as criticism of all standards that posit expectations for today's children that their parents cannot meet. Many such expectations are justifiable, even essential. But exactly which ones? Again, we have to avoid not only nonsense but the quite understandable temptation for adult experts in a particular field to suggest (even fervently believe) that every-

one should master skills they possess but that are patently unnecessary for competent life in a democracy.

However, there are standards to which adults in a democratic society should be held. Some time ago, the Government Accounting Office estimated that schools in our nation require more than $200 billion in repairs. Acknowledging this, the incumbent Presidential candidate pledged that the federal government would get the repair process started with some $5 billion. That pledge was quietly ignored when a balanced budget was designed. My own youngest daughter teaches in a classroom with a roof that leaks during every rain. Pots are placed around the room to catch water. This has been going on for years. Perhaps a good start on national standards would require policy makers to establish and achieve defensible standards for their own contributions to the improvement of education. To establish standards for itself and to encourage widespread, thoughtful conversation for the entire citizenry is the best role for the federal government at this time — perhaps at any time.

1. Diane Ravitch, *National Standards in American Education* (Washington, D.C.: Brookings Institution Press, 1995).

2. Ibid., p. 12.

3. Ibid.

4. Ibid., p. 13.

5. See Paul Lauter, "Race and Gender in the Shaping of the American Literary Canon: A Case Study of the Twenties," *Feminist Studies*, vol. 9, 1983, pp. 435-64.

6. See Nel Noddings, "Does Everybody Count?," *Journal of Mathematical Behavior*, vol. 13, 1994, pp. 89-104.

7. See the tribute to Albert Shanker in *Education Week*, 14 May 1997, p. 44.

8. For further discussion of the debate over goals and standards, see Dayle M. Bethel, ed., *Compulsory Schooling and Human Learning: The Moral Failure of Public Education in America and Japan* (San Francisco: Caddo Gap Press, 1994); Blythe McVicker Clinchy, "Goals 2000: The Student as Object," *Phi Delta Kappan*, January 1995, pp. 383-92; Evans Clinchy, ed., *Charting a New Course* (New York: Teachers College Press, 1996); and Ron Miller, ed., *Educational Freedom for a Democratic Society* (Brandon, Vt.: Resource Center for Redesigning Education, 1995).

9. John Dewey, *Experience and Education* (1938; reprint, New York: Macmillan, 1963), p. 67.

10. See Mortimer Adler, *The Paideia Proposal* (New York: Macmillan, 1982).

11. But see Mike Rose, *Possible Lives: The Promise of Public Education in America* (Boston: Houghton Mifflin, 1995). Rose shows that courses in trade-like subjects can be powerful cognitively, instrumentally, aesthetically, and even morally.

12. "Hypocrisy Distorts the Standards Debate," *Rethinking Schools*, Spring 1997, p. 2. K

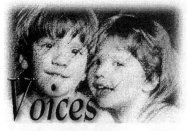

Voices

Many children are denied the opportunity to use their full learning potential by current educational techniques. Budget cutbacks affecting the arts and physical education not only eliminate enrichment classes, but may actually eliminate classes that help visual or kinesthetic learners learn. Our present system is geared to verbal learning, and if your children are not verbal learners, they don't fit the system. Most testing methods are limited to a linear, sequential format geared to verbal content. Visual or kinesthetic students often are labeled "slow learners."

— **Maureen Murdock,**
Spinning Inward

Spinning Inward: Using Guided Imagery With Children for Learning, Creativity and Relaxation. Boston: Shambhala, 1987.

Educational Standards
To Standardize or to Customize Learning?

BY CHARLES M. REIGELUTH

Standards, properly conceived, are just one necessary, but not sufficient, part of a comprehensive redesign of a very complex education system, Mr. Reigeluth notes. If not properly conceived, standards can do far more harm than good.

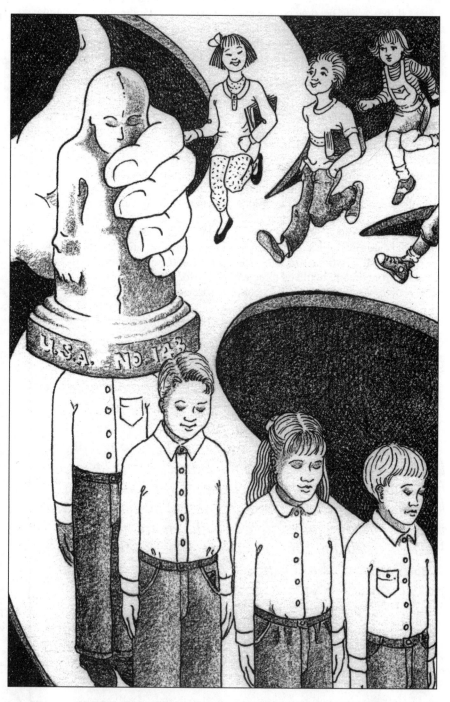

THE EDUCATIONAL standards movement has gained much public visibility. The topic has been extensively covered in the *Kappan* (June 1995), in *Educational Researcher* (November 1996), and in *Educational Leadership* (March 1995). Rigorous educational standards have been strongly advocated by many people, both within and outside the education establishment, including the participants at the recent National Education Summit, who were primarily U.S. governors and business leaders. And many states have passed or are considering legislation establishing educational standards. Clearly, this is an important issue that is likely to affect all who have a stake in public education.

Partly for this reason, there are also many cautionary voices about educational standards. Some voices ask us to consider whether standards should be mandatory or voluntary. Some raise the questions of who should define the standards (e.g., the government or professional associations such as the National Council of Teachers of Math-

CHARLES M. REIGELUTH is a professor of Instructional Systems Technology, School of Education, Indiana University, Bloomington (reigelut@indiana.edu).

ematics) and on what level (national, state, or local). Other voices express concern that the standards movement will lead to test-driven instruction[1] or will impede the move toward thematic or interdisciplinary instruction. And still others caution that higher academic standards are necessary but not sufficient for improving public education.[2]

Differing Conceptions Of Standards

The picture grows even more complicated because different people have different conceptions of standards. For example, Darrell Sabers and Donna Sabers identify "hire" standards (those set by business leaders to ensure that students are employable), "higher" standards (government leaders' more rigorous standards to maintain world-class status for the U.S.), and "high" standards (educators' expectations for high levels of student achievement).[3] Anne Lewis identifies content standards, performance standards, opportunity-to-learn standards, and world-class standards.[4] And the variety of conceptions goes on.

These differing conceptions of standards stem from the differing reasons that people want standards. Business leaders with whom I have spoken in Indiana seem most interested in ensuring that the high school graduates they hire are able to read, write, and compute. They expect to provide job training but not basic skills education. "Hire" standards seem to be conceptualized as minimum standards to ensure competence in basic skills for all students, and they are regarded more as mandatory than as voluntary.

In contrast, government leaders seem more interested in improving U.S. students' world rankings, which requires far more than ensuring the attainment of basic skills. For example, the New Standards (a joint effort of the National Center on Education and the Economy and the Learning Research and Development Center) seem intended as a tool for education reform to help schools "work as systems whose parts are focused on coherent, consistent, publicly articulated goals" because "a centrally articulated set of goals, even if vaguely stated, plays important roles: It organizes the development of exams and curriculums, informs textbook writing, and determines the direction of teacher training."[5]

On the other hand, many educators seem more interested in standards as a vehicle for professionalizing teaching. As Matthew Gandal of the American Federation of Teachers put it, "The basic premise here is that once these standards and monitoring practices are up and running, teachers and schools can be freed from traditionally burdensome rules and given the flexibility to determine the best ways to help their students achieve at higher levels."[6] Still other people have other purposes for advocating standards.

Two Uses of Standards

Given all these purposes and conceptions of educational standards, as well as the cautionary voices about them, what is a reasonable stance to take on standards? To address this question, it is helpful to understand that standards can be used in two very different ways that represent very different views of education, each of which can be applied to any of the purposes described earlier. They can be used as tools for standardization — to help make all students alike. Or they can be used as tools for customization — to help meet individual students' needs. Sabers and Sabers lament, "Unfortunately, most of the discussions about standards have centered on their importance. Less effort has been expended on what they should be, and little thought seems to have been given to the consequences of their implementation."[7] This article addresses both questions in terms of the broader issue of standardizing or customizing education.

Consequences of Uniform Standards

At the National Education Summit in 1996 educational standards were characterized as tools for standardization, a view that also prevails in many of the articles on standards. Martin Covington states, "After reading the Summit statement one is left with the impression that achievement standards are best thought to be imposed equally on all children, irrespective of ability or circumstance."[8] This seems particularly ironic, given that many business leaders are evolving their companies from standardization to customization.[9] The terms "uniform standards" and "common standards" are often applied to this conception of standards. But what are the likely consequences of conceiving of educational standards in this way?

First, because students differ greatly in ability (ranging from severely learning disabled to highly gifted), as well as in mastery of learning skills, prior knowledge, home environment, and so forth, it seems likely that standards that are challenging for some students will be easy for others. Therefore, uniform standards cannot be uniformly challenging (rigorous) for all students and cannot attain the frequently stated goal of standards: to accelerate student performance.

Second, as Covington puts it, "If students cannot now measure up to old, presumably less demanding standards, increased demands seem pointless."[10] To the extent that uniform standards are applied, even with high-stakes accountability, they will most likely lead to more frustration for students and teachers and more high school dropouts, unless great emphasis is placed on improving educational processes. This will require considerable investment in professional development (intensive rather than piecemeal), in powerful learning resources (largely technological), and in systemic change (largely in the roles of teachers, learners, and administrators). Yet there is little talk about seeing that such investments accompany the new standards, and without them the new standards may well do more harm than good.

A third consequence of higher uniform standards — especially if high-stakes accountability is attached to them — is that teachers will feel forced to devote more time to whatever the standards call for, regardless of whether or not they, their students, and their students' parents believe that those standards are important. This will make the education system less flexible at a time when many policy makers and educators alike are calling for more flexibility. The Education Commission of the States, which advises state legislatures and the same governors who attended the National Education Summit, has pointed out:

> The demands on public education are changing in many ways: demographically, economically, politically. To adapt to these changes, public education must be flexible. In a more ordered and less demanding time, it made sense for American states and localities to seek the efficiencies of a uniform model of education. . . .
>
> While flexibility is no panacea, it offers several advantages over a more rigid system of education. Autonomy allows schools to be more responsive to parents' wishes and students' needs.[11]

Similarly, given their frequently exclusive emphasis on academic achievement, higher uniform standards will probably mean that less time will be devoted to the important nonacademic missions that schools serve.[12] The 1996 Phi Delta Kappa/Gallup poll of public attitudes toward the public schools revealed considerable support for nonacademic purposes of public schools.[13]

Daniel Goleman has made a persuasive case that a small investment in emotional- and social-development programs in the public schools can have a powerful influence on reducing violence, teen pregnancy, drug dependence, depression, and many other social problems that end up costing us far more than such programs, and he describes schools in which successful efforts of this nature have been designed and implemented.[14] There is a danger that a focus on academic standards with high-stakes accountability will impede the development and spread of such programs, even though the public feels they are important.

Uniform standards may be appropriate for business — a manufacturer wants all its microwave ovens to meet specified standards of quality. That's good. But to what extent do we want all students to be alike? Of course, there are certain basic skills we want all students to master, but should all students be required or expected to attain them at exactly the same age or grade level? To use a travel analogy, standards for manufacturing are comparable to a single destination for all travelers to reach, whereas standards for education are more like milestones on many never-ending journeys whereby different travelers may go to many different places. We must be careful not to overgeneralize what works well for business.

Based on a careful analysis of consequences, it seems that uniform or common higher standards could have considerable negative consequences for public education. But standards could instead have considerable positive consequences. How must they be operationalized for this to happen?

Principles for Using Standards To Customize Education

Martin Covington helps to capture a critical factor in the ways standards can be operationalized: "The urging of tougher achievement standards on American schools [is] a recommendation that is part of a broader strategy of *intensification* . . . that is, simply continuing to do what has been done for years, but more of it — lengthening the school day, requiring more homework, and the like."[15] For standards to have a positive effect on meeting student needs, we must think of them as serving a purpose other than the intensification of the currently predominant standardization approach to education.[16]

If the goal of the standards movement is to accelerate learning for *all* students, especially low-achieving students, then we must recognize that different students learn at different rates. Yet our current system is characterized by grade levels with classes and classrooms in which all students typically learn the same thing at the same time. By holding time constant, we force achievement to vary among students, with the consequence that the low-achieving ones gradually accumulate deficits in learning that handicap them in their future learning endeavors. Our current time-based system serves the function of sorting students, and we have developed norm-based testing (grading on a curve) and tracking as additional tools to that end. A focus on sorting students may have met an important need during the industrial age, when we needed large numbers of people for assembly-line jobs, but it is antithetical to helping all students achieve "hire, higher, or high" standards. So the very structure of our education system works against the goals of the standards movement.

To refocus our education system on meeting high standards, however you conceptualize them, we must no longer hold time constant; we must allow students the time they need to meet each standard. But to hold back the faster learners while the slower ones reach the standard would be to lower the standards for those students. So we must look for alternatives to our current mindset that can conceive only of classes and classrooms in which all students learn the same thing at the same time.

We need customization to replace standardization, in order to have an education system that is focused on learning (attaining high standards) rather than on sorting.[17] This does not mean that the basic standards for faster learners should be different from those for slower learners; rather it means that we should not expect all students to meet the standards within the same time frames. Further rationale for

To refocus our education system on meeting high standards, we must no longer hold time constant.

this conclusion is provided by differences in developmental rates for learners of the same age, differences in opportunities to learn outside of school, differences in prior knowledge and skills, differences in interests, and many other factors.

Depending on how they are conceived, standards can be used to foster either a standardized approach to education (a sorting-focused system) or a customized approach (a learning-focused system). The following are some principles that reflect a role for standards in a learning-focused (customized, learner-centered, results-oriented) approach to education.

Standards as levels of attainment. Standards should represent levels of attainment, with many different levels in each area of competence. As Gandal put it, "We can establish challenging standards without sacrificing rigor by developing multiple levels of achievement for each content standard."[18] These levels of achievement are similar to the notion of different performance standards for a given content standard. And different content standards also frequently represent different levels of complexity. Students, then, advance to progressively higher standards in different areas of competence.

Standards without timetables. Standards should not be tied to age levels or time in any way. This idea represents the greatest departure from common or uniform standards. Some standards may be common in the sense that all students should eventually attain them (e.g., basic skills), but no standards should be common in the sense that all students should be required to attain them at the same age. Moreover, many standards should not be required of all students; they should represent areas in which students may pursue their interests and develop their unique talents. Options are as important a feature of automobile manufacture as standards are. As Covington states:

> Striving for excellence — that is, maximizing the intellectual potential of each student — is the most legitimate of all academic goals and, happily, the one on which all interested parties can most likely agree. However, this kind of excellence is best promoted when achievement standards are applied flexibly, according to the gifts and experiences of each child, not imposed uniformly in procrustean ways across all children. . . . Standards and standardization are not the same thing, nor can equivalency substitute for excellence.[19]

Standards in all areas. Standards should be identified in all areas of learning and human development — nonacademic as well as academic. They should pertain to civic concerns as well as workplace preparation. They should address the needs of communities as well as those of students. As Mary McCaslin put it, "Achievement is *one* aspect of being a student; failure to recognize the larger arena within which achievement is pursued is to risk attainment of Summit goals."[20] The National Education Summit concluded that "standards can be effective only if they represent what parents, employers, educators, and community members believe children should learn and be able to do."[21] For standards to be effective in a learning-focused education system, this statement should be qualified so that these stakeholders do not come to believe that a certain attainment is important for all children. Several observers have expressed concern that "the sheer bulk of some of the [new education standards] will make it difficult for schools to put together a coordinated curriculum."[22] However, for a learning-focused, customized education system, such a high level of specification will help educators to generate a variety of educational resources and to keep track of learners' differing attainments, though technological tools will be important for managing this diversity.

Choice within limits. Gary Natriello has advocated that standards be "challenging yet attainable to students who differ in ability."[23] How can this be accomplished? Teachers, parents, and students should be allowed to decide when a given standard is appropriate ("challenging yet attainable") for a child during the child's development, within certain limits. Those limits should be in accordance with the general principle that attainments highly valued by the community or the state (such as mandatory basic skills) should be pursued in a timely fashion. Teachers, parents, and students should also be allowed some degree of choice as to which standards to pursue, beyond those deemed essential by the community or the state.

Learning-focused instructional processes. Standards must be accompanied by instructional processes that allow children to continue to work on the attainment of a standard until it is reached. Standards must be tools for "success for all students," not tools to propagate the traditional focus on sorting students. Even in business, the focus is on preventing defects in a product and immediately correcting those that do occur. As Rhona Weinstein put it, "Without appropriate pedagogy as well as systemic support, tough standards and punitive accountability will hold children and teachers accountable without providing the means to successfully meet those standards."[24]

So what would an appropriate pedagogy and systemic support look like? To enable children to continue to work on a standard until it is reached, the pedagogy must be flexible enough to allow different students to be working on different standards at the same time. This means that the teacher's role must change from being a "sage on the stage" to being a "guide on the side" — a coach, a mentor. For this approach to work, there must be much more reliance on team-based learning, self-regulated learning, and advanced technology as tools for customized learning. We have much to learn to fully develop the potential of this kind of pedagogy, yet important inroads have already been made.[25]

As Weinstein indicated, to be successful, this kind of pedagogy must be accompanied by systemic support. It may not be useful to think in terms of teachers working alone in self-contained classrooms with the day divided into periods (or even blocks) and age-based grade levels. Again, we have much to learn about how to redesign the "system" to support a learning-focused pedagogy. But when we look at schools that have been successful in helping all students reach higher standards, such as Central Park East[26] and Weld County School District 6 in Greeley and Evans, Colorado,[27] we find that a statement of standards was not among the most important factors; a learner-centered (customized) focus was, including a learning-focused pedagogy and systemic support.

Unfortunately, much of the discussion of standards seems to assume a "magic bullet" mentality that overlooks the considerable complexity and systemic interdependencies that will strongly influence our ability to help all students reach higher standards of excellence.

Performance-based measures. A standard should, if possible, be specific enough to be measurable. But we must recognize that some standards cannot truly be measured until many years after schooling takes place, such as certain standards in civic education or in parenting. And there are some standards for which any cost-effective measure will inevitably be unreliable, such as standards for attitudes about, say, the importance of reading or the arts. Nevertheless, aside from these relatively rare problems, a standard should be specific enough to be measurable. But how specific is specific enough?

Sabers and Sabers propose that "too much specificity drastically limits the domain of behaviors and tasks relevant to the measurement of success."[28] Is this always a bad thing? Certainly for some types of learning it is useful to maintain a broad domain of behaviors and tasks that can indicate success. But are there not other types of learning for which it is important to limit the domain to some extent, perhaps more so in a customized system than in a standardized system? It seems reasonable that different types of learning should have different degrees to which the domain of behaviors and tasks is limited, with some appropriately being considerably limited. And to the extent that the domain is not very limited for a standard, there should be a variety of kinds of performance-based measures for determining whether or not the standard has been met.

Certification of standards. Given that there exists a wide variety of standards within a wide variety of areas, and given that students have different needs, interests, and talents, it seems reasonable that different types of degrees or certificates should be offered for different combinations of standards. An extreme for customizing the certification of standards met would be a personal portfolio, which provides such an overwhelming amount of information that no two students' "certification" would be exactly alike. The opposite extreme is our current high school diploma, which tells you so little about what a given student has actually learned that it makes most students look alike. But there could be intermediate degrees of certification that are in essence "package deals" that indicate that the student has reached certain determined standards in certain determined areas.

Positive incentives for meeting standards. Standards should be accompanied by positive, not negative, incentives. Monetary sanctions and rigid controls in particular are likely to produce the opposite of the desired effect of elevating the standards that students are able to attain.[29]

Limitations of standards. Elliot Eisner has pointed out that "standards do not represent the most important ends we seek in education. . . . We seek work that displays ingenuity, complexity, and the student's personal signature."[30] So we should find ways to represent those grander ends in our specifications of what is important to teach and assess. Eisner talks much about the value of criteria in lieu of standards for assessing (and presumably coaching the attainment of) these important educational ends.

The Broader Context

It seems that, in spite of many different conceptions of standards, there is consensus that the major purpose of standards is to accelerate student learning and performance. But this can be done only by getting students to spend more time actively mentally engaged in learning. Perhaps the two most important conditions for active mental engagement are the intensity of motivation to learn and the quality of the instructional support for learning. And, as was discussed above, common, uniform standards are actually likely to be counterproductive with regard to both of these conditions. To support the goal of accelerating learning and performance, we need standards that support customization rather than standardization in education.

But even such standards are not sufficient to create either of the conditions for active mental engagement. Also needed are significant stakeholder-designed changes in the use of time, talent, and technology — time in the form of allowing students the time they need to reach each standard; talent in the form of changing the roles of students, teachers, and administrators (which requires a sustained program of professional development); and technology in the form of providing teachers and students with more powerful tools for learning. These changes in turn need to be supported by changes in the ways schools, school districts, and state education agencies are organized, administered, and governed, so as to provide appropriate systemic supports. As David Cohen put it, "Standards should be understood as one tool for helping the entire education system to learn and improve, not as the kingpin of change or as the occasion to decide for our time what the content of education should be and what level of achievement will be acceptable."[31]

Standards, properly conceived, are just one necessary, but not sufficient, part of a comprehensive redesign of a very complex education system, as the exemplary effort in Weld County School District 6 in Colorado aptly demonstrates. If not properly conceived, standards can do far more harm than good. As Martin Maehr and Jane Maehr put it, "Emphasizing standards is an all too ready, all too quick solution to a much more complex issue."[32] We must recognize this complexity, use standards to support customization rather than standardization, and address all the interrelated parts of the system (e.g., instructional processes, assessment, and systemic supports). Otherwise, the standards movement will inevitably end up as yet another wave of reform that came and went without any positive impact on student learning.

1. Theodore Sizer, "Making the Grade," *Washington Post Education Review*, 2 April 1995, p. 12.
2. See, for example, Angela R. Taylor, "Conditions for American Children, Youth, and Families: Are We 'World Class'?," *Educational Researcher*, November 1996, pp. 10-12.
3. Darrell L. Sabers and Donna S. Sabers, "Conceptualizing, Measuring, and Implementing Higher (High or Hire) Standards," *Educational Researcher*, November 1996, pp. 19-21.
4. Anne C. Lewis, "An Overview of the Standards Movement," *Phi Delta Kappan*, June 1995, pp. 744-50.
5. Lauren Resnick and Kate Nolan, "Where in the World Are World-Class Standards?," *Educational Leadership*, March 1995, p. 7.
6. Matthew Gandal, "Not All Standards Are Created Equal," *Educational Leadership*, March 1995, p. 16.
7. Sabers and Sabers, p. 21.
8. Martin V. Covington, "The Myth of Intensification," *Educational Researcher*, November 1996, p. 24.
9. See, for example, Michael Hammer and James Champy, *Reengineering the Corporation* (New York: HarperBusiness, 1993).
10. Covington, p. 24.
11. Education Commission of the States, "About ECS" (http://www.ecs.org).
12. Mary McCaslin, "The Problem of Problem Representation: The Summit's Conception of Student," *Educational Researcher*, November 1996, pp. 13-15.
13. Stanley M. Elam, Lowell C. Rose, and Alec M. Gallup, "The 28th Annual Phi Delta Kappa/Gallup Poll of the Public's Attitudes Toward the Public Schools," *Phi Delta Kappan*, September 1996, p. 56.
14. Daniel Goleman, *Emotional Intelligence: Why It Can Matter More than I.Q.* (New York: Bantam Books, 1995).
15. Covington, p. 24.
16. Rhona Weinstein, "High Standards in a Tracked System of Schooling: For Which Students and with What Educational Supports?," *Educational Researcher*, November 1996, pp. 16-19.
17. For more about the differences between an education system focused on sorting and one focused on learning, see Charles M. Reigeluth, "The Imperative for Systemic Change," in idem and Robert J. Garfinkle, eds., *Systemic Change in Education* (Englewood Cliffs, N.J.: Educational Technology Publications, 1994), pp. 3-11.
18. Gandal, p. 20.
19. Covington, pp. 24-25.
20. McCaslin, p. 13.
21. Thomas L. Good, "Educational Researchers Comment on the Educational Summit and Other Policy Proclamations for 1983-1996," *Educational Researcher*, November 1996, p. 5.
22. Chris Pipho, "Calling the Play-by-Play on Standards," *Phi Delta Kappan*, February 1996, p. 398.
23. Gary Natriello, "Diverting Attention from Conditions in American Schools," *Educational Researcher*, November 1996, p. 7.
24. Weinstein, p. 18.
25. For a broad sample of what has been learned, see Charles M. Reigeluth, ed., *Instructional-Design Theories and Models*, vol. 2 (Hillsdale, N.J.: Erlbaum, forthcoming).
26. Deborah Meier, *The Power of Their Ideas* (Boston: Beacon Press, 1995).
27. Tim Waters, Don Burger, and Susan Burger, "Moving Up Before Moving On," *Educational Leadership*, March 1995, pp. 35-40.
28. Sabers and Sabers, p. 20.
29. Education Commission of the States, op. cit.
30. Elliot Eisner, "Why Standards May Not Improve Schools," *Educational Leadership*, February 1993, p. 22.
31. David Cohen, "What Standards for National Standards?," *Phi Delta Kappan*, June 1995, p. 756.
32. Martin L. Maehr and Jane M. Maehr, "Schools Aren't as Good as They Used to Be: They Never Were," *Educational Researcher*, November 1996, p. 23.   **K**

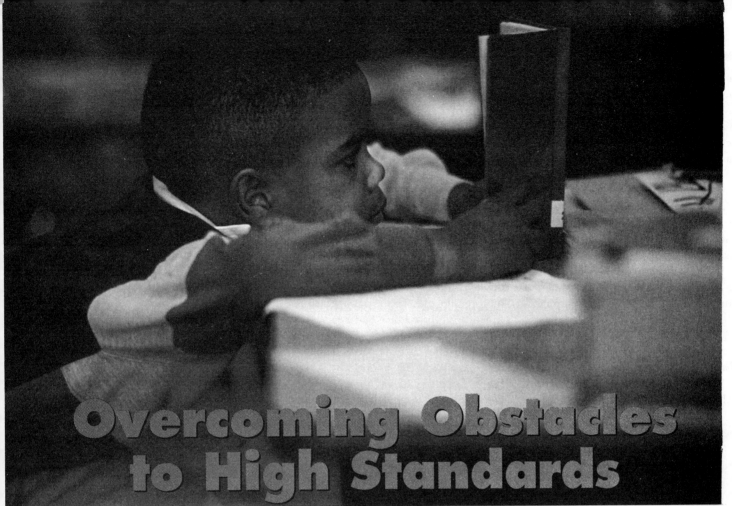

Overcoming Obstacles to High Standards

Jeffrey High

Schools must make some major adjustments
in order to raise the learning bar for all students.

JIM GRANT AND BOB JOHNSON

Wouldn't it be wonderful if we could create and implement high standards for the politicians, pundits, corporate executives, and others who demand that we impose high standards on America's students? I wonder how many of them would do the hard work required to "measure up" and "make the grade."

Here in the real world, however, meeting demands for high standards—and accepting responsibility for making sure that every student meets those standards—means that we need to overcome some major obstacles.

Jim Grant is founder and executive director of the Society for Developmental Education in Peterborough, New Hampshire.

Bob Johnson is a senior associate with the Society for Developmental Education.

Obstacle 1:
Children's Problems

If the quality of children's lives were held to high standards outside of school, imposing such standards within schools would be far easier and make much more sense. Unfortunately, as many as 20 percent of America's students now live in poverty and are likely to be deprived of adequate nutrition and health care. In addition to having hunger and sickness interfere with their education, many of these children and others may also be suffering from various forms of neglect and abuse, which make them all the more unlikely to become enthusiastic learners and high achievers. Moreover, in some areas as many as half of all students do not live with both parents, which can also lead to emotional and financial instability, as well as the sort of

transience that prevents them from having a positive educational experience.

The end result is that rather than having one or two serious problems, many of today's students have multiple, co-occurring problems that undermine their "personal infrastructure." Yet, they are supposed to meet the same high standards as more fortunate children who suffer from none of these problems.

A Solution: Diverse Services for Diverse Students. Knowing that these problems are not about to disappear and may, in fact, increase, we should be ready to provide the full range of services needed to stabilize and educate a diverse student population. And because the roots of many of these problems lie outside the school, this may require coordination with social service providers and community organizations that have not been part of our traditional educational system.

Within our schools, we need to recognize that many students struggling with severe social and emotional problems may need additional support to deal with their problems and meet high academic standards. Of course, it would be convenient if all this additional support could be squeezed into the school day along with everything else. But since that is not likely to be the case, the services we provide must include time-flexible options that allow us to accommodate different students' needs for additional learning.

The Traditional Grade Structure

While the student population in many schools has changed dramatically dur-

ing recent years, a large number of those schools continue to adhere rigidly to the lockstep model Horace Mann brought to America in the 1840s. Designed for an agrarian era in which students were released to do farm work during the summer, this antiquated system continues to dole out education in 36-week increments, often penalizing individual students who need additional learning time.

The problems created by this structure are compounded by the equally rigid and obsolete processes often used to determine grade placement. Schools across America still base initial placement decisions on the number of candles on a child's birthday cake at a particular cutoff date—as early as July in one state and as late as December 31 in another. This arbitrary process ignores factors that can

help determine whether a child will experience success or failure in school. As a result, many students are placed in the wrong grades and will not be ready to meet high standards in the upper grades unless they spend an extra year in one of those grades.

A Solution: Flexible Time Options. Just as most elementary schools now recognize the importance of accommodating students' different *learning styles*, a growing number are also recognizing the importance of accommodating different *learning rates*. As the National Commission on Time and Learning pointed out in 1994, "Research confirms common sense. Some students take three to six times longer to learn the same thing." Despite some claims to the contrary, reliable research also confirms the conventional wis-

Michael Tony

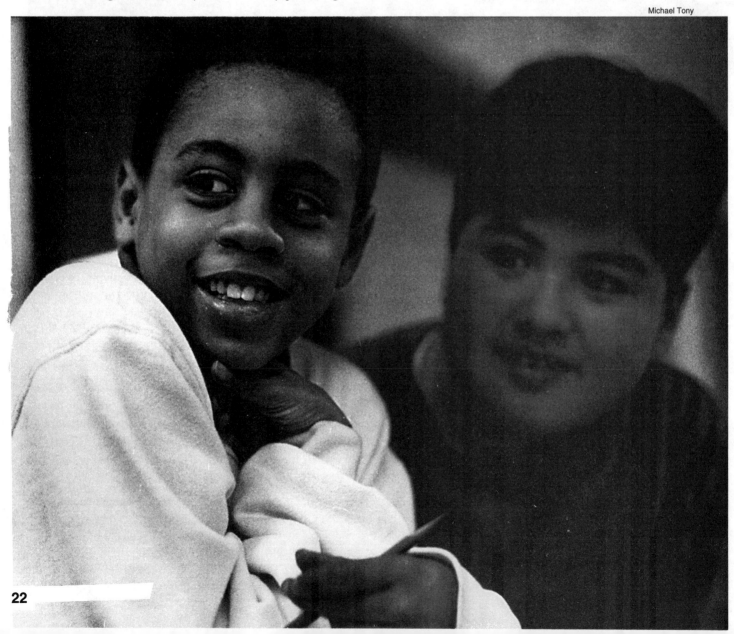

dom that the youngest children in a class are less likely to achieve school success than the oldest ones.

For all students to achieve success and meet high standards, today's schools need a range of time options to match their needs. Along with traditional grade-level classes and additional-year options, schools need transition classes between grades, multiage classes, and looping programs in which teachers move up through the grades with their students. Otherwise, students will continue to be promoted without having learned required grade-level material, even though this sort of social promotion is incompatible with high standards.

Obstacle 3:
"The Upholstery Curriculum"

I like to describe the curriculum now being used in many elementary schools as the Upholstery Curriculum because it's well padded and covers everything. In recent years, elementary school teachers have been told that they not only can but *must* teach their students about proper nutrition, drug and alcohol abuse, good and bad touching, saving the environment, gun safety, and other topics that many grown-ups have not yet mastered. When I started teaching in an elementary school a few decades ago, we were required to teach *none* of those topics—which left us more time to teach reading, writing, and arithmetic.

Mandates from on high are responsible for much of this curriculum overload. The politicians, bureaucrats, and special-interest groups that keep coming up with new ways to fix society's ills seem to have forgotten about time constraints. They also don't seem to have noticed that many of their mandates conflict with—or cancel—other mandates!

A Solution: Curricular Deflation. Just as the Federal Reserve Board watches for signs of economic inflation and strikes swiftly when they appear, we need to monitor our curriculum closely to make sure it matches our students' capabilities, our school day, and our school year. In most cases, this may require us either to reduce the volume of material being

"...IN TOO MANY CASES, THE STANDARDS ARE CREATED BY PEOPLE WHO DON'T...SPEND MUCH TIME IN ELEMENTARY SCHOOLS."

taught or to expand the amount of time in which to teach it.

While a complete moratorium on new mandates would be one of the most dramatic education reforms in recent decades, the reality is that new mandates will probably keep appearing, and we will have to keep adjusting the curriculum and teaching schedules accordingly. However, the need to prepare students to meet high standards may provide a convincing rationale for rejecting new add-ons and providing additional learning time for students.

Obstacle 4:
Ideology-Driven Educational Strategies

In recent years, a number of "experts" have proclaimed that they have the one and only correct approach to some vital aspect of education. Some whole-language purists want us to ban all direct phonics instruction, and certain inclusion advocates insist that we have to keep disruptive and violent children in our classrooms. Promoters of "developmentally appropriate" practices demand that we prohibit any student from spending an extra year of learning time in a readiness class, a transition class, a multiage class, or a repeat grade.

Extreme ideological positions like these have kept many educators from

meeting the needs of their diverse student populations. As a result, test scores have dropped, special education designations have increased, and parents have lost faith in our schools.

A Solution: Child-Compatible Educational Strategies. We need to base our decisions on what actually works for our students, rather than on an ideological "one size fits all" position that ignores individual needs and differences. Firsthand knowledge, experience, and common sense can help us find a combination of strategies and techniques that support the full range of students in our own schools, rather than rely on "experts" who cite highly selective or subtly manipulated data from other times and places to justify their ideological positions.

A balanced, moderate approach allows us to recognize, for example, that some children need direct phonics instruction and others don't; some children thrive in a regular classroom and others don't; and some children can successfully complete the curriculum during the school year, while others need additional learning time. Recognizing and meeting the different needs of our diverse students is the best way to help them meet high standards. Trying to make them conform to a rigid academic model is a waste of everyone's precious time.

In an ideal world, we would start the process of creating and implementing high standards for our students with detailed knowledge of where they are now, and then raise the standards in a continual but realistic way directly linked to improvements in student performance, as well teaching methods and materials.

Unfortunately, in too many cases the standards are created by people who don't know our students and don't even spend much time in elementary schools. This top-down approach runs the risk of creating standards that do not reflect the realities found in many schools. The best way to help our students meet high standards, therefore, is to recognize that they come from many different starting points and need many different routes to reach success.   □

PASSING ON FAILURE

*Social promotion is not the
way to help children who have
fallen behind.*

BY SANDRA FELDMAN

A S YOU know, I was recently elected president of
the American Federation of Teachers. Some of
you also know me as a local union leader in a "small
town" called New York City, where I've spent countless hours in schools talking to teachers and kids. I
know the problems of poor urban districts *very* well.
So it doesn't seem strange when a place like New York
decides to have a big literacy push to make sure that
all our students leave third grade able to read. It's an
idea we've supported for some time.

But it knocked my socks off when I heard the President of the United States, in his State of the Union address, hold out as a *national* goal that every child will
be able to read well by the end of third grade.

Frankly, I was embarrassed. How is it that the President of the wealthiest, greatest nation in the world has
to talk about universal third-grade literacy as a national
goal? And what did that actually mean, given that
American kids, on average, were in the top tier on the
1992 International Assessment of Reading, and that
our fourth graders were at the very top this year in science in the Third International Mathematics and Science Study?

What it means, really, is that a substantial portion of
our poor kids—and in America more than 20 percent
of kids are poor—can't read as they should. And when
you can't read properly, you can't learn as you should
in other subjects, either.

Now poor children, especially urban children, are
people I know well. Very well. Not only was I one of
them, but I've spent my entire adult life among them. I

*Sandra Feldman is president of the American Federa-
tion of Teachers. She delivered this speech at the National Press Club in Washington, D.C., on September
9. The results from the national survey on school district promotion policies and practices are drawn
from a new report prepared by the AFT Educational
Issues Department, as are the sidebars that accompany this article. For copies of the full report, see or-
dering information on p. 8.*

know what problems they have and the burdens they
bring to school. And I also know that the schools they
attend, rather than getting more, get less. But I also
know that, short of situations of serious damage,
urban kids are perfectly capable of reading well and
doing well in school in general.

So how does it happen that a child gets beyond
third grade without solid skills in reading or math?
How could it happen that a youngster could reach
twelfth grade, let alone graduate from high school,
without solid skills in reading, writing, and math? How
did it happen that colleges have to offer remedial
courses and businesses have to spend millions teaching new employees basic skills?

Good questions.

Now, we in the AFT spend a lot of time listening to
our members, so we had a pretty good sense of the answers. And one of the persistent answers we were
hearing was "social promotion"—the practice of sending students on to the next grade even though they
weren't really ready.

But we wanted to check on what we were hearing.
So, as part of our ongoing push for higher standards of
conduct and achievement, we decided to conduct a
national survey about student promotion policies. I am
here today with the results of this AFT survey, the first
such national survey ever conducted. We collected
promotion policies from eighty-five districts across the
country, including the forty largest. And we now have
much clearer answers about why the richest nation on
earth has to set a goal of all children reading well by
the end of third grade and about why a youngster can
graduate from high school without a solid foundation
in the basic skills necessary to lead a productive life.

What did we find? We found that no district has an
explicit policy of social promotion. That was odd.
Were our members wrong? Could Chicago and other
districts that are now banning social promotion be
banning something that doesn't exist?

Not at all.

Because we also found that just about every district

ILLUSTRATED BY ROBERT BARKIN

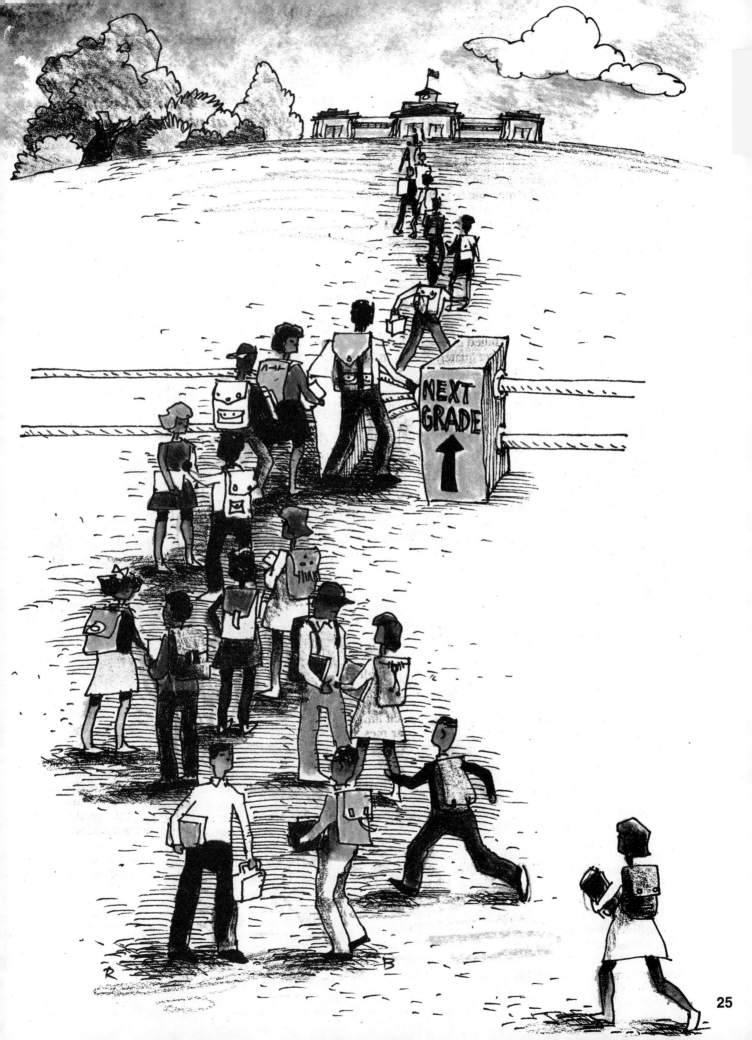

NEXT
GRADE
↑

Social Promotion: Everyone Loses

AS CRITICS point out, social promotion is an insidious practice that hides school failure and creates problems for everybody:

■ *For kids,* who are deluded into thinking they have learned the knowledge and skills necessary for success, who get the message that effort and achievement do not count, and most important, who often are denied access to the resources and support programs they need because their failure is not acknowledged by the system.

■ *For teachers,* who must deal with impossibly wide disparities in their students' preparation and achievement that result from social promotion, and who face students who know that teachers wield no credible authority to demand hard work.

■ *For parents,* who are lulled into thinking that their children are being adequately prepared for college, for civic responsibility, and for the world of work.

■ *For the business community,* which must invest millions of dollars in teaching new employees the basic skills they did not learn in school.

■ *For colleges and universities,* which must spend a sizeable portion of their budgets on remedial courses to prepare high school graduates to do college-level work, and for the professors who must lower their standards in order to accommodate an ill-prepared student body.

■ *For taxpayers,* whose support of public education is eroded by evidence that a high school diploma is not necessarily a guarantee of basic literacy and numeracy.

■ *For society,* in general, which cannot afford, in both economic and civic terms, a growing proportion of uneducated citizens who neither benefit from, nor contribute to, the commonweal.

In most districts, there are no agreed-upon standards defining what students should know and be able to do at various grade levels.

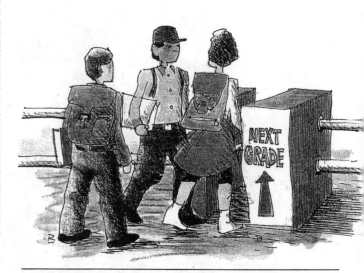

has an *implicit* policy of social promotion. Almost all districts say that holding students back must be the option of last resort—which is a clear message to promote socially—and many of them also put explicit limits on retaining students—which is another clear message to promote socially.

For example, about one-half of the districts restrict the number of times a student can be retained. In Orange County, Florida, only one retention is permitted in elementary school. Houston restricts retention to once in kindergarten through fourth grade and once in fifth through eighth grade.

Still other districts essentially forbid retaining certain children, like students with limited English proficiency or learning disabilities, saying that these students are to be moved along according to "a pace that is appropriate to their abilities"—whatever that means.

Another major answer our survey revealed about why a student can leave third grade without reading well or graduate from high school without solid knowledge and skills is that, in most districts, *there*

are no agreed-upon standards defining what students should know and be able to do at various grade levels.

As a result, there are no clear criteria for whether or not a student should be promoted. Instead, we see vague policies like Clark County, Nevada's: To be promoted, a student's "progress should be continuous and student advancement through the curriculum should be according to the student's demonstrated ability."

What does *that* mean?

Or take the policy of the Long Beach, Calif., School District: Promotion depends on a student's ability to "demonstrate sufficient growth in learning required basic skills." But what is "sufficient?" The policy is silent. And is "sufficient growth" the same as mastery? The policy gives no clue.

So how *are* promotion decisions made? We found that, in most districts, a student's grades in class and on standardized tests, along with teacher recommendations, form the basis for promotion decisions.

Sounds sensible. But think about it: In the absence of clear, grade-by-grade standards for what students should know and be able to do, class grades are based on different things and, therefore, vary greatly. Some teachers grade based on student mastery; other emphasize effort; still others look at mastery or effort relative to perceived student ability; and still others may use different combinations of these. And the result is that some students arrive in the next grade unprepared for work at that level, even though they may have gotten A's and B's.

Standardized tests are also not a good guide to promotion decisions. First, they are not generally reliable when young children are involved. And second, they often aren't aligned with the curriculum—that is, with what the students have been taught.

That brings us to teacher recommendations, presumably the third leg of the three-legged stool that constitutes promotion decisions. But our survey revealed that this third leg is very shaky indeed: While teachers *participate* in promotion decisions in the majority of districts we surveyed, they have little *authority* over the decision. They have final authority at the elementary or middle school level in only *two* districts, and final authority at the high school level in only *one* district. In fact, more districts give parents final authority over a student's promotion than they do teachers!

In the majority of districts, final authority for promotion decisions rests with the principal. And here, once again, we see the effects of not having clear standards for students. Because in the absence of standards, teachers who grade strictly may have little support—and grades become negotiable. Principals can overturn a teacher's recommendation or change her grades. And, frequently, they do, either because they don't want the school to look bad or because of parent or district pressure. Sometimes, it's because the resources aren't there to hold over too many children.

In fact, in a separate poll of teachers we conducted some time ago, we found that, although teachers are opposed to social promotion, they, like many principals, feel uneasy about retention because usually there are no options for the students—no program that's different and helpful, not even summer school, in many cases. And children who are retained without any extra help or different programs often continue to do poorly. It's a terrible bind.

AND THAT brings me to the next major finding of our survey: In the majority of districts we looked at, promotion policies are generally silent about providing special help to students who fail, or who are at risk of failing, or who are socially promoted.

Only about 15 percent mention tutoring; and only about 13 percent mention alternative programs and strategies, such as transitional classes, extended instructional time, customized instructional programs or other support services. About one-half of the promotion policies mention summer school, but discussions with school officials and union leaders indicate that in many instances funds to support summer school have been cut drastically, if not eliminated. In some districts, students must pay to attend summer school!

Now, some of you may be thinking, "Special programs may be nice, but they're costly. Isn't the solution simple? Clearly, if we don't want social promotion—and we don't—then retention is the answer."

....Which brings me to the last major finding from our survey: Ironically, and painfully, it turns out that not only is social *promotion* rampant, retention is, too. Despite the restrictions on holding back students, retention is used as often as it can be. Accurate figures are hard to get, but it is estimated that 15 percent to

Teachers' Role in Promotion Decisions

THE ROLE teachers play in social promotion decisions is complicated. Teachers do not like social promotion, but they are ambivalent about retaining students. Ninety-four percent of teachers in a recent survey* agreed with the statements: "...promoting students who are not truly prepared creates a burden for the receiving teachers and classmates. Automatic promotion inevitably brings down standards and impedes education." Yet, 54 percent of those same teachers indicated that they had promoted unprepared students in the past year. Why? Our polls indicate:

■ Teachers do not have the authority to retain students.

■ Teachers succumb to pressure from principals and parents to promote students that the teachers consider to be unprepared. Six in 10 teachers indicate that teachers in their school are pressured by principals and other administrators not to retain students, while 52 percent say parental pressure is a problem.

■ Teachers fear that when students are retained, they will cause behavior and discipline problems in class.

■ Teachers know that there is already a significant amount of retention occurring in schools.

■ Teachers believe that the educational research indicates that retention is both harmful and ineffective.

■ Teachers believe that there are insufficient educational alternatives to social promotion or retention for youngsters who do not master the grade-level material. They see their dilemma as having to choose between two unsatisfactory alternatives. Teachers often know that retention may result in students' repeating the same material, taught with the same instructional strategies that were ineffectual for those students in the first instance. To recommend retention in such a situation is not only a violation of all that teachers know about how children develop and learn, but it also lends support to what teachers perceive as a fundamental problem—the failure on the part of the administration to develop and support alternatives and prevention programs for children at risk of failure.

*Peter D. Hart Associates. *Academic Standards and Student Discipline: AFT Teachers Assess Their Schools*, 1996.

Why Students Fail

A VERY SMALL percentage of children fail because they do not have the innate capacity to acquire the complex knowledge and skills required for functioning in today's information age. The vast majority of children are unsuccessful in school for other, more complicated reasons.

■ Some children don't prosper in school because they are immature or otherwise unready for school.

■ Some don't learn because we feed them with an empty spoon; they are not provided a rich curriculum and/or instructional practices that support high achievement.

■ Others don't acquire the necessary knowledge and skills because of excessive absenteeism.

■ Some students achieve at minimal levels because they make little effort to acquire knowledge—either because they do not view academic achievement as crucial or instrumental to their goals, there are no consequences to failure, or other things, such as money or physical prowess, are more highly esteemed.

■ Still others are the victims of ill-conceived theories about children and how they learn that result in failure—and in practices on the part of teachers, administrators, parents and students, and the wider society, that sustain low achievement.

■ Some students don't learn because they have no incentive (positive or negative) to engage them in the educative process.

■ And still others fail because of a combination of the reasons identified above.

Policies to help underachieving students learn must address these underlying causes of failure. For some students, creating a negative incentive may be enough. Sending them a clear signal that learning counts, that failure to perform will result in retention may be sufficient to inspire this small number of students to devote attention to their studies. For a few others who have been absent, repeating the grade may make sense, since they were not exposed to the material in the first place. And for some children, particularly those with little or no access to high-quality early childhood programs, repeating the early grades may make sense. But for the vast majority of underachieving students, systemic change is required if success is to be achieved. Policies and practices have to be developed that address the problems of a lack of standards, undemanding curriculum, underprepared teachers, and administrative indifference to whether learning takes place. These policies must address what unique educational experiences and support services are necessary for children who fail or are at risk of failure. Absent attention to these issues, we are doomed to continue the ineffective pendulum swing between social promotion and retention.

19 percent of U.S. students are held back in the same grade each year. And in many large urban districts, upwards of 50 percent of the students who enter kindergarten are likely to be retained at least once before they graduate or drop out.

Now, a number of school districts—Chicago most prominent among them—have ended social promotion, and many more will follow suit. They are to be congratulated; ending social promotion is the right thing to do.

But just going to a policy of retention won't work. The fact is, neither social promotion *nor* retention is the answer—if the answer we're seeking is getting kids to achieve. In fact, throughout the 20th century, we've swung like a pendulum between these two policy approaches to student progression—and neither policy has done the job.

Now, if I had a gun to my head and had to choose between retaining or promoting a student who had not mastered the requisite material to be prepared for the next grade, I would choose retention over promotion.

But there *are* better choices. What are they? First, we need to take an "intensive-care" approach to students who are falling behind—*well before* we're at the point of promotion or retention decisions—by quickly identifying these students and concentrating every possible resource on getting them back on track quickly.

For example, Cincinnati's reform efforts include *immediate* intervention, such as providing students with in-class, small-group instruction or multi-age grouping and also offering tutoring and summer school on top of that. For students in grades three, six and eight who still do not meet promotion standards but are at an age at which it is inappropriate to remain with younger students, there is something called "Plus Classes"—Three Plus, etc.—that have fewer students than regular classes do and an intensive, different approach to teaching students the specific knowledge and skills they haven't yet mastered.

In Albuquerque, the principal and parents must be notified early if retention is anticipated, and a special support program is designed for each child in danger of failing. Albuquerque also stipulates that no student can be retained without a specific intervention plan detailing the student's needs and how they will be met.

Second, we have to adopt rigorous standards that are clear to parents, teachers, and students. The stan-

Neither social promotion nor retention is the answer.

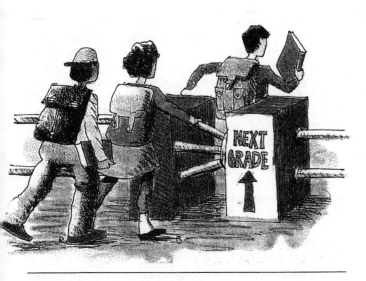

dards should be accompanied by grade-by-grade curricula and assessments that make it possible for teachers to know *in time* when children are in trouble so they can seek *timely* intervention.

Corpus Christi is farthest along with this, combining clear and rigorous standards with an end to social promotion and an emphasis on intervention. Results of the first two years are encouraging: Scores on state reading, writing, and math tests are up significantly in all grades—which proves our youngsters *can* do what's required of them.

In fact, the students would have told us this. In their own way, they've been asking adults to take a stand on

standards; they've been asking to be taken seriously. Listen to a teenager from wealthy Westchester County, N.Y., quoted in a Public Agenda report: "It's so dumb. You don't even have to try in my school. So I think if they did raise the standards, I probably would be a harder worker." And listen to a California teenager: "I think adults don't take us seriously enough. We're really smarter than they think. It's how far and how they push us ... I think a lot of kids—even those getting D's and stuff—can do a lot better." How right the kids are.

Third—and I want to say this loud and clear—we must place well-educated, well-trained teachers in every classroom, but especially in the classrooms of our neediest and most vulnerable children. And we have to make it a top priority, both in schools of education and in districts' professional development programs, to *insist* that all teachers of young children are fully proficient in teaching reading.

Teacher preparation is woefully inadequate in this crucial area, especially when it comes to preparing teachers who will be teaching our most at-risk youngsters. And many of our experienced teachers, too, need ongoing support in teaching phonology, phonetics, orthography, and other language skills—because we know a lot more now about teaching reading, but that research hasn't reached the classroom.

I use those fancy words like "phonology" deliberately. Because I want to remind everyone of the sophisticated knowledge and skill it takes to teach reading to a group of twenty-five or thirty wiggling, restless children, many of whom have never before been exposed to the printed page. They're depending on their teacher to unlock the mysteries of eye-to-brain coordination, of decoding and comprehending squiggles on a page that result in the joy and pleasure of reading. It is daunting.

And it's as dumb and cruel to expect someone—even a brilliant young AmeriCorps type—to go in and do that with at-risk kids without proper training as it would be to think one of us could take out another's appendix, armed only with good will, a workshop, and the advice from a few books.

THESE RECOMMENDATIONS—clear standards, special *timely* help for children who need it, and additional reading training for teachers—can be put in place immediately. In some instances, we'll see immediate results; in others, results won't be evident for a couple of years, but progress will be evident immediately, not only in terms of students—as well as teachers—getting the help they need, but in the strong signal that will be sent to parents and the public that school districts will be deploying every available resource to ensuring that all kids, and not just our more advantaged kids, will read and generally achieve well by the time they leave third grade and that all students, and not just our more advantaged students, will graduate from high school with the requisite skills to go to college or get a decent job.

But perhaps our most significant recommendation—the one that will ultimately make the biggest difference—is not something we in school districts can do tomorrow—unless we get state and federal help. And that is to make available high-quality pre-school and

Explicit Standards Give Definition to 'Earned' Promotion

CLEAR ACADEMIC standards are essential to higher achievement and success for all. As Lewis Carroll's Cheshire Cat said: "If you don't know where you're going, any road will take you there." Without explicit grade-by-grade standards for students, anything goes, and anything is accepted—and sometimes even mediocre or poor work is rewarded as excellent.

Commonly shared grade-by-grade standards for students are essential. These standards

■ support academic rigor and ensure fairness by defining the expectations for success for all students;

■ eliminate the need for every teacher to set his or her own standards for grading and promotion decisions, or for requesting special services for students who are falling behind;

■ give teachers the authority to demand that students work hard, without the risk of appearing arbitrary or mean;

■ make academic expectations public and, therefore, accessible to students, parents, and the community;

■ furnish the basis for professional development for teachers as they come to consensus about what evidence of student learning is appropriate, how to spot problems in achieving the standards, and what strategies enhance student progress toward meeting the standards; and, most important

■ provide the basis for monitoring and managing student learning and making decisions about promotion, retention, and the need for additional educational services.

kindergarten programs for all children—and if not for all children, then definitely, urgently, immediately, for our neediest children.

Let me point to the example of France, which not only has high student achievement but also the smallest gaps in achievement between advantaged and disadvantaged youngsters. A major reason for that is a system of preschools that was originally started for the children of working mothers and immigrant families to make up for the children's lack of academic readiness. And because France did not treat these preschools as a poverty program and gave these children the best, the preschool programs proved to be so effective that middle-class, full-time mothers are sending their kids, and the demand has made the pre-schools practically universal.

Look at what we're suggesting: A good preschool *educational* experience; special help like tutoring and extended day and extended year when children are falling behind; high standards, a challenging curriculum, and tests that measure what's supposed to be taught; qualified, well-prepared teachers .... This all exists in schools across America. But not in all schools where we're working to educate our neediest youngsters. Not in all of our large urban districts. Far too few of them, relative to the need.

So the big question is, can we make it happen there? I believe we can. I know that in many places we are. We see achievement getting better; we see standards being raised; we see investment being made and scarce resources being spent more wisely. But we have to step it up. Our urban kids face terrible problems, and they need extra help. Instead, they get less. And then either they or their teachers, or both, are blamed for failure.

Too many adults in our society have given up on our poorest youngsters. Instead of raising hell and making sure poor kids get the common-sense things they need, the things middle-class kids in middle-class schools take for granted, we get political leaders and opinion makers calling for vouchers and privatization, as if those radical schemes will provide what every other advanced civilized nation in the world provides for *all* its kids: safe, orderly, well-supplied schools with high standards and highly educated, well-trained teachers.

Many of you are aware that, within the past few weeks, two polls came out showing growing public support for vouchers. They got a lot of press, and they deserved to. But what didn't get any press is something else in those polls, something that is far more significant. And that is that parents and the public want first and foremost for their public schools to be fixed. They believe that better discipline and more rigorous academic standards that are faithfully adhered to would be a far more effective reform than vouchers. And they are correct. To the extent that support for vouchers has grown, it is because of frustration with the pace of getting better discipline and higher standards in our schools, particularly in our poorest schools. Too many of our leaders, too many of the people in charge of our schools, still aren't taking the public's message seriously enough.

Friends, our society needs a lot of things. Those who want to eliminate all government regulation or a government role in education should be reminded of what "government" means in a democracy. It means us. It means "the people." It means the public. And if that is too abstract, let them ponder the 25 million pounds of meat with the E.coli bacteria that the "government" just had to have recalled.

We survived that. We would not survive the demise of a public education system. And we can't survive unless we have the best public school system in the world—including and especially for our toughest, roughest, neediest students, who are also, underneath it all, many of our sweetest, greatest kids.

I have seen it happen. I know it can be done.

There is nothing wrong with our kids that adults can't cure. And there is nothing wrong with our schools that we can't fix. We must—and can—prevent failure before it occurs. We must—and can—intervene swiftly and effectively if it does. And stopping the empty, useless cycle of social promotion and retention has to be high up on our agenda. □

Various Ways to Reduce Grade Level Retentions

- Provide universal preschool programs

- Adapt Reading Recovery® type strategies

- Expand head-start enrollments

- Provide a full-day kindergarten program

- Provide summer school (for at-risk children)

- Expand Title I support services

- Create looping classrooms

- Create multiage classrooms

- Provide accelerated learning opportunities

- Adopt the Success for All®
Reading program

- Provide remedial math and literacy services

- Private tutoring (outside of school)

- Change the school entrance date (to at least September 1)

- Modify the school calendar, i.e.,
    - Extend the school year
    - Lengthen the school day
    - Space school vacations out over the school year

- Change to a child-compatible curriculum

- Eliminate grade-level promotional gates

- Eliminate all-group standardized testing **before** grade four

---

Options to Eliminate Grade Level Retentions

- Stay at home (one year) *

- Extra year of pre-school *

- Home schooling *

- Pre-kindergarten program (for young fives)

- Pre-first grade (young sixes)

- Pre-second grade (young sevens)

- Pre-third grade (young eights)

- Remain 3 years in a two year multiage continuous progress classroom

*   These options are usually available only to financially advantaged parents/guardians.

CAUTION, LOOK BEFORE YOU LEAP!

Some students may be placed at-risk when remaining in the same grade for a second year

1. A student whose parent(s)/guardian(s) are opposed to an additional year of learning time through grade level retention

2. An unmotivated student

3. An emotionally disturbed student (Note: Some students exhibit emotional problems from being in over their heads.)

4. A student with a behavior disorder (Note: Some students exhibit behavior problems as a result of being in over their heads.)

5. Some children who are raised in poverty

6. A student who has a history of excessive absenteeism (15-20 days per year)

7. A student who is below average in ability (slower learners – 70-89 IQ)

8. A student who is already one year older than his/her peers

9. A student who is considered too "street wise" for his/her age

10. A student who has a multitude of complex problems

11. A child with a long history of having a very low self-esteem (Note: In many, if not most, cases students in the wrong grade exhibit signs of low self-esteem.)

12. A child from a highly transient family (Three moves in five years)

13. Some linguistically different students

14. Some students who are physically large for their age.

Note: Some of these students may show some level of improvement when retained as a result of the stress of being in the wrong grade being removed. These are cautions and not a rigid list of students to eliminate from consideration for an additional year of learning time

---

Students Who Most Likely Will Benefit From Grade Level Expansion:

1. a child whose parent(s)/guardians strongly support having their child remain in the same grade or program another year

2. a student who is chronologically too young for his/her present grade level placement

3. a developmentally young child who has been inadvertently assigned to the wrong grade or program

4. a student who is in the average or above average ability range

5. a student who has indicated he/she wants to remain in the same grade or program another year

6. a student who has never had an extra year of time in any form and is <u>not</u> already one year older than his/her classmates

7. a child who doesn't appear to have serious learning problems or other extenuating circumstances other than being a late bloomer

8. a student with good school attendance

9. a student who is not highly transient

10. a child who is physically small for his/her age

Common Sense Tips to Make an Informed Grade Level Retention/Promotion Decisions for Individual Students

1. Always present parent(s)/guardian(s) with multiple placement options from which to choose. Children with very different beginnings need very different beginnings!

2. Always explore alternatives to grade level retention first. Think of grade level retention as the intervention strategy of last resort. *

3. Parent(s) should never be pressured to retain a child against their wishes. Forced retentions simply do not work. *

4. Don't cause students to be two years older than their classmates. Students two or more years over-age are most likely to drop out of school.*

5. Always make high stakes decisions with an ad hoc child study team, i.e., parents, teacher, principal, counselor, etc. *

6. Don't substitute grade level retention in place of special education intervention. They are two very different interventions.

7. Do not make a grade level retention decision based on a single factor, i.e., standardized tests, chronological age, reading level, etc. *

8. If a student needs more time in grade, do it during the early childhood years (K-3). *

9. Don't hesitate to change a child's placement mid-year (grade re-placement).

10. Only retain an upper grade student if you have his/her unconditional support.

11. Provide retained students remedial support services when needed. Many developmentally young students also have learning problems. *

12. When possible, allow the child to stay with the same teacher a second year. Take the child's feelings into account when making this decision.

13. Parents must be allowed the right to cast the deciding vote to retain or not to retain their child. *

14. Create and adopt flexible grade level retention guidelines versus a rigid grade level retention policy. A no retention policy is an extremist position leaving no room to make case by case individual decisions. Such an absolute position denies the existence of students placed in the wrong grade.

15. Remember, grade level retention research is reported as an average of a group. An individual retention is a very personal one child, one family at a time decision, and is NOT a group activity.

16. Bear in mind that keeping students in a grade or program another year without changing the curriculum and instruction will most likely produce dismal results.

17. Don't overstate the benefits of retention. Be modest in your claims.

18. Remember, people stigmatize people. (A stigma is an adult "gift" to children!)

19. The social promotion fad of recent years is not without consequences and generally creates a host of other problems (i.e., an increase in students who are labeled LD, ADD, BD, ED, ect.)

20. Taking an extra year of learning time in a transition class is not the same experience as grade level retention. This is not "another form of retention!"

21. Remaining an extra year in a multiage continuous progress classroom is not considered grade level retention. This is not "another form of retention!"

22. All students will come to school ready to learn by the year 2000. A noble goal that is unlikely to happen. Until this goal is met it is likely that different students will need different amounts of learning time to participate successfully in school.

Important points to include in your school system's grade level retention guidelines.

Jim Grant

Some Schools Enforce Some or All
of the Following Retention Rules:

1. All potential retentions must be reported to the principal's office by March 15

2. Former Reading Recovery® students are not allowed to be retained in grade

3. Retained students are automatically excluded from the Reading Recovery® program

4. Students identified as learning disabled or ESL are not allowed to be retained (No Double Dipping)

5. Retained students are not allowed any form of special eduction services (No Double Dipping)

6. No grade level retentions permitted at the kindergarten and first grade levels

7. Students who take on an additional year of learning time in a transition program or remain an extra year in a multiage program are officially noted as retentions in the school register and are reported to the state as a grade level retention

8. All students shall be socially promoted. There will be no additional learning time available in the form of an extra year for any student for any reason

9. Teachers are not allowed to acknowledge the concept of "wrong grade placement" with parents and are asked not to suggest retention

10. Once class rosters are set, no student can have their placement changed

Note: Most rules are based on politics, economics or administrative convenience rather than education principles

Jim Grant

Incoming Third Graders Should:

→ Read well enough to comprehend age appropriate content-area texts

→ Be able to work independently

→ Be comfortable working in a cooperative learning group

→ Be able to sustain a 25-30 minute teacher-directed lesson

→ Have good number sense and be ready to learn the multiplications table with ease

→ Be able to transfer information from textbooks/chalkboard to paper/pencil

→ Begin to write in cursive without mixing manuscript

→ Begin to tell time to the minute (no digital watches)

→ Make the transition from temporary to dictionary spelling

→ Possess the emotional maturity to handle the "workload" required of third graders

Contrary to what research says,
children **do not** catch up at grade three.

4-Year-Olds

Signs & Signals of Preschool Stress

	Often	Rarely	Never
At Home — How often does this 4-year-old child:			
1. not want to leave Mom/Dad			
2. hide shoes so as not to have to go to preschool			
3. complain about stomachaches or headaches			
4. have bathroom "accidents"			
5. come home exhausted			
6. have nightmares			
At Preschool — How often does this 4-year-old child:			
1. have difficulty separating from Mom/Dad			
2. cling to the teacher, showing a high degree of dependency			
3. not participate in "cooperative" play — instead, his or her play is "isolated" (child plays alone) or "parallel" (playing next to other children but not with them)			
4. not like other children			
5. show "young" fine-motor coordination while cutting, gluing, drawing, etc.			
6. demonstrate a lack of awareness of appropriate behavior in the classroom			
7. not catch on to "classroom" routines, which more mature classmates adapt to easily			
8. find it difficult to select activities and stick with them			
9. become "outspoken" and/or want to leave when asked to perform a task that is too difficult			
In General — How often does this 4-year-old child:			
1. cry easily			
2. lack self-control or self-discipline (biting, hitting and kicking)			
3. appear to be "shy"			
4. revert to thumbsucking, nail biting or "baby talk"			
5. become aggressive during games and other activities involving the taking of turns or sharing			

Note: All children display some stress signs at times. Severe stress is indicated when a child consistently displays several stress signs over an extended period of time.

Adapted from "*I Hate School! Some Common Sense Answers for Parents Who Wonder Why. Including the Signs and Signals of the Overplaced Child*" by Jim Grant. © Modern Learning Press, Rosemont, NJ 08556

5-Year-Olds

Signs & Signals of School Stress

	Often	Rarely	Never
***At Home* — How often does this 5-year-old child:**			
1. not want to leave Mom/Dad			
2. not want to go to school			
3. suffer from stomachaches or headaches, particularly in the morning before school			
4. dislike school or complain that school is "dumb"			
5. complain that the teacher does not allow enough time to finish his or her schoolwork			
6. need to rest, but resist taking a nap			
7. revert to bedwetting			
***At School* — How often does this 5-year-old child:**			
1. show little interest in kindergarten "academics"			
2. ask if it's time to go home			
3. seem unable to hold scissors as directed by the teacher			
4. worry that Mom/Dad will forget to pick him or her up after school			
5. have a difficult time following the daily routine			
6. talk incessantly			
7. complain that schoolwork is "too hard" ("I can't do it,") or "too easy" ("It's so easy I'm not going to do it,") or "too boring"			
8. interrupt the teacher constantly			
9. seem unable to shift easily from one task to the next			
10. seem overly restless during class and frequently in motion when supposed to be working at a task			
***In General* — How often does this 5-year-old child:**			
1. become withdrawn			
2. revert to thumbsucking or infantile speech			
3. compare herself negatively to other children ("They can do it but I can't.")			
4. complain that he/she has no friends			
5. cry easily and frequently			
6. make up stories			
7. bite his or her nails			
8. seem depressed			

Note: All children display some stress signs at times. Severe stress is indicated when a child consistently displays several stress signs over an extended period of time.

Adapted from "*I Hate School! Some Common Sense Answers for Parents Who Wonder Why. Including the Signs and Signals of the Overplaced Child*" by Jim Grant. © Modern Learning Press, Rosemont, NJ 08556

6-Year-Olds

Signs & Signals of School Stress

	Often	Rarely	Never
At Home — **How often does this 6-year-old child:**			
1. complain of before-school stomachaches			
2. revert to bedwetting			
3. behave in a manner that seems out of character to the parent			
4. ask to stay home			
At School — **How often does this 6-year-old child:**			
1. want to play with 5-year-olds			
2. want to play with toys during class time			
3. choose recess, gym and music as favorite subjects			
4. feel overwhelmed by the size and activity level in the lunchroom			
5. have a high rate of absenteeism			
6. try to take frequent "in-house field trips" to the pencil sharpener, bathroom, school nurse, custodian, etc.			
7. mark papers randomly			
8. "act out" on the playground			
9. reverse, invert, substitute, or omit letters and numbers when reading and/or writing (This is not unusual for properly placed students)			
10. complain about being bored with schoolwork, when in reality he or she cannot do the work			
11. have a short attention span — unable to stay focused on a twenty minute reading lesson			
12. have difficulty understanding the teacher's instructions			
In General — **How often does this 6-year-old child:**			
1. cry easily or frequently			
2. tire quickly			
3. need constant reassurance and praise			
4. become withdrawn and shy			
5. develop a nervous tic – a twitching eye, a nervous cough, frequent clearing of the throat or twirling of hair			
6. return to thumbsucking			
7. lie or "adjust the truth" about school			
8. revert to soiling his or her pants			
9. make restless body movements, such as rocking in a chair, jiggling legs, etc.			
10. dawdle			
11. seem depressed			
12. act harried/hurried			

Note: All children display some stress signs at times. Severe stress is indicated when a child consistently displays several stress signs over an extended period of time.

Adapted from "*I Hate School! Some Common Sense Answers for Parents Who Wonder Why. Including the Signs and Signals of the Overplaced Child*" by Jim Grant. © Modern Learning Press, Rosemont, NJ 08556

Attributes of a Slower Learner *

Please check all attributes that apply to: _____ Date: _____

Student's name

Caution: Do not use this information to identify, diagnose or label any student a slow learner. This information is for discussion purposes only. The determination of a child's index of intelligence should only be assessed by trained personnel.

How often have you observed this student exhibiting the following behaviors:	Often	Sometimes	Rarely	Never
Frequently cannot recall detail(s) from memory				
Questions/comments reveal a lack of comprehension of new concepts				
Has difficulty following directions				
Becomes easily frustrated and upset when he/she doing his/her homework				
Takes an inordinate amount of time to complete his/her work				
Becomes confused when there are changes in routines or plans				
Becomes easily distracted when attempting school work				
Has difficulty focusing on a specific task				
Has difficulty sustaining attention to verbal explanations				
Complains about too much schoolwork				
Complains about not having enough time to do his/her school work				
Becomes easily confused about the rules to games				
Tends to be a spectator rather than a participant in activities				
Follows the lead of others; has difficulty remembering classroom routines				

Note: None of these attributes of a slower learner are absolutes; many students may display a few attributes of a slower learner at times. Serious concern may be warranted when a student exhibits multiple attributes of a slower learner. If the "often" column is checked repeatedly, the child study team should create and implement an Individual Retention Plan or Individual Promotion Plan (depending on its placement decision) to assure support for this student.

Certain attributes of a slower learner may also be indicative of other problems or conditions such as Attention Deficit Disorder, depression, school-related stress, learning disabilities, or developmental immaturity. If you believe this student is a slower learner, referral for a comprehensive evaluation should be requested immediately to determine the nature of this child's problem or condition.

Name(s) of the individual(s) who provided this information:

_____ Title/Position _____ Date _____

_____ Title/Position _____ Date _____

(*70–89 IQ)

Reproducible Page
For Classroom Use

Adapted from *The Retention/Promotion Checklist*, by Jim Grant and Irv Richardson. Peterborough, NH: Crystal Springs Books, 1998.

Signs of Attention Deficit Disorder

Please check all signs that apply to: _____ Date _____
Student's name

Caution: Do not use this information to identify, diagnose or label any student as having ADD. This information is for discussion purposes only. A diagnosis of ADD/ADHD should only be made by a medical doctor.

How often have you observed this student exhibiting the following behaviors:	Often	Sometimes	Rarely	Never
Calls out in class when asked not to				
Forgets items				
Daydreams or "spaces out"				
Has difficulty focusing on a single task				
Becomes impatient				
Has difficulty delaying gratification				
School work is done with little care				
Exhibits poor fine motor control in handwriting				
Loses things (toys, clothes, books, etc.)				
Tends to be in constant motion				
Is easily discouraged				
Lacks self-control				
Appears disorganized				
Exhibits inattentiveness				
Has difficulty completing all aspects of a task				
Easily distracted by external stimuli				

Note: Many students may display some of these signs at times. Serious concern is warranted when a student exhibits multiple signs of ADD over an extended period of time. Some of these signs of ADD may also be indicative of other problems or conditions such as depression, emotional difficulty, developmental immaturity, or lower than average ability. If the "often" column has been checked repeatedly, then the student should be referred for a comprehensive evaluation.

Name(s) of the individual(s) who provided this information:

_____Title/Position _____Date _____

_____Title/Position _____Date _____

Reproducible Page
For Classroom Use

Spotting a Possible Learning Disability

Please check all traits that apply to: _____ Date _____
Student's name

Caution: Do not use this information to identify, diagnose or label any student as learning disabled. The use of this information is for discussion purposes only. A diagnosis of learning disabilities should only be made by a psychologist in conjunction with a pediatrician or family doctor.

How often have you observed this student exhibiting the following traits:	Often	Sometimes	Rarely	Never
Has difficulty recalling acquired knowledge				
Requires a number of repetitions of taught materials (rate of acquisition and knowledge retention are lower than those of age-appropriate peers)				
Depends on others to organize work for him/her				
Seems unable to discriminate between important facts and details or unimportant facts				
Seems unable to remain attentive and focused on classroom learning				
Experiences difficulty with language expression				
Experiences difficulty with receptive language				
Motivation for school work is low				
Struggles with social interaction				
Experiences difficulty applying information in new contexts				
Requires work load and time allowances to be adapted to specific need				
Exhibits poor social judgement				
Is easily confused by changes in schedule				
Is easily confused by verbal innuendo; misreads body language				

Note: Many students exhibit some of these traits at various times. Serious concern may be warranted when a student consistently displays many of these traits over a long period of time. If the "often" column is checked repeatedly, then referral for a comprehensive evaluation by a child psychologist should be requested to determine if this child has learning disabilities.

Certain signs of learning disabilities may be indicative of other problems or conditions such as Attention Deficit Disorder, depression, lower than average ability, behavior problems and school-related stress. None of these learning disability traits are absolutes.

Adapted from the work of Gretchen Goodman with permission. This chart was taken from the book *Our Best Advice: The Multiage Problem Solving Handbook,* by Jim Grant, Bob Johnson, and Irv Richardson.

Name(s) of the individual(s) who provided this information:

_____ Title/Position _____ Date_____

_____ Title/Position _____ Date_____

Reproducible Page
For Classroom Use

Signs and Signals of Depression

Please check all signs and signals that apply to: _____ Date _____
Student's name

Caution: Do not use this information to identify, diagnose or label any student as being depressed. This information is for discussion purposes only. Diagnosis and subsequent treatment for depression should only be provided by a medical doctor.

How often have you observed this student exhibiting the following signs or signals:	Often	Sometimes	Rarely	Never
Expresses a dislike for school				
Cries easily or frequently				
Has a pervasive mood of sadness				
Tends to be a loner with few friends				
Tends to be non-participatory in school activities				
Seems disengaged, unattached				
Seems not to care about his/her personal hygiene				
Tells you he/she has trouble sleeping				
Appears irritable, angry, or sullen				
Lacks enthusiasm about things in general				
Makes negative statements about the future				
Has excessive absenteeism				
Complains about being tired in spite of adequate sleep				

In extreme cases of depression, a child may exhibit self-destructive behaviors such as:

Bulimia/Anorexia	☐ Yes ☐ No	Talking about suicide ☐ Yes ☐ No
Pulling out hair	☐ Yes ☐ No	Alcohol/drug abuse ☐ Yes ☐ No
Digging/scratching/cutting of skin	☐ Yes ☐ No	Other _____

A yes to any of the above areas indicates a top priority referral for this student.

Note: Many students display a few signs and signals of depression at times. Serious concern is warranted when a student displays multiple signs of depression over an extended period of time. If the "often" column is checked repeatedly, then this student should be referred to the school guidance counselor for services.

Certain signs and signals of depression may also be indicative of other problems or conditions such as social difficulty, poor self-concept, lower than average ability, school-related stress, emotional difficulty, behavior problems, Attention Deficit Disorder, and learning disabilities. None of these signs and signals of depression are absolutes.

Name(s) of the individual(s) who provided this information:

_____ Title/Position _____ Date _____

_____ Title/Position _____ Date _____

The Retention/Promotion Checklist   **Reproducible Page** *For Classroom Use*   © 1998 Crystal Springs Books • 1-800-321-0401

Auditing Your Retention/Promotion Policy

This audit will help you evaluate your current retention/promotion practices and create a policy that is effective, beneficial for children, and ethically and legally defensible. A model policy addresses the following factors, circumstances and practices.

Please check the boxes that indicate your current policy or practices.

Characteristics of a Comprehensive Retention/Promotion Policy	True for our school system	Not true at this time for our school system
1. While the placement of students is the legal prerogative of the superintendent of schools, retention/promotion decisions are mutually agreeable to both school officials and the parent(s)/guardian(s).		
2. Retention/promotion decisions are made based on the recommendations of an ad hoc child study team that includes:		
A. The principal		
B. The teacher(s)		
C. Parent(s) and/or guardian(s)		
And may include:		
D. A counselor		
E. Learning specialist(s)		
F. Social worker(s)		
G. A psychologist		
H. Other: _____		
3. When appropriate, the child study team creates and implements an Individual Retention Plan (IRP) or Individual Promotion Plan (IPP)		
4. Retention/promotion decisions consider the following factors or circumstances:		
A. Academic attainment/needs		
B. Social maturity		
C. Emotional maturity		
D. Physical size/development		
E. Ability level		
F. Primary language		
G. Learning disabilities		
H. Gender		
I. Attendance		

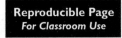

Reproducible Page
For Classroom Use

	True for our school system	Not true at this time for our school system
J. Transiency		
K. ESL		
L. Student motivation		
M. Chronological age		
N. Student attitude		
O. Parent support		
P. Overall health and wellbeing (vision, hearing, physical disability, malnutrition, chemical damage, trauma, poverty)		
Q. Other: _____		
5. A retention decision is never based on a single indicator such as reading level or standardized achievement tests.		
6. When possible, retention takes place in the early years (pre-school through grade three)		
7. Retention of students after grade three is approached with extreme caution.		
8. Retained students are given additional support services when needed. (Without appropriate services the positive impact of retention is substantially reduced.)		
9. A student is not placed in a grade where he or she is more than 1 year older than his/her classmates.		
10. Students are not given an additional "extra year of learning time" if they:		
A. Stayed home an extra year		
B. Have already been retained in grade		
C. Spent an extra year in a day care or preschool setting		
D. Remained an extra year in a multiage classroom		
E. Took an extra year in a transition grade/program		
11. Retention is not used:		
A. As a punishment		
B. To motivate a student academically		
C. In place of special education services		
D. To "red shirt" a student for athletic or academic purposes		
E. To address transiency-related problems		
F. To supplant remedial instruction		
G. In place of ESL services		
H. To compensate for excessive absenteeism (15 or more days per school year)		

Reproducible Page
For Classroom Use

What Parents Want from Teachers

What do parents think about their children's teachers? Two school districts are trying to find out—in ways that will encourage stronger home-school connections.

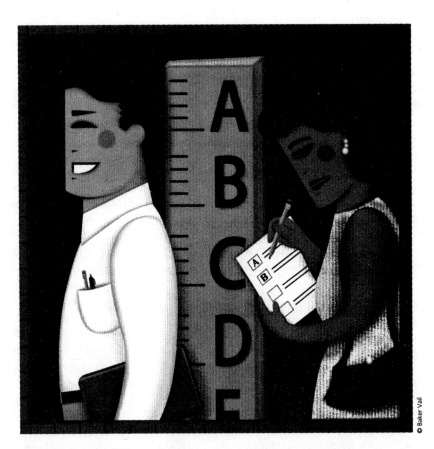

Parent surveys provide the basis for ongoing discussions at each school, often about curriculum.

Parents in Anchorage, Alaska, and Rochester, New York, have been rating the teachers of their children. This is something new—and some teachers may perceive getting a report card from parents as threatening. But increasingly, parents and community members are grading schools and are seeing themselves as customers. Such reports can be a good thing. Educators can make the most of them, getting credit for what they do well and making sure that the report cards help both teachers and parents work together to improve student learning (see box, p. 39).

In my work with schools across the United States, I have identified three consistent parent concerns: how well teachers *know and care* (1) about teaching, (2) about their children, and (3) about communicating with parents. Here, I use the basic list of questions from the Anchorage and Rochester (1997) report cards. For each question, I outline specific strategies, used in the MegaSkills Parent Involvement Program, that every teacher can use to get higher ratings from parents—not just in Anchorage or Rochester, but anywhere. I have found that teachers can use these questions and reports to spark their own creative ideas (see Rich 1997).

...About Teaching

■ *Does this teacher appear to enjoy teaching and believe in what he or she does in school?* Teachers need to smile . . . often. We need to share stories, not only about our interests and successes, but about funny things that happen in school. A good laugh together between teachers and parents is a strong bond.

■ *Does the teacher set high expectations and help children reach them?* Set and share with parents specific learning goals for their children. Start with easily measurable goals, such as a certain number of books to read and papers to write. Involve children in setting these goals and keeping track of their own progress.

■ *Does the teacher know the subject matter of the class and how to teach it?* This can get sticky, because everybody went to school once. Teachers must be academic sharers—explaining the curriculum, teaching methods, and how parents can reinforce learning at home.

■ *Does the teacher create a safe classroom where children are encouraged to pay attention, participate in class, and learn?* Invite parents to see the class in action. Ensure that you have many ways to get students to participate daily—by birth dates, letters in names, and all those good old stand-bys.

■ *Does the teacher deal with behavior problems fairly and consistently?* Have a set of rules that everyone understands. Include only those that can be enforced with reliable, consistent consequences. Kids

> *Before making assignments, ask yourself: "What does this really teach? Would I want to do this?"*

and parents should know the rules as well as you do.

■ *Does the teacher assign meaningful homework? Are the assignments clear? Is enough time provided? Is homework returned in a timely manner?* Before making assignments, ask yourself: "What does this really teach? Would I want to do this?" Ask children to rephrase the assignment in their own words. Share your homework schedule with parents, and check with them at conferences, through random phone calls, and through informal surveys.

■ *Does the teacher make clear what my child is expected to learn?* Parents, like students, need to know what is expected—and what excellent, average, and poor work looks like. Ask for their input on these expectations. Then make sure everyone knows the standards. Such publicized expectations are

helpful for students trying to improve their own work—before they turn it in.

...About Their Children

■ *Does the teacher understand how our child learns and tries to meet these needs?* Teachers must remember details about all the students in the class. It helps to keep a file on every student and place little notes in the files every now and then. This specific information is priceless during phone calls or conferences.

■ *Does the teacher treat my child fairly and with respect?* Here, again, classroom rules help ensure fairness. When we identify each child's abilities and build on them, we show respect. When we do the same for the family, we build a bridge from the classroom into the home.

■ *Does the teacher contact me promptly with any concerns about my child's academic and behavioral performance?* No parent wants to learn at the end of the year that there are problems that started mid-year. Use all means to contact parents, even hard-to-reach parents. Keep notes on when and how you made these efforts.

■ *Does the teacher provide helpful information during conferences?* Use those trusty files on each child for both praise and problems. When we share those problems, we need to have a solution or two ready and ask for parents' ideas.

■ *Does the teacher tell me how my child is doing in class?* All parents want to hear that their children are doing wonderfully and that they are above average. While we can't promise this, we can keep parents informed and, especially, discuss what they can do to help. Avoid that old classic, "Your child can do better," unless you have concrete suggestions that parents can try.

...About Communicating with Parents

■ *Does the teacher provide clear information about class expectations?* Here's where a written set of expectations can provide information about the curriculum, goals for class achievement, standards for quality of work, and the classroom behavior code. Be brief and as specific as possible. At the fall open house, give each parent a copy and ask for questions.

■ *Does the teacher use a variety of communication tools to report progress and student needs?* Use many ways to get your points across. You may lecture, send notes, e-mail, telephone,

> *Teachers must be academic sharers— explaining the curriculum, teaching methods, and how parents can reinforce learning at home.*

hold conferences—and it's still hard. At the elementary level, attach memos for parents to the school menu. In kindergarten, attach them to jackets. At the secondary level, it's a lot harder. It's helpful to have parents' work numbers and addresses.

■ *Is my child's teacher accessible*

and responsive to me when I call or want to meet? Teachers can be accessible without being on call. Parents need to know what days and hours teachers will be available. How much easier and more efficient this will be when every teacher has a telephone in the classroom! Some teachers give out their home telephone numbers; others do not. This is a personal choice.

■ *Does the teacher work with me to develop a cooperative strategy to help my child?* Make sure that parents know that everything about education is cooperative—that you expect them to work with you in mutually supportive ways. This is the big message that has to get across early—and often.

Moving Forward

The changes resulting from parent report cards in Rochester and Anchorage are yet to be determined. (The Rochester surveys, begun in early 1998, will be analyzed later this school year.)

The Anchorage surveys were begun two years ago. The state legislature instructed schools to find out from parents which issues were most significant to them. What evolved in Anchorage was a systematic set of surveys—for elementary, middle, and secondary schools. Each school could add additional items to the basic set of questions.

Fred Stofflet, Director of Curriculum and Evaluation for the Anchorage Public Schools, reports that getting people to return the surveys was difficult. Overall, there was about a 50-percent return rate, with the highest response at the elementary level.

What the surveys provide, he says, is the basis for ongoing discussions at each school, often about curriculum.

Educators can make the most of parent reports, getting credit for what they do well and making sure that both teachers and parents work together to improve student learning.

The surveys also get at differences between what adults and children say. In the area of school safety, for example, adults and students had differing perceptions; and that, says Stofflet, helped identify an area that needed attention.

Stofflet says that in Anchorage,

Sample Survey Questions for Parents

The Anchorage School District survey form asked parents to rate teachers from *A* (strongly agree) to *E* (don't know) on 16 statements, such as the following:

■ Understands how my child learns and tries to meet known needs.

■ Sets high expectations and helps my child to reach them.

■ Treats my child fairly, with respect, and understands that all children are special.

■ Knows the subject matter of the class and how to teach it.

■ Has regular contact with me about my child's conduct and performance.

In addition, the survey asked parents to write about what they liked best (and least) about their child's program, and to provide any other comments.

---

teachers' initial concerns have evaporated. Even though information from the surveys was used in their evaluations, teachers came to understand that the purpose of the surveys was to find out what was on parents' and students' minds and to deal with issues before they become problems.

Surveys and activities such as these may seem insignificant, compared to other weighty issues surrounding education reform (see Langdon 1997). But reform is not somewhere "out there." It's in every classroom and in every home. ■

References

Anchorage School District. (1997). *Teacher Evaluation Document*. Anchorage: Alaska Board of Education.

Langdon, C. (1997). "The Fourth Phi Delta Kappa Poll of Teachers' Attitudes Towards the Public Schools." *Phi Delta Kappan* 79, 3: 212–220.

Rich, D. (August 6, 1997). "Seven Habits of Good Teachers Today: What This 'Good Teacher' Didn't Know." *Education Week* 16, 41: 53, 57.

Rochester Teachers Association. (September 17, 1997). "Parents in N.Y. District to Critique Teachers." *Education Week* 17, 3: 3.

Dorothy Rich is Founder and President of the Home and School Institute, the MegaSkills Education Center of the Home and School Institute, 1500 Massachusetts Ave., N.W., Washington, DC 20005 (e-mail: hsidra@erols.com). For more Information, visit the MegaSkills Web site (http://www.MegaSkillsHSI.org).

THE UNVARNISHED TRUTH ABOUT PARENTS

By Jim Grant

*A recovering principal reveals
the real secrets behind successful
parent management*

I'M JIM, AND I'M A RECOVERING PRINCIPAL. IF you are now or have ever been a principal, you're probably saying, "Oh, my Lord, you mean you never fully recover?" No, you never do. That's the reality. There's another reality, too: If you're reading this article to learn six sweet ways to have a parent conference go nicely, turn the page, because I want to clear away the brush and open the pathway. I want to talk about the real stuff. I want to talk about a secret—the collapse of society—and I want to talk about the condition the kids are in when they come to us. I want to talk about the tremendous pressure parents are under. And I want to talk about your job description and how it's changed dramatically. Then I want to give you some commonsense tips that have worked for me in trying to elicit parent support for their children's education.

Whenever I travel around the country and hold parent meetings, parents inevitably will say, "Schools aren't like they used to be." Well, that's not quite true. Schools are like they used to be—which is part of the problem. We still have the same lockstep, time-bound curriculum that we've had for the last 147 years; we still collect and group kids according to their chronological age.

What isn't the same is society and family life. Both have changed dramatically. Divorce rates are high; as a result, many kids coming to school today are from broken homes. Does that change their outlook? Absolutely.

Next, there's the blended family—a kind of yours, mine, and ours. We have more kids coming to school today from blended families. Ask yourself this question: Have you ever encountered children from the same family who are so different from one another that you've actually considered doing a DNA test to see if there has been a swap? Blended families share resources and bedrooms and parents—and all that sharing means a whole new set of dynamics that many parents simply aren't geared to deal with—things like family incomes that are below the poverty line, inadequate housing, lack of basic needs, and a good measure of household anger.

We have larger class sizes than we've had in the past—and we have a higher number of high-maintenance children.

And what are parents asking us to do in response? They're asking us to adopt a new edition of a basal reader and to increase testing so we can test our way out of this mess.

Ask anybody from New Hampshire. In New Hampshire, farmers made a startling discovery: They found that if they wanted to fatten their cows they should feed them, not weigh them. I'd argue that we need to take that philosophy and apply it to kids: If you want to educate children, you do it by teaching, not testing.

I started my teaching career in Dublin, N.H., in 1967. I taught one year, and that year was so wonderful, I decided to go back for a second dose. The last Friday of November in my second year of teaching, I heard a knock at the door; it was the friendly neighborhood assistant superintendent. At the time, I had accumulated 11 contact months with children.

Jim Grant, executive director of the Society for Developmental Education, served as a teacher-principal in New Hampshire for two decades.

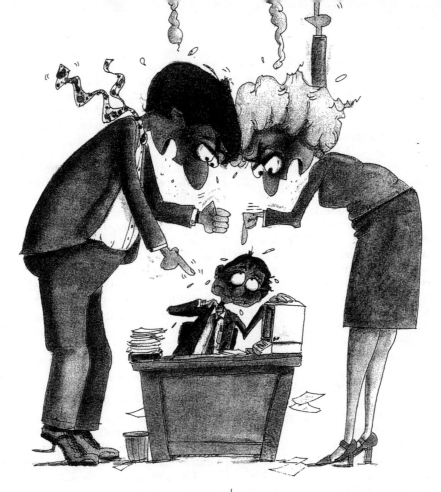

The assistant superintendent swung the door open with a bang and wiggled his finger at me. I was a good boy: I obeyed his finger and walked toward him, and as I approached him, he said, "We've watched you for a year." I got defensive. I said, "I've been a good boy. I have never so much as skipped one page in the basal like Ray has." (You always tattle when you're in trouble.) He said, "Jim, we like the way you work with kids, we like the way you work with staff, and we love the way you work with parents. We're going to give you a chance to experience upward mobility and professional growth. We're going to make you the principal of Temple Elementary School."

Now, I don't look very smart, but I'm good at mathematics, so I knew that if I accepted the job at Temple, I would be the fifth principal there in 24 months.

"The parents kill principals up there," I said. "Thank you for thinking of me, but I'm not going."

He said, "You don't have tenure."

I said, "I meant to ask you, When am I going to start?"

So at 8:00 Monday morning, I went to the Temple Elementary School and took over the reins. When I got there, what did I find? I found many, many problems—and had my first taste of a principal's fantasy life. After only three days on the job, I began fantasizing about how exciting it would be to be a superintendent of an orphanage where there were no parents.

The first day of school I met the only man that Will Rogers hadn't met. (Will Rogers wouldn't have liked him either.) His name was Ken. The next day I met his wife, Barbie, who had a black belt in telephone skills.

You probably have parents like Ken and Barbie who try to live through their children. It helps them with the guilt they bear for putting their kids in day care before the kids were born. Their attitude is: "I haven't been able to stay home and raise my child, so I'm going to expect you to make sure the child is put in all the right programs."

And they particularly want him in which program? The *gifted* program, of course. No, don't test him; take their word for it. He's gifted. Why, even the pediatrician said that when this kid was 4 years old and all the other kids knew the four-letter words, Harvey could rhyme them.

We have other parents with unreal expectations as well. You and most of your colleagues probably get to school by 6:00 a.m. Have you ever encountered parents who think you couldn't possibly mind if they drop Willy off a little early? Listen, you're there anyway, right? And by the way, is there any chance that you could feed him breakfast and lunch, and could you send dinner home with him?

As principals today, we have many families who have gone through some sort of chemical dependency, emotional problems, employment problems, fear of losing their homes, or not having any home at all. All that changes a person's perspective. Children are coming to school bolder—and with more brass—today than ever before, too. Have you ever had a child lecture you, "I don't want to scare you, but my dad says if my grades don't improve, somebody is going to get it"?

Or, to keep a child safe, have you ever agreed to take the child home for a weekend? Today, we sometimes have to be innkeepers. How about being subpoenaed to testify as a character witness in a divorce case? It happens. And how about the divorce decree? Because you have nothing else to do, it's easy for you to remember every third Wednesday Uncle Bill picks up Skippy.

And have you ever been addressed as "Daddy? I mean Mr. Smith"?

Our classrooms are under a tremendous amount of pressure. We've got to go public. I blame a lot of our issues on principals and teachers. We have not gone public with our concerns; we have not told the public what you and I are up against daily.

Now, I'm going to tell you something that you know—and that you have to take public. We have a skyrocketing number of children we call "gray-area" kids. I say this in a loving way. These kids aren't needy enough to qualify for Title I or Reading Recovery or special-education services. But I don't care how you slice it: These are high-risk, high-impact kids—kids with asthma, kids born to teen mothers, low birth-weight babies, and more. Are these "tweeners" recognized in the eyes of the federal or state law? No. There's little help for these kids. They fall between the cracks.

D O YOU FIND THAT SOMETIMES YOU WAKE UP in the middle of the night and think you're supposed to be attending a meeting? Twenty years after I graduated from college, I would wake up thinking I was missing a test. And then, you know, in my last year of teaching, I would wake up and say, "Shouldn't I be in an IEP meeting?"

Schools today have more paperwork and more staff meetings than ever before. Teachers want shared decision making. Is there a cost attached to it? Yeah, it's called meetings. Teachers have to take on more and more responsibility for nonacademic things.

And what do you do as a principal? You say to your staff the first day of school, "We're going to have high standards, and we're going to improve reading, writing, and math skills. But I'm also going to ask you if you would be willing to sneak in a few very important curriculum components, just a few of them. I'm going to ask you to do manners education, alcohol and drug education, head-lice prevention, sex education, plant-a-tree campaign, poison prevention, handgun safety, earthquake safety, flood safety, tornado safety, hurricane safety—nay-nay from strangers, stay away—nutrition education, electrical hazard, fire safety, aluminum recycling, divorce education, deaf education, and AIDS education. (And don't you dare get me in trouble by mentioning gays, sex, or blood.) Then there's emergency numbers, safety programs, stop-drop-and-roll when gunfire breaks out in the playgrounds, suicide prevention, and be kind to animals. What about be kind to kids?

Forget that; there isn't time. And, by the way, teachers, there will be no materials or training forthcoming.

And that's not all. Do you ever have parents send a sick child to school? Have you ever gotten a note saying, "Our Charlie was puking and pooping all night, and he's way, way too sick to stay home. Keep him in at recess"?

THE CARE AND FEEDING OF PARENTS

So what can you do to promote good linkages between schools and parents? I'm going to start off by saying that when you're doing a parent conference, watch your body language. Do any of you have a teacher or a parent who actually comes into your personal space? You probably don't like it. Don't inflict such an invasion on anyone else. So the No. 1 rule is don't invade a parent's space. No. 2 is, don't let an in-the-face parent invade your space; it's so distracting, it is hard to collect your thoughts.

You'll also want to know when not to make eye contact. In some cultures, eye contact is a threat, so be aware of cultural distinctions.

Don't come across as being aloof. Have you ever had a superintendent who was aloof? If you come across as aloof, then it sends the message, "You're not taking me seriously." You don't want parents thinking that.

Be open and friendly, and, please, develop a sense of humor and use it. Humor defuses tension. Humor takes a difficult situation and makes it easier. Humor means you're human. I always had a standard greeting for anyone who came to my office. A parent would say, "I'm here to see you," and I would say, "Come on in my office so I can quickly determine if I'm happy to see you." And all the parents would laugh. Except for Ken.

Please, don't be a finger-pointer. Do you like having a finger shaken at you? No. And don't put your hands on your hip; it makes you seem arrogant. Some principals put a desk between themselves and parents for protection, but I don't recommend it.

Be open to meeting in a neutral zone, such as a coffee shop, or on the parent's turf. Meeting in their domain shows some respect.

Whatever you do, don't use education jargon. It puts barriers between you and parents. They want to hear things in English, not edu-babble.

Know when to end a meeting. And when you do end your meeting, always try to restate what's been said or decided. Some parents have selective amnesia, so just before the meeting breaks up say, "Could I ask you to just listen, and let me restate? What we agreed to is this, this, that, and the other. OK. And as long as we agree to that, that's what I kind of put in the little record that I'm keeping here." Always try to document the outcome of your meeting.

If you need a witness, get one.

Another tip: Don't overwhelm parents. A parent who might be uneducated—or easily intimidated—will probably be blown away if you have 100 experts lined up for the conference. Try to reduce the number of people who might be attending.—J.G.

You're facing other pressures as well. If you have a classroom of 25, you do 25 parent conferences. But it's not uncommon to do 36 parent conferences today due to broken homes—so much for having a private life.

Ever been forced into the role of head-lice constable? When Ken and Barbie moved to my school, the first thing on their son's agenda was to sit next to someone and catch head lice. And when Ken called me up, he said, "My kid caught head lice," I said, "Yes." He said, "I want this stopped immediately." I said, "OK."

Have you ever had a parent accuse you of calling his child a liar? Don't ever do it again. OK. Just tell that parent that you suspect the child is suffering from Truth-Deficit Syndrome.

Oh, the roles you play as a principal: field-trip financier, grocery purchaser, bank loan officer for teachers and some parents, staff referee (you mediate between the phonics-first and the whole-language people). Custodian? Designated driver for sick kids who need to go home? Snow shoveler? Welfare officer?

School chaplain? That's right, it's the principal who often must help children deal with a child's death or take a child home when a parent has died.

What principal, on two minutes' notice, has not had to be a substitute teacher?

And is there a principal anywhere in the United States who hasn't had a parent call and ask, "Could I ask you to pop back to school, flip the dumpster over, and find Betty Ann's dental appliance?"

It's a tough job. But somebody has to do it.

WHEN PARENTS COME TO VISIT, DO THEY OPEN the classroom door at 10:00 a.m. and say to the teacher, "Are you busy?"

You see, for a parent, perception is reality. Parents come to school, and there is no seating chart. They'll come and say, "I need to get something out of Charlie's desk," and you say, "Well, you're in the right room," but face it: You can't find the desk. So you have to explain to the parents that you hire high-level substitutes who don't need a seating chart because they can ask children their names. Have you had parents speak to you about too much activity in the classroom? They pop in and say, "What the deuce is Skippy doing? I've been in the room for an hour watching, and all Skippy has been doing is wandering here and there."

What does the principal say? "Skippy's taking an in-house field trip."

Parents see whole-language teaching strategies, and they ask, "Where's phonics?" When I was in school, the teacher used to give us three hours a day of sitting there looking at phonograms, barking and grunting, "eh, ah, eh, ah, eh, ah." That was real teaching, they thought.

Is your building locked during school hours, and do you have a sign on the door saying, "Visitors report to the office"? So are parents visitors or are they parents? In some ways, we've created an unfriendly atmosphere.

Parents look askance at other newfangled strategies as well. Take noncomparative reporting, for example. What do parents want? They want the bell curve. "When I was a kid," they say, "if you didn't do your work, you flunked." Parents today want winners and losers. They want comparative reporting. They want unfair competition.

Authentic assessment. Whole language. Cooperative-learning groups. Full inclusion of differently abled students. Multiage classrooms. Parents sometimes equate multiage classrooms with the open classrooms of the '60s. To us, the multiage classroom is not unstructured; it is *differently* structured. But to some parents, it's a free-for-all.

So where do you find common ground? Are you and parents just by nature on opposite sides? First of all, the research is very clear about certain things: (1) If parents become your partners, everyone benefits; (2) when parents are involved in the school, their children actually do better academically and have a better relationship with their parents; and (3) children actually do more things with the parents, and they have a more positive attitude about school, when they know the parents support the school.

Parents benefit as well. According to the research, parents who are involved in their children's education have more self-confidence and more positive feelings about themselves. And this is really a wonderful by-product: When parents are connected to the school, they will actually seek out ways to grow academically themselves, taking a course, attending a lecture, listening to a cassette tape, whatever. It's all education. They have a more positive feeling about the school and the personnel, and they are willing to work for the school.

ONE MASSACHUSETTS SCHOOL SYSTEM MADE NAtional news not long ago. The system had to put a cigarette-style warning label on report cards to encourage parents not to abuse their children physically when they looked at the report card. That came as a surprise to the news media, but it doesn't come as a surprise to me—or to you. I've had cases in which a mother would come in and say, "I live with a man of violence; I need some help. If Johnnie doesn't get A's and B's, he is in serious trouble." What did I do? I had two report cards, one that stayed with us and the other that would go home—to protect Johnnie.

But, please, be inventive with your options. True story: I once had a foster child enrolled in my school. The child had a tooth that was broken and rotted, but, when I talked with the foster parents, they refused him dental care. What did I do?

I got a substitute in my room, and I went dentist-hopping. Finally, I found a dentist to pull this child's tooth. A little later I got a call from the superintendent, who said, "Put your spanking suit on, and get down to see me. I just got a call from the foster parents that you pulled a kid's tooth without parent permission."

So I said, "OK." I went to the superintendent's office, stood where the superintendent told me to stand (he was one of those guys), and listened to his diatribe. "I'm furious with you," he said. "You could have put the district in liability."

Then he said to me, "I've just got to ask you one more question: What stupid dentist in his right mind would pull a kid's tooth without parent permission?"

"Oh," I said, "that was Don Johnson, the chairman of the school board."

Parental Engagement That Makes a Difference

Parental involvement in schooling can lead to real academic benefits for children—but some parent behaviors are more effective than others.

*H*ome-school partnerships command a lot of attention these days. Well-intentioned educators are recommending an infusion of energy toward increasing parental participation in schools. The federal government has issued documents to help schools organize parent participation programs (for example, Rutherford et al. 1997). Major reform efforts and educational interventions list parental involvement as an important ingredient. Scholarly writing on the topic abounds, and various publications offer guidance to schools or describe exemplary programs.

What does research say about the role of parental

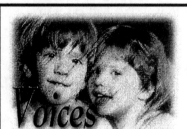

*C*hildren have more need of models than of critics.

— *Joseph Joubert*

From *The Heart and Wisdom of Teaching: A collection of thought-provoking quotations for teachers.* Compiled by Esther Wright, M.A. TEACHING FROM THE HEART © 1997 by Esther Wright.

involvement—at home and in school—in supporting youngsters' academic achievement? Unfortunately, the mountain of material about parent-school partnerships yields few if any empirical data about the impact of parental involvement on students' academic achievement. But a different set of research studies provides much information that educators should consider. Empirical data show that *specific parenting practices* are related to students' academic achievement. It is important to understand how, and to what extent,

"parental engagement behaviors" bolster student learning.

The Importance of the Home Environment

Until the early 1960s, sociologists believed that school performance and intelligence were immutably connected with socioeconomic status and family structure. However, building on the ideas of Benjamin Bloom, Dave (1963) and Wolf (1964) demonstrated that differences in children's performance could be explained instead by specific conditions and parental behaviors, including parents' roles as language models, parents' press for achievement, and provisions for general learning.

Clark (1983) added significantly to our understanding through an intensive study of 10 African-American students from poor homes, half of whom were successful academically and half of whom were not. The researchers discovered that parents of high-achieving students had distinct styles of interacting with their children. They created emotionally supportive home environments and provided reassurance when the youngsters encountered failure. They viewed school performance as being accomplished through regular practice and work. They accepted responsibility for assisting their children to acquire learning strategies, as well as a general fund of knowledge.

Research reveals that parental *engagement at home* and *engagement at school* are not equally important to children's learning. At the same time, extensive research reviews find that the home environment is among the most important influences on academic performance (Wang et al. 1993).

Parental Engagement at Home

Researchers have identified three types of parental engagement at home that are consistently associated with school performance:

■ actively organizing and monitoring the child's time;
■ helping with homework; and
■ discussing school matters with the child.

A fourth set of activities that is germane, particularly for younger children, consists of parents reading to and being read to by their children.

The exact form that each of these takes may differ from one family to another, but research shows that each is important. In fact, studies of student resilience

 Finn, Jeremy (May 1998). "Parental Engagement that Makes A Difference." *Educational Leadership* 55, 8: 20-24. Reprinted with permission of the Association for Supervision and Curriculum Development. Copyright © 1998 by ASCD. All rights reserved.

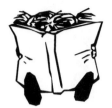

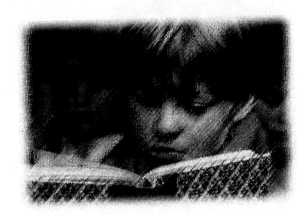

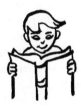

whether or not they have been assigned homework; and they make certain that a place and time are allocated for homework. In addition, school performance is better among students whose parents know where they are, who they are with, and when they plan to come home. These parents also exercise reasonable control over nonschool activities—television viewing, in particular.

Involvement with homework. Homework offers an opportunity for parents to show an interest and to take a direct role in their youngster's schooling. Making certain that homework is completed, discussing the specifics of assignments and papers, explaining the assignments, checking accuracy, and actively helping children complete

> *The most efficient time to set a child on a positive path is at a young age.*

assignments have all been found to be related to children's academic performance (Ho and Willms 1996, Clark 1983, Finn 1993, Lamborn et al. 1992). If a parent is not familiar with the content of the schoolwork, the acts of asking questions about an assignment and examining completed work still underscore the importance attached to skill development.

In some instances, parents may serve as tutors to their children. Peterson (1989) notes that the familiarity of the home environment, in contrast to the structure of the classroom, can become a comfortable setting for tutoring. In a survey of parents of elementary schoolchildren, Epstein (1983) found that more than 85 percent spent at least 15 minutes daily tutoring their children when the teacher requested it. Of course, tutoring requires some degree of subject-matter knowledge and some knowledge of teaching strategies.

Discussing school matters. Children whose parents converse regularly with

indicate that many of these same behaviors explain why some students succeed academically despite the adversities posed by poverty, minority status, or native language (Finn 1993, Masten 1994, Peng and Lee 1992).

Managing and organizing time. Clark's original study found that parents of successful students actively helped them organize their daily and weekly schedules and checked regularly to see whether they were following the routines. Other studies have shown that children who are involved in regular

routines at home tend to have better school performance (for example, Astone and McLanahan 1991, Taylor 1996).

Monitoring children's use of time is identified as important in all studies of parental engagement (for example, Astone and McLanahan 1991; Ho and Willms 1996; Crouter et al. 1990; Lamborn et al. 1992). Research shows that parents of academically successful students make sure they are informed about their youngsters' activities in school, their school performance, and

them about school experiences perform better academically than children who rarely discuss school with their parents (Astone and McLanahan 1991, Ho and Willms 1996, Finn 1993). Other research suggests that the *nature* of parent-child discussions is also important. Parents should be willing to hear about difficulties, as well as successes, and play a supportive role, encouraging persistence when schoolwork or relationships at school are problematic (Clark 1983, Lamborn et al. 1992, Steinberg 1996). Research supports joint parent-student decision making when the situation permits, such as choosing what project to undertake or, in later grades, what courses to take (for example, Lamborn et al. 1992, Taylor 1996). This level of interest is associated with higher student engagement, as well as academic achievement.

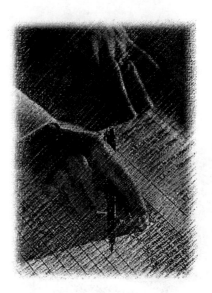

Literacy and reading at home. Studies from Wolf and Dave to the present have shown a positive relationship between a literacy-laden home and students' school performance. The presence of newspapers, magazines, books, a dictionary, and a computer or word processor helps to create a positive home setting. Even when these resources are in short supply, reading to a child and asking the child to read to the parent are crucial activities for the development of literacy. A great deal of research confirms a strong relationship between parents reading to their children and the development of reading proficiency (see Anderson et al. 1985 for a summary). Further, there is an important connection between children's reading to their parents and reading achievement—especially if the parents guide and correct the young readers (Tracey 1995).

Unfortunately, many households,

Teachers may pay more attention to students whose parents are involved in the school.

especially low-income or minority homes, have few books in total and even fewer that are appropriate and interesting to children (Edwards 1992; Baker et al. 1997). Children from these homes arrive at school with surprisingly little experience with books. At the same time, many parents feel they lack, or actually do lack, the skills to guide their children's reading or schoolwork (Edwards 1995; Hoover-Dempsey et al. 1995). Some parents who attempt to read with their youngsters make beginners' mistakes, such as reading an entire story just to get through it when part of a story would suffice; focusing so much on mechanics that their child's motivation is diminished; and taking a punitive attitude when the child makes errors.

School-sponsored programs, although not universally available, have been highly successful in improving these situations. At least one program provided books for children to take home twice a week (Toomey 1992). A large number of school-parent reading

programs have been reviewed by Topping (1986), Edwards (1992), and Tracey (1995). Better programs have proactive components to recruit parents, improve their literacy skills, help them develop a regular structure for home-based literacy, help them overcome obstacles to literacy activities in the home, and convince them that their children can become successful readers.

Most research on parental engagement at home, with the exception of studies of parent-child reading, has involved students at the junior high level. There are good reasons to believe that the same parental engagement behaviors are important for younger children. Psychologists and educators agree on the importance of setting habits early on that persevere throughout childhood and beyond. Early behavior that is dysfunctional tends to be sustained and to increase over the years (see Finn 1993); the most efficient time to set a child on a positive path is at a young age.

Parental Engagement in School

The opportunity for parents to stay intensively involved in school diminishes as students become increasingly independent and as peers come to have greater influence (Epstein 1984, Steinberg 1996). At the same time, parents can continue to be in-school participants by visiting the school; attending school events, performances, and athletics; and initiating contact with teachers and administrators.

It may be surprising that research has *not* consistently documented links between parents' in-school engagement and student achievement. Steinberg (1996) found a small but statistically significant correlation of achievement with parents' attendance at school programs, conferences, and extracurricular activities. The author noted that teachers may pay more attention to students whose parents are involved in the school, which may in turn explain the relationship. But others (for example, Finn 1993, Ho and Willms 1996, Taylor 1996) found little or no relationship between grades or achievement scores and parental visits to school, volunteer work, attendance at school events, and so on. Interestingly, several studies found that the relationship between parent-teacher contacts and academic achievement is negative; obviously, contacts increase when a student experiences academic or behavior problems (Milne et al. 1986; Ho and Willms 1996).

Given this research base, it is natural to ask why there is so much pressure to increase parent-school partnerships. Much has been written about different ways in which parents and schools can work together to facilitate academic outcomes. For example, Epstein and Dauber (1991) list basic health and safety responsibilities of parents and of schools; volunteering and attending school functions; parental involvement in learning at home, as recommended and supported by school staff; parental involvement in decision making; and encouraging parents and schools to become involved in community organi-

zations that can support families and children's learning. Like other research, the data presented by Epstein and Dauber show that parents who are involved in some of these activities tend also to be involved in others, but not that these activities are related to children's school performance. These types of activities require real time commitments—time not always available to a single or working parent (Moles 1987). A parent who does not have the time for in-school involvement may, out of frustration, not consider more helpful activities that can take place at home.

For these reasons, we must ask whether it is prudent to emphasize increased parent-school connections at this time. Although there can certainly be no harm in promoting parental involvement, and although parents who

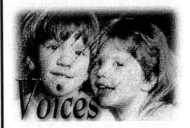

Children are mirrors. When they are in the presence of love, that's what they reflect. When love is absent, they have nothing to give out.

— *Anthony DeMello*

From *The Heart and Wisdom of Teaching: A collection of thought-provoking quotations for teachers.* Compiled by Esther Wright, M.A. TEACHING FROM THE HEART © 1997 by Esther Wright.

exhibit one sort of engagement are likely to practice others, the only answer research provides about the unique benefits of engagement in school is "the jury is still out."

What of the Disengaged?

In his work on child-rearing practices, Steinberg (1996) described parents who are "disengaged"—that is, who are authoritarian in their interactions with their children, who fail to provide guid-

ance or structure in the family setting, and who fail to provide the emotional support needed when the child encounters problems. Steinberg found that children whose parents are disengaged have the *poorest developmental patterns,* lacking psychological maturity, social competence, and self-esteem. The problems encountered by these youngsters, in school and out, multiply throughout the school years.

The research reviewed here points to specific attitudes and behaviors that, if implemented by parents, are associated with improved academic performance. These practices have been classified by Hoover-Dempsey and others (1995) as (1) providing structure—structuring routines at home, and coordinating with school when problems arise; and (2) active involvement—monitoring the

youngster's expenditure of time, teaching and explaining concepts, reviewing homework, and providing support when the child experiences difficulties. These authors and others give guidelines for parents who wish to increase their support for their children's academic work, and many effective programs are available for parents who would like assistance. Although the research evidence on participation in school is mixed, the evidence about parental engagement at home is persuasive. Disengagement is incapacitating.

Studies reviewed here (Epstein 1983, Toomey 1992) indicate that schools can foster the specific behaviors at home that promote student performance. In view of this, educators should pay particular attention to one ingredient of home-school partnerships. Most programs include an "outreach" effort to encourage parental involvement, both at home and at school. Educators should encourage this function, at least, of parent-school partnerships. ■

References

Anderson, R.C., E.H. Hiebert, J.A. Scott, and I.A.G. Wilkinson. (1985). *Becoming a Nation of Readers: The Report of the Commission on Reading*. Washington, D.C.: National Institute of Education.

Astone, N.M., and S.S. McLanahan. (1991). "Family Structure, Parental Practices and High School Completion." *American Sociological Review* 56, 3: 309-320.

Baker, L., D. Scher, and K. Mackler. (1997). "Home and Family Influences on Motivations for Reading. *Educational Psychologist* 32, 2: 69-82.

Clark, R.M. (1983). *Family Life and School Achievement*. Chicago: University of Chicago Press.

Crouter, A.C., S.M. MacDermid, S.M. McHale, and M. Perry-Jenkins. (1990). "Parental Monitoring and Perceptions of Children's School Performance and Conduct in Dual- and Single-Earner Families." *Developmental Psychology* 26, 4: 649-657.

Dave, R.H. (1963). "The Identification and Measurement of Environmental Process Variables That Are Related to Educational Achievement." Unpublished doctoral diss., University of Chicago.

Edwards, P.A. (1992). "Involving Parents in Building Reading Instruction for African-American Children." *Theory into Practice* 31, 4: 350-359.

Edwards, P.A. (1995). "Combining Parents' and Teachers' Thoughts About Storybook Reading at Home and School." In *Family Literacy: Connections in Schools and Communities*, edited by L.M. Morrow. College Park, Md.: International Reading Association.

Epstein, J.L. (1983). *Study of Teacher Practices of Parent Involvement: Results from Surveys of Teachers and Parents*. Baltimore: Johns Hopkins University, Center for Social Organization of Schools.

Epstein, J.L. (1984). *Effects on Parents of Teacher Practices in Parent Involvement*. Baltimore: Johns Hopkins University, Center for Social Organization of Schools.

Epstein, J.L., and S.L. Dauber. (1991). "School Programs and Teacher Practices of Parent Involvement in Inner-City Elementary and Middle Schools." *The Elementary School Journal* 91, 3: 289-305.

Finn, J.D. (1993). *School Engagement and Students at Risk*. Washington, D.C.: National Center for Education Statistics.

Ho, E.S., and J.D. Willms. (1996). "Effects of Parental Involvement on Eighth-Grade Achievement." *Sociology of Education* 69, 2: 126-141.

Hoover-Dempsey, K.V., O.C. Bassler, and R. Burow. (1995). "Parents' Reported Involvement in Students' Homework: Strategies and Practices." *The Elementary School Journal* 95, 5: 435-450.

Lamborn, S.D., B.B. Brown, N.S. Mounts, and L. Steinberg. (1992). "Putting School in Perspective: The Influence of Family, Peers, Extracurricular Participation, and Part-time Work on Academic Engagement." In *Student Engagement and Achievement in American Secondary Schools*, edited by F.M. Newmann. New York: Teachers College Press.

Masten, A. (1994). "Resilience in Individual Development: Successful Adaptation Despite Risk and Adversity." In *Educational Resilience in Inner-city America*, edited by M.C. Wang and E.W. Gordon. Hillsdale, N.J.: Erlbaum.

Milne, A.M., D.E. Myers, A.S. Rosenthal, and A. Ginsburg. (1986). "Single Parents, Working Mothers, and the Educational Achievement of School Children." *Sociology of Education* 59, 3: 125-139.

Moles, O.C. (1987). "Who Wants Parent Involvement? Interests, Skills, and Opportunities Among Parents and Educators." *Education and Urban Society* 19, 2: 137-145.

Peng, S.S., and R.M. Lee. (April 1992). "Home Variables, Parent-Child Activities, and Academic Achievement. A Study of 1988 Eighth Graders." Paper presented at the annual meeting of the American Educational Research Association, San Francisco.

Peterson, D. (1989). *Parent Involvement in the Educational Process*. (Eric Digest Series No. EA 43). Eugene, Ore.: Eric Clearinghouse on Educational Management. Eric Document Reproduction Service No. ED 312 776.

Rutherford, B., B. Anderson, and S. Billig. (1997). *Parent and Community Involvement in Education*. Washington, D.C.: U.S. Department of Education, Office of Educational Research and Improvement.

Steinberg, L. (1996). *Beyond the Classroom*. New York: Simon and Schuster.

Taylor, R.D. (1996). "Adolescents' Perceptions of Kinship Support and Family Management Practices: Association with Adolescent Adjustment in African-American Families." *Child Development* 32, 4: 687-695.

Toomey, D. (April 1992). "Short and Medium Run Effects of Parents Reading to Pre-School Children in a Disadvantaged Locality." Paper presented at the annual meeting of the American Educational Research Association, San Francisco. Eric Document Reproduction Service No. ED 346 439.

Topping, K.J. (1986). *Parents as Educators*. London: Croom Helm.

Tracey, D.H. (1995). "Children Practicing Reading at Home: What We Know About How Parents Help." In *Family Literacy: Connections in Schools and Communities,* edited by L.M. Morrow. College Park, Md.: International Reading Association.

Wang, M.C., G.D. Haertel, and H.J. Walberg. (1993). "Toward a Knowledge Base for School Learning." *Review of Educational Research* 63, 3: 249-294.

Wolf, R.M. (1964). "The Measurement of Environments." In *Invitational Conference on Testing Problems,* edited by A. Anastasi. Princeton, N.J.: Educational Testing Service.

> *It is important to understand how, and to what extent, "parental engagement behaviors" bolster student learning.*

Jeremy D. Finn, Professor of Education at State University of New York at Buffalo, is Visiting Scholar at the Center for Research in Human Development and Education during the 1997–98 academic year. He may be reached at Temple University, Center for Research in Human Development and Education, 915 Ritter Hall Annex, Philadelphia, PA 19122-6091 (e-mail: Jfinn@nimbus.temple.edu).

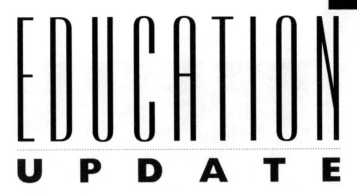

ASSOCIATION FOR SUPERVISION AND CURRICULUM DEVELOPMENT

Volume 40
Number 2
March 1998

Looping—Discovering the Benefits of Multiyear Teaching

On the first day of school, the 2nd graders in Stephanie Jones' class run eagerly into the room to greet their teacher and one another. They quickly put away their lunches, jackets, and school supplies. As the bell rings, Jones invites the students to sit in a circle. They compare what they have written in their journals over the summer and then get started right away on a new writing assignment.

Students in Jones' class are able to start learning on the first day of school because they were all 1st graders in Jones' class the previous year. "Last year on the first day of school, the kids were crying and wouldn't let go of Mom and Dad," she relates. "I spent the morning learning the students' names and teaching them how to introduce themselves to one another. The second half of the day we spent going over bus schedules and procedures."

Buying Time

Jones is one of four teachers at Maple Dale Elementary School (Cincinnati, Ohio) who are involved in looping. Looping—which is sometimes called multiyear teaching or multiyear placement—occurs when a teacher is promoted with her students to the next grade level and stays with the same group of children for two or three years.

"After a year with my students, I felt like I was just beginning to know them," Jones explains. She first learned about looping three years ago from an article in *Education Update*. "It seemed that there was no down time in looping, so I would have more time for teaching."

"September 1 of the second year of looping is the 181st day of school for those in the class," says Jim Grant, who directs the Society for Developmental Education and codirects the National Alliance of Multiage Educators. Teachers who loop have fewer transitions to make at the beginning of the school year and can introduce curriculum topics right away at the start of the second year, he explains.

"Looping places kids in a developmental continuum," says Carol Cummings, staff development coordinator for the Raising Healthy Children Project at the University of Washington (Edmonds, Wash.). "It can take from three to six weeks at the beginning of the school year to establish classroom routines and expectations." By allowing students and teachers to remain together, says Grant, "looping literally buys time." ▶

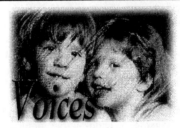

Did is a word of achievement;
Won't is a word of retreat;
Might is a word of bereavement;
Can't is a word of defeat;
Ought is a word of duty;
Try is a word each hour;
Will is a word of beauty;
Can is a word of power.

From *Teacher's Inspirations: Motivational Quotes for You and Your Students* © 1990, Great Quotations, Inc.

Looping

▶ continued from page 1

A Richer Curriculum

More time for teaching translates into a richer curriculum, say teachers. Since she began looping, Jones says, the most significant way her curriculum has changed is the addition of more social learning at the beginning of the 1st grade. Because she knows she'll have extra time in the second year, Jones spends the first several weeks building a sense of community. Once students have the skills to cooperate and communicate, she says, "you reap the benefits in the second year."

With their extra time in the second year, Jones and her students pursued topics they were interested in. During a heritage unit, the class studied quilts. Their fascination with tessellation led them to an in-depth study of math, science, and the work of Dutch artist M.C. Escher. Using a computer, students created their own designs and made quilts out of paper.

Sara Oldham, a 1st and 2nd grade teacher at Shelton Elementary School in Golden, Colo., appreciates that looping, in addition to giving her more teaching time, permits her to address topics when children show they are ready for them.

Oldham discovered looping when she and two other teachers at her school decided to investigate multiage configurations for their school. "The more I learned, I found I liked some aspects of multiage," she says. "But I didn't want such an age span in my class. In a single grade I think you have enough of a developmental span in the class."

Oldham views the 2nd grade curriculum as an extension of what happens in 1st grade. "Students read and write in 1st grade every day, and they do in 2nd, too, only it's more sophisticated."

Although Oldham is responsible for covering 1st and 2nd grade curriculums, she can address topics when she thinks students are ready for them. For example, math standards for place value and money are in the 1st grade curriculum, says Oldham. But "I've taught 1st grade long enough to know that money is a hard concept for 1st graders to understand."

At the end of 1st grade, Oldham introduces money to her students and then asks parents and children to practice using money over the summer. She resumes studying it in the 2nd grade, by which time most of the students have practiced exchanging money and getting change.

Because looping allows teachers to decide when to introduce curriculum topics, Oldham suggests that teachers who loop keep records of what they have taught during the first year so they don't repeat themselves. "Sometimes I'll pull out a book and a child will say, 'We read that last year.'"

Meeting the Needs of Each Student

Another benefit of looping cited by teachers is the opportunity to get to know students over two years. After a year, Oldham says, she has learned a lot about each student's skills and strengths. During the summer, "I think about certain children who are having behavior or academic problems and ask myself, 'What can I do to help this child?'" With looping, "you don't have to start from scratch with each child."

Grant believes that building a bond between teachers and students is at the heart of looping: "Teachers have tried everything and now they are getting back to the basics, which is that strong student, parent, and teacher relationships are important."

These strong relationships help all students, but are especially important to students with special needs, say experts. In her class, Oldham has a child who is paraplegic, three ESL students, and two hearing-impaired students. The parents of the wheelchair-bound and hearing-impaired students chose the looping program because they believed the teacher should know a lot about their children's needs, says Oldham.

"This helps both the students and the teacher because the teacher can get used to having the child's aide in the room and students get used to seeing their friend in a wheelchair or brace." By being together for two years, the students feel more comfortable with their peers and will take risks, she explains.

Postponing High-Stakes Decisions

At the same time that looping helps teachers meet special needs of students, it also allows them time to consider the best interests of the children. "Looping allows teachers to postpone high-stakes decisions," says Grant. "If a teacher thinks a child may need a special education referral or an ADD diagnosis—decisions that could dramatically affect the life of the child—they can put it off for a year until they can better observe the child."

Jones remembers a child in her 1st grade class who was having social and academic problems and was physically small for his age. Although she thought repeating 1st grade might give him a chance to mature, she worried that he would feel punished. "On the first day of 2nd grade, I started with him where he'd left off the previous year. That year he took off." He passed all proficiency tests and began to interact more comfortably with his peers, she says. "He skyrocketed and was at grade level by the end of 2nd grade."

Young children are not the only students who benefit from the strong teacher-student relationships and individual attention provided by looping, say experts. Patricia Crosby, a 7th and 8th grade language arts and social studies teacher at Robert J. Coelho Middle School in Attleboro, Mass., cites

---

ADDRESSING PARENT AND TEACHER CONCERNS

Parents considering placing their child in a looping class usually voice three concerns, says Jim Grant of the Society for Developmental Education and the National Alliance of Multiage Educators. And teachers interested in looping often ask the same questions as parents, he says. In his own words, Grant lists and responds to these concerns:

1. What if there is a personality conflict between a child and teacher?
The answer is to move the child to another class. This is what in done in traditional, non-looping classrooms, too. The goal is always to facilitate student learning.

2. What if my child has to stay with a bad teacher for two years?
It is the school administrator's job to make sure that no inadequate teacher teaches in the school, let alone loops, for more than one year. Besides, it's the best teachers who are looking for new challenges who usually volunteer to loop. Because it's a lot of work, the best teachers usually end up looping.

3. What if the class is dysfunctional?
Sometimes a class may have too many high-needs kids or be top-heavy with kids with summer birthdays. Most schools try to balance each class by gender, abilities, needs, culture, race, and linguistic ability. This should be the same for looping classes. ●

many of the same benefits of looping as her colleagues in elementary schools. In addition to those benefits, Crosby states that the trust a student has in a teacher can become even more important as children become adolescents. "They ask you questions they don't always think they can ask their parents," she says. "And because you know them so well you can observe any changes in behavior that might indicate problems, such as drug or alcohol abuse."

"Looping is a K–8 thing right now," says Grant, "but it could work at the high school level. Think how great it would be. Adolescence is a tough time. Many young people's lives have been saved because they found a mentor in high school whom they were able to form a bond with through having him or her as a teacher for more than one class."

Helping At-Risk Students Succeed

Jan Jubert, a 1st and 2nd grade teacher at Lac du Flambeau Public School in Lac du Flambeau, Wisc., agrees with Grant that looping provides opportunities for students who might otherwise fall through the cracks of the education system. Of her 15 students, most come from low socioeconomic backgrounds and have been identified as at-risk. Additionally, one child in Jubert's class is deaf and requires an interpreter, and the students' ability levels range from learning disabled to gifted and talented. Jubert believes that equal opportunity, which requires equal education, will enable the children to set and reach their life goals.

"Children today join gangs because they want to feel they are part of a group and feel accepted," says Jubert. "Looping makes children feel secure. At-risk kids are starving for this." Because many parents work two jobs or are single parents, she explains, students need to feel a bond with one another and with adults. "It takes the entire first year to build a level of trust," she says.

By staying with a teacher who really knows them and whom they trust, students are given time and high-quality instruction to succeed, says Jubert. Because she has more time to teach and to consider the needs of each child, Jubert says, she covers more material, offers more hands-on activities to her students, and designs activities using multiple intelligences theories that will help children learn the way they learn best.

Jubert believes that looping has helped her reach her goal to make a difference for her students. She cites high attendance, increased test scores, improved self-esteem,

and a love of learning as the results. "The children love to be at school. They come in at 6 a.m. and stay as long as they can or until the bus leaves."

Parent Involvement

Not only do students who loop enjoy school more, but teachers say that parents of those students feel more comfortable talking to teachers. "Increased parent involvement is a nice by-product of looping," says Grant.

Because families get to know teachers, parents relax in the second year, Oldham says. Some parents feel uncomfortable in schools or may not have had a positive education experience themselves, explains Oldham. "For those parents who tend to be a little more reserved, looping helps them because they know the teacher and communication can take place on a deeper level. Especially if a child is struggling, the teacher and parents can work closely together."

"Knowing that parents and I will be in a partnership for two years changes our ideas about what our relationship will be," says Jones. To lay a foundation for parent-teacher communication, Jones routinely invites parents to visit the class and calls parents with positive remarks and reports about their child during the first year of the loop. By the second year, "the parents know your expectations for their child," she says. "Sometimes, the parents have different expectations than you, and the parents speak more frankly in the second year."

Fostering a good relationship between parents and the teacher benefits the child in the end, says Jones. "Because parents are comfortable with the teacher, the teacher learns how to help parents and parents learn how to help the teacher."

Making Smooth Transitions

For students, leaving a looping class can be scary, says Oldham. To help prepare them, students in grades 1–3 work on projects together throughout the year so the children can meet other students and teachers. In December, for example, they decorated cookies and took them to local nursing homes.

As the end of the school year approached last year, Jones knew that the children in her class would be divided into six 3rd grade classes. With another 2nd grade teacher she held writing workshops during the last month of school so the students could get to know one another. Still, this wasn't enough, she says, because she would see her former students clinging together on the playground during recess this year. In response, she and

her colleagues have instituted "Fabulous 1st Graders" assemblies once a month so students can interact.

Despite its benefits for students, teachers, and parents, Grant concedes that looping isn't for everyone. "The entire school shouldn't adopt looping. One teaching model won't work for everyone."

He warns that looping by itself will not cause student achievement scores to skyrocket. Jubert agrees, saying, "Looping is not a cure-all and it may not be for everyone. It is a means rather than an end."

Nevertheless, Jubert calls looping "the most rewarding opportunity to help children I've ever engaged in." For her, looping has allowed her to "see the children be the best they can be—to see them read, cooperate and work together, and to see joy in them as they learn." ●

—Karen Rasmussen

RESOURCES

The Looping Handbook
By Jim Grant, Bob Johnson, and Irv Richardson
Published by Crystal Springs Books, this publication contains a wealth of definitions, explanations, ideas, case studies, and examples for those interested in or involved in looping. To order, call 800-321-0401.

Multiage Classrooms—ASCD Professional Inquiry Kit
ASCD
1250 N. Pitt St.
Alexandria, VA 22314 USA
800-933-2723
The kit contains eight folders and one videotape to help teachers learn more about multiage practices, including looping. ASCD is also producing a video on multiage education, which will be available this year in late spring.

The Society for Developmental Education
Ten Sharon Rd.
Peterborough, NH 03458 USA
800-924-9621
<http://www.socdeved.com/>
SDE offers workshops and conferences on looping and multiage practices. Publications on these topics may be purchased from the Society's division, Crystal Springs Books, at the same address. ●

Deciding to Loop

A decision to loop can be as simple as a principal saying to you, on the last day of school, "Mrs. Hartwell ran off to Bogata with the bus driver; can you move up a grade next fall? You can take your class with you!"

It can be that simple; but if you're the one initiating the concept in your school, a little planning is required, especially if you want to optimize the benefits of looping.

First you need to find another teacher, either in the grade above you or below you, who shares your enthusiasm for potential long-term relationships with his or her students, and who enjoys working with the students' parents on an in-depth basis.

You need to read the literature that exists on looping and long-term teacher-student relationships, then approach your principal with the concept. Once you get the support from your principal, contact a school that has been looping for a few years (a number of schools are profiled in this book), and arrange for a visit. Be prepared to ask lots of questions:

- Did you enjoy having the same children for two or more years?
- How have the children benefited from two or three years with you?
- How have the parents responded?
- How has your relationship with the parents changed?
- Did you enjoy working with the same group of parents for two or more years?
- How much work did changing grade levels involve? Do you feel that it was a positive experience? Why?
- How did you adapt to dealing with children at different developmental stages? Did you enjoy it? (This is an important consideration. Second graders and third graders can express themselves very differently, depending on where they're at in terms of development. Some teachers may enjoy second graders immensely, but find teaching third grade a thoroughly harrowing experience.)
- What problems did you encounter? How did you solve them?
- What would you do differently if you could start all over again?
- Do you want to loop again?

Jan Jubert, a first-second grade looping teacher in Lac du Flambeau, Wisconsin, says,

> I wish I'd known skills, when I started out, on setting expectations and standards of behavior, little tricks of the trade to get the children learning more quickly and working well with each other, and becoming more self-directed.

Excerpted from *The Looping Handbook: Teachers and Students Progressing Together,* by Jim Grant, Bob Johnson, and Irv Richardson. Peterborough, NH: Crystal Springs Books, 1996.

Jubert has developed strategies for developing cooperative and caring behaviors and for spiraling learning using multiple intelligences and other instructional techniques, right from the beginning of the school year. These strategies give her first grade students a jump start on their education, which follows them through their two-year stay with her.

The Two-Teacher Partnership

When entering a looping relationship with another teacher, you need to work out an agreement which covers all possible events. What happens if you get to the end of the first year and one of you decides you don't want to loop — either the teacher due to move up doesn't want to teach that particular class of children for a second year, or the teacher at the higher grade level decides to stay at that grade level? What happens in the second year if the teacher who has looped from first to second grade, for instance, decides she wants to stay in second grade?

All eventualities should be explored and resolved before the fact; it would be wise to put the agreement in writing and bring the principal in on the decision.

Avoiding Dissension at the Outset

Whenever teachers are involved in any education change, the door is wide open for criticism. By being aware of issues that can arise among staff members, most problems can be averted.

- Be careful not to create an elitist program by placing all of the school's gifted students in the looping classroom.
- Nothing splits a staff more quickly than unequal class size. Make sure your looping classroom has the same class size as other classrooms at the same grade level. (At the same time, be protective of your own class in terms of size. You shouldn't be required to carry more than your share of students.)
- Place the same number of special-needs students in your multiyear program as any other classroom at the same grade level — not fewer, and definitely not more.
- When students transfer out of your classroom be sure to take your turn receiving new students.
- Giving your classroom a regal-sounding name, i.e., *The Wonder Years* or *The Platinum Program*, will almost always give fellow staff members the feeling that you think your program is somehow superior to theirs.
- Publicly comparing the benefits of being in your two-year program versus being placed in a 36-week classroom always divides the staff. Always represent your program as one of several fine options at your school.

Staff Development

While looping is about as inexpensive as an educational reform can be, it's wise to allocate some funding for staff development. Workshops on looping, child development and developmentally appropriate practices, authentic assessment, cooperative learning, theme-based instruction, multiple intelligences, and learning centers, as well as training in grade-specific curriculum requirements, will help a teacher make the most of her two or three years with her students.

Balancing Your Class Population

Mid-spring is when most schools put together their class rosters, and administrators considering beginning a looping program should start thinking about balancing next year's class population at this time.

Any classroom can benefit from a little foresight in terms of class composition; but when you're thinking of keeping the same group of children together over a two- or three-year period, creating a balanced class becomes even more important. Try to balance your class in terms of:

- gender
- ability levels
- racial and cultural background
- economic background
- linguistic background
- special needs

Providing a diverse, yet manageable class population will allow you to optimize the learning that takes place between students in any classroom, and that will only expand in a close-knit, caring, multiyear environment.

You also need to be careful not to overload your class with high-maintenance or special-needs kids. Because multiyear arrangements help the children who need help the most, there may be a tendency on the part of the administration to give the multiyear classrooms more than their share of these children.

As teachers, we are all going to have to accept the fact that we will be having lots of children coming to school with lots of problems, from now on. But these children need to be distributed evenly among all the classrooms in the schools, so that one or two classes aren't impacted more heavily than others, to the detriment of the students in those programs.

Before You Begin —

Familiarize yourself with the curriculum for all grade levels you foresee teaching, should you decide to loop. Your curriculum will probably be a hybrid of a single-grade, single-year curriculum and a mixed-age, continuous progress curriculum; you will want to meet the curriculum requirements of each grade level, but provide yourself with the flexibility to extend learning over the two-year period for students who may need a little extra time and work on some content areas.

Teacher Char Forsten says that one of the main benefits of looping is

> . . . to be able to teach to the students' strengths, while looping back to help their weaknesses. Sometimes you can only work so long on a topic before you realize that a certain child has had enough, and if you push it, you're going to lose him. With looping you have time to go on to other things, and then loop back and address the child's needs later.

You may already be using learning centers and theme-based instruction in your classroom; if not, now may be the time to explore some of these instructional strategies. They are well-suited to the kind of close-knit, cooperative environment natural to a multiyear classroom.

HOW LOOPING WORKS	NOTES:

WHAT IS LOOPING?

WHAT ARE DIFFERENT LOOPING CONFIGURATIONS?

- **Two-Year**

- **Three -Year**

- **Team Teaching**

- **Multiage**

- **School Within a School**

- **Interbuilding**

- **Half-Day Kindergarten**

WHAT IS THE RATIONALE FOR LOOPING?

- **Curriculum**

- **Learning**

- **Benefits**

WHAT STEPS SHOULD BE FOLLOWED WHEN CONSIDERING A CHANGE TO LOOPING CLASSROOMS?

- **Exploring & Understanding Looping**

- **Considering & Developing an Action Plan for Implementation & Assessment**

- **Identifying & Addressing Personal Needs & Concerns**

WHAT IS MY NEXT STEP BEYOND THIS SEMINAR?

Char Forsten

LOOK BEFORE YOU LOOP!
OUTLINE FOR AN ACTION PLAN

POSSIBLE EXPLORATION ACTIVITIES:

- Form Study Group(s);
- Read & Share Books & Articles;
- Make School Visits/Interviews;
- Attend Seminars/Training;
- Try Out Multiyear Practices.

ASSESS YOUR SITUATION:

- Determine Administrative, Staff, & Parent Support;
- Consider Process for Change;
- Develop an Action Plan & Tentative Time Line:

PLANNING CONSIDERATIONS: (Note your plans or write N/A)

- Looping Partner(s) -
- Looping Team -
- Grade Assignment(s) -
- School Year -
- Grade Level Mentor -

- Materials -
    Personal -
    Core -

- Room (Physical Space) -

- Student Selection & Placement -

- Parent Involvement -
    Information Night -
    Notification -

- Opt Out Clause
    Decision Making Process - (Child Study Team)

- Curriculum

- Staff Development Needs -

- Looping Assessment/Evaluation Tools -

Char Forsten

LOOPING CONSIDERATIONS		
Benefits	**Comments**	**Concerns**
More Effective Use & Control of Instructional Time & Curriculum		Planning & Managing a Multiyear Classroom
Better Understanding of Learners		Learning a New Curriculum
Patient with Individual Readiness & Growth in Learning		Class Imbalance
Fewer, Less Stressful Transitions		Transition from Multiyear Classroom
Building Significant Relationships for Significant Learning & Improved Academic Performance		Dealing with Personality Conflicts
Fewer SPED Referrals & Retentions		Masking a Learning Disability
Improved Parent Relationships		Knowing When & How to Involve Parents

Char Forsten

PLANNING CONSIDERATIONS:

Instructional Design: Looping

Teacher Contract Assignment: (Example) "Grade 1 With Looping"

	Prior Grade: PROS/CONS	Present Grade:	Next Grade: PROS/CONS
Curriculum:			
Learners:			
Expectations:			
Staff:			

LOOPING: TWO-YEAR ACTIVITIES & THE SUMMER BRIDGE

♥ Team Building Activities

♥ Before & After Projects:

1. Growth Charts & Graphs
2. Interactive Murals
3. Time Lines & Time Capsules
4. Hello & Good-bye -- A Multicultural Study

♥ Anthologies / Yearbooks / Scrap Books / Photo Albums/ Class Logo / Slogan / Song

♥ The Summer Bridge:

1. Calendar Activities
2. Reading Logs
3. Writing Journals
4. Projects
5. Scavenger Hunts/Real World Connections
6. Correspondence
7. Extensions/Maintenance/Review
8. Get-Togethers

Char Forsten

M.Y. Middle School

Sample Letter: Fall

September 25, 1998

Dear Parents,

How often have you wished your children could remain with their teacher(s) for more than one year? During the past year, we have been investigating an instructional design called "looping." This means that the same class of students is taught by the same teacher or team of teachers for two consecutive years.

There are compelling reasons to consider looping. We would like to share these with you on October 1st, (Wednesday evening) at 7:00 p.m. in the school library. We also want to listen to any questions and concerns you might have about looping.

At M.Y. Middle School, we are pleased that a number of teachers are presently studying this concept and are interested in implementing this 2-year cycle of teaching, beginning next school year.

We look forward to meeting with you and discussing this student-centered concept of spending two years with the same teacher. If you cannot attend, please feel free to call me for information. Thank you!

Sincerely,
(Principal)

My child's name: _____

My child's grade next fall: _____

_____ I would like my child to be <u>considered</u> for placement in a looping classroom, beginning the 1999-2000 school year.

OPT OUT CLAUSE: *(I understand that if my child is selected to be in a looping classroom, he/she will have the same teacher for 2 consecutive school years. I also understand that at the end of the first school year, either the school or I can choose a more appropriate placement for my child without consequence.)*

_____
Parent Signature   Date

M.Y. Elementary School

Sample Letter: Spring

May 22, 1998

Dear Parents,

I couldn't let the school year draw to a close without commenting on what I believe is a very unique class. It's been an exciting and productive year!

I am also writing to let you know that your child will progress to second grade with me in a "*looping configuration*." "A WHAT?" you might ask. *Looping* or *student/teacher progression* is a concept that allows me to teach students over a two-year time period.

The benefits of having the same teacher for two years are quite extraordinary. Your child and I have developed a relationship that can only continue to grow. We have begun to establish trust and understanding that is the foundation to a powerful learning atmosphere. Also, consider the academic growth that can take place immediately upon arrival in the Fall, because students are already familiar with everyday classroom procedures. These benefits are just to name a few! It is and can be a very exciting option.

There are pros and cons to every issue, though. One con could be that you/your child is not comfortable with me or my teaching style. If that is the case, please let me or D. Principal know as soon as possible so we can place your child appropriately next year.

If you have questions/concerns, please feel free to call me or the principal. Thank you! I look forward to seeing you in the Fall!

Sincerely,
(Teacher)

PARENT QUESTIONNAIRE*

Dear Parent or Guardian:

The staff is about to begin the student placement process for next year. We value your thoughts about your child's needs and would like you to share your impressions with us. Please answer the following questions about how you perceive your child in school.

As a staff, we devote our expertise and time toward creating classroom assignments that ensure balance for optimal teaching and learning. If you would like your thoughts considered in our placement process, please return this questionnaire to the school no later than March 15. Thank you for your help!

CHILD'S NAME: _____   DATE: _____

Circle statements that apply to your child:

1. likes frequent change.
2. prefers to work alone.
3. likes teacher direction.
4. has difficulty with transitions.
5. likes predictability.
6. prefers group work.
7. likes to be independent.
8. adapts easily to change.

Please write any other information you would like to share about your child: _____
_____
_____
_____
_____

_____
parent's name

LOOPING SURVEY*

Please circle A for Agree, D for Disagree, or U for Unsure in response to these questions about your child being with the same teacher for two years:

My child enjoyed being with the same teacher for two years.	A D U
My child enjoyed being with the same classmates for two years.	A D U
Starting the second year was less stressful for my child.	A D U
The second year was less stressful for me as a parent.	A D U
I had a better understanding of my child's education after two years with the same teacher.	A D U
At the beginning of the second year, my child understood what was expected of him/her.	A D U
The teacher better understood my child's strengths and needs the second year.	A D U
The summer between the two years was less stressful for my child.	A D U
I felt more comfortable communicating with my child's teacher the second year.	A D U
If I had it to do over, I would choose looping for my child.	A D U
I would recommend looping to other parents.	A D U

Comments: _____
_____
_____

*Adapted from surveys from a collection of sources

PARENTAL INVOLVEMENT ASSESSMENT

Strategy	Happening	Not Happening	Could Happen	Not Likely
1. Parent/Teacher Partnership: 3-Way Conferences Contracts Summer Bridge Other-				
2. Home/School Partnership: Parent/Teacher Organization Volunteer Program Family Night Other-				
3. Home/School Communication: Homework Hotline- Newsletters Parent Handbook Surveys/Questionnaires Other-				

Comments:_____
_____
_____
_____

Resources for Parent Involvement

1. Baskwill, Jane. *Parents and Teachers: Partners in Learning.* Toronto, Ont.: Scholastic, 1990.

2. Davies, Anne et al. *Together Is Better.* Winnipeg, Canada: Peguis Publishers, 1992. (Comprehensive book on three-way conferences among students, teachers, & parents)

3. Ohle, Nancy and Lakin Morely. *How to Involve Parents in a Multicultural School.* Alexandria, VA: ASCD, 1996.

4. Stenmark, Jean Kerr et al. *Family Math.* Lawrence Hall of Science, University of California, 1986. (Terrific ideas for "family math night" activities at school.)

WEBSITES:

The PTA
http://www.pta.org

Great site for parents and teachers wanting methods of working with parents. Contains lots of information on how parents can help their children learn.

U.S. Department of Education
http://www.ed.gov/pubs/pubdb.html

A database of U.S. Department of Education publications in ERIC. Offers great ideas for ways schools and parents can work together.

Char Forsten

A STUDENT PLACEMENT PROCESS

Goal: To create balanced, teachable classes where optimal teaching/learning practices can occur. Unless there is an agreed-upon, educational reason to do otherwise, each class should reflect the profile of the student population of the school.

Decision-Making Considerations for Staff & Administrators:

- Classroom Configurations - Does your school have choices in classroom configurations? (multiage, looping, teams, conventional, etc.) What criteria will you use to place students in different configurations?

- Parent Roles - Will parents have a role in the placement process? Will you survey parents for information about their children or for placement in particular configurations?

- Classroom Balance (Equity) -- How will you place students so that a balance is achieved according to gender, ability, class size, grades (if multiage), special needs, learning disabilities, & diversity, etc. Each classroom should reflect a profile of the entire population being placed.

- Changes in Classroom Assignments - How will requests for change be handled after the placement process is completed? To ensure balance, a guideline could be: Any requests for changes in assignments receive final approval from administrator & staff members affected by change. (This point needs to be addressed in your placement guidelines. Two messages are sent to staff members involved in the process if class lists are randomly changed: their time & recommendations are not respected.

- Opt Out Clause - Will "opting out" at the end of the first year be an option in your plan? How will this be handled? What circumstances will warrant a decision to not continue with a particular classroom or configuration?

- Incoming/New Students - How will new students be placed in classrooms? You might establish a "Getting to Know You" time period for the first two weeks of the school year, or a set time period for incoming students once the school year has started. This will allow observation & decision-making time to make alternative recommendations.
  Note: Some teachers might opt to begin the year with a greater number of students, with the condition that new students will be placed in other classrooms. This reduces chances for disruption of instruction and classroom dynamics, especially when teachers are teaching in a multiage or other modified setting.

PLACEMENT EXAMPLE:

The grids on the following page are visual summaries of 3 classes that were created by teachers during the spring student placement process. Typically, teachers spend many hours thoughtfully placing their students for the next year, and without a visual organizer, class imbalance can occur quite easily. When student assignments are placed on the grids, it becomes a visual organizer, and teachers can implement a revision process to create balance in all of the placement factors being considered by your particular school. Examine the 3 grids for balance. What do you find?

Char Forsten   Society for Developmental Education   1-800-924-9621

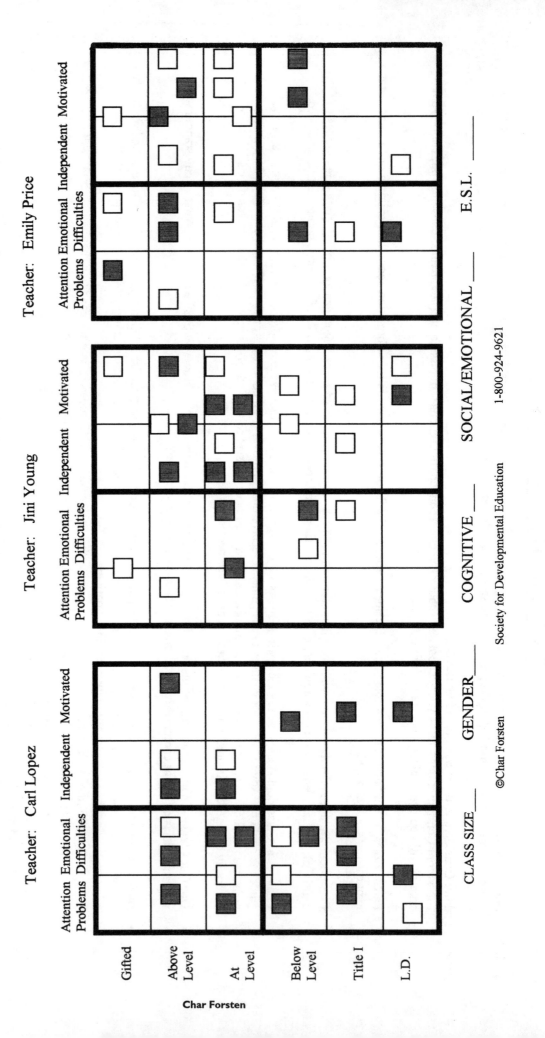

PLACEMENT: GRADE 3   1998 - 99 SCHOOL YEAR

KEY: Boys - ■   Girls - □   E.S.L. - ✓

Teacher: Carl Lopez   Teacher: Jini Young   Teacher: Emily Price

CLASS SIZE_____   GENDER_____   COGNITIVE_____   SOCIAL/EMOTIONAL_____   E.S.L. _____

©Char Forsten   Society for Developmental Education   1-800-924-9621

72

Char Forsten

"PERMANENT" SUBJECT & REFERENCE CENTERS

Sample Room Plan

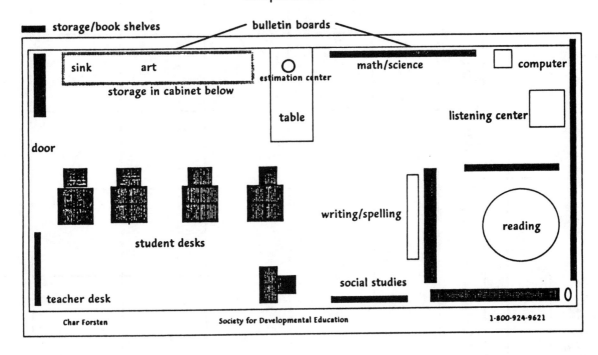

Char Forsten   Society for Developmental Education   1-800-924-9621

U.S.A. TODAY

Date: Special:
Day of School Year: Fraction:
News:

Class Math:
- Math Whiz Kids:
- Marvelous Multipliers:
- Math Maniacs:

Class Reading:
- *Fantastic Mr. Fox:*
- *Charlotte's Web:*
- *Cricket in Times Square:*

Spelling:
- Mighty Spellers:
- Spelling Bees:
- Spellbound:

Writing:

Social Studies:

Science:

Challenge:

Other:

Reminders:

Math Center: OPTIONS

1. Free Choice
2. Number Facts Game
3. Number Facts Tape
4. Equation Game
5. Thinkersize
6. Tessellations
7. Geoboards
8. Tangrams
9. Calculator
10. Assigned Center

PRE-PLANNING ORGANIZER

THEME:

	READING	WRITING	MECHANICS SPELLING	SOCIAL STUDIES	MATH	SCIENCE	MUSIC	ART	PE
Standards/ Test Elements:									
Concepts/ Content:									
Skills:									
Multiple Intelligences:									
Real World Connections:									

*Recommendation: Enlarge chart on photocopier before using.

© Char Forsten

Society for Developmental Education

1-800-924-9621

STRATEGIES FOR TEACHING MIXED-ABILITY LEVELS

- Incorporate Multiple Intelligence Theory

- Teach to Individual Strengths

- Emphasize Understanding

- Use Flexible Grouping Strategies

- Plan Adequate Time Blocks

- Use Manipulative Materials

- Provide Challenge for All Students

- Use Learning Centers

- Plan a Variety of Assessment Techniques

Char Forsten   Society for Developmental Education   1-800-924-9621

Teaching Full Circle:

Organizing Your Instruction & Incorporating Multiple Intelligences

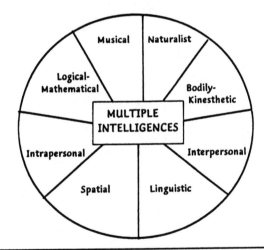

Multiple Intelligences*

As you plan your instruction, incorporate activities that teach to the strengths of a wide range of intelligences among your students. Use this chart to help in your planning:

Logical Mathematical - Numbers, Logic, Puzzles, Scientific Method
Linguistic - Reading, Writing, Speaking, Storytelling, Poetry
Musical - Singing, Music Appreciation, Imagery, Composing, Music Software
Spatial - Charts, Graphs, & Diagrams, Painting & Drawing, Photography, Geometry
Bodily-Kinesthetic - Movement, Skits & Plays, Hands-On Activities, Manipulatives
Interpersonal - Cooperative Groups, Simulations, Conflict Resolution, Clubs
Intrapersonal - Private Space, Journals, Independent Study, Self-Awareness
            Activities
Naturalist - Ecology, Nature, Outdoor Activities, Global Themes, Real World
            Connectio

*Gardner, Howard. *Frames of Mind: The Theory of Multiple Intelligences,* 1983.
_____*Multiple Intelligences: The Theory in Practice.* Basic Books, 1993.

Char Forsten

Modifications + Accommodations = Adaptations

Modification - Objectives are changed for individual learners and noted on report card/student record. Less content & volume of work are expected from the student to help the learning process.

Accommodation - Students learn the same curriculum in different ways. Extra time, alternative test-taking settings, & varied instructional strategies are examples of accommodations.

Process:

- Why is the student a struggling learner?

- What are the goals for the student?

- Are modifications recommended?

- Which accommodations might be effective?

- Follow-Up: Are the adaptations working?

STRUGGLING LEARNERS

" RISK" FACTOR(S):	ACTION PLAN	NOTES
LD		
ADD		
Language		
Emotional		
Unmotivated		
Slow Learner		
Reluctant, Lacks Confidence		
Disorganized		
Negative Attitude		
Lack of Parental Support		
Illness/Absenteeism		
Social Skills		
Lack of Responsibility, Self-Discipline		
Different Learning Style:		

Char Forsten

STRATEGIES THAT BUILD CONFIDENCE

- **Plan Individual Modifications**

- **Accommodate Different Learning Styles**

- **Encourage Child to Change Self Perception**

- **Teach Positive Self Talk**

- **Encourage Child to Take Risks**

- **Make Mistakes OK**

- **Focus on Improvement**

- **Note Contributions & Recognize Achievement**

- **Make Materials Attractive, Concrete, & Helpful**

- **Acknowledge Difficulty of Task**

- **Set Time Limit on Tasks**

- **Teach One Step at a Time**

*Permission from Richard S Dufresne, MSW Peterborough, NH   (Adapted from *Cooperative Discipline*, by Linda Albert)

Char Forsten   Society for Developmental Education   1-800-924-9621

LEARNING CONTRACT

Name: _____   Date:_____

I will show what I know by:	✓ Plan Complete	✓ Project Complete
____ writing a report		
____ making a booklet		
____ building a model		
____ doing a demonstration		
____ presenting a slide show		
____ videotaping a lesson		
____ telling a story		
____ writing a play		
____ making a map or chart		
____ painting a mural		
____ writing music		
____ writing & reciting a poem		
____ making a game		
____ teaching a younger student		
Other: _____		

Char Forsten

Adaptations = Modifications + Accommodations	Notes
Music	
Movement	
Art	
Drama/Role Playing	
Simulations	
Learning Contracts	
"Previews of Coming Attractions"	
Modifications:	
1 - 2 - 3	
"Less Is More"	

Page Protectors

Color Transparency Overlays

Highlighting Tape

Post-It™   Note Tape

Post-It™ Notes

Focus Frames

Focus Strips

Wikki Stix®

Student Invention: _____
Inventor: _____
Presentation Date: _____
Patent Symbol: _____

Char Forsten

FOCUS FRAME

DIRECTIONS: Use the "Focus Frame" pattern below to cut out pieces of posterboard or another type of heavy weight paper. Cut along the dotted line of frame section "A." Insert "B" into section "A" to form a movable box. Slide the "Focus Frame" to adjust for amount of space needed.

Student slides focus frame to fit the present problem,

eliminating unnecessary information or distractions →

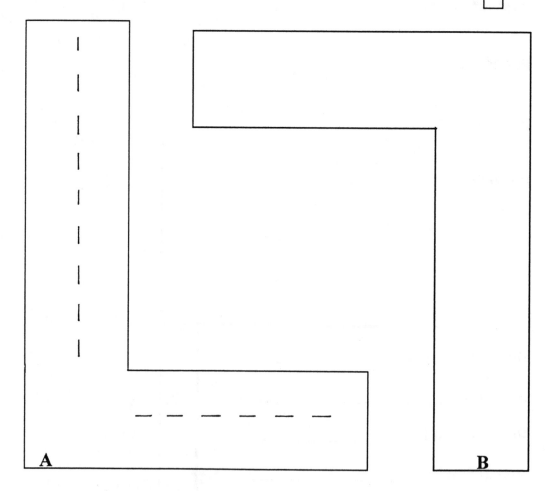

1	2	3	4	5	6	7	8	9	10	11	12
2	4	6	8	10	12	14	16	18	20	22	24
3	6	9	12	15	18	21	24	27	30	33	36
4	8	12	16	20	24	28	32	36	40	44	48
5	10	15	20	25	30	35	40	45	50	55	60
6	12	18	24	30	36	42	48	54	60	66	72
7	14	21	28	35	42	49	56	63	70	77	84
8	16	24	32	40	48	56	64	72	80	88	96
9	18	27	36	45	54	63	72	81	90	99	108
10	20	30	40	50	60	70	80	90	100	110	120
11	22	33	44	55	66	77	88	99	110	121	132
12	24	36	48	60	72	84	96	108	120	132	144

FOCUSING ON THE FACTS

Directions:

1. Locate 2 sheets of colored acetate (each a different color);
2. Cut out 2 different colored strips of acetate, using the above patterns;
3. Choose a "fact family," such as *4 X 7 = 28* on the multiplication chart. Lay one colored strip along the 4's row, and the other colored strip down the 7's column.
4. The product or dividend appears at the intersection of the 2 strips.

Char Forsten

Spelling Level: _____
    Program: _____
    Progress: C P N /
    Effort: C P N /
Comments: _____
_____

Listening:
   Follows Directions: C P N /
   Shows Understanding: C P N /
   Enjoys stories   C P N /

Comments: _____
_____

Speaking:
   Expresses Self Clearly: C P N /
   Uses Good Diction: C P N /
   Joins Discussions: C P N /

Comments: _____
_____

Writing:
   Writes interesting leads: C P N /
   Sequences ideas: C P N /
   Develops Theme: C P N /
   Uses "voice" in Stories: C P N /
   Uses grammatical rules: C P N /
   Uses legible penmanship: C P N /
   Writes strong endings: C P N /

Comments: _____
_____

Social/Emotional Growth:
   Is Cooperative: C P N /
   Accepts Responsibility: C P N /
   Accepts Rules & Limits   C P N /
   Uses Self-Control: C P N /
Comments: _____
_____

Reading Level: _____
Reading Program: _____
   Selects Books at Level: C P N /
   Reads Independently: C P N /
   Reads for Meaning: C P N /
   Self-Corrects: C P N /
   Shows Understanding: C P N /
   Sustains Silent Reading: C P N /
   Enjoys Reading: C P N /
   Reads Different Genre: C P N /
Comments: _____
_____

Math Concept(s): _____
_____

Approximate Level: _____
   Number Facts: C P N /
   Number Sense: C P N /
   Addition: C P N /
   Subtraction: C P N /
   Multiplication: C P N /
   Division: C P N /
   Geometry: C P N /
   Measurement: C P N /
   Problem Solving: C P N /
Comments: _____
_____

Social Studies/Science Theme(s): _____
   Participates: C P N /
   Understands Concepts: C P N /
   Effort: C P N /
Comments: _____
_____

Study & Work Habits:
   Stays on Task: C P N /
   Completes Assignments: C P N /
   Works Neatly   C P N /
   Works Independently: C P N /
   Stays Organized   C P N /
Comments: _____
_____

BIBLIOGRAPHY / RECOMMENDED BOOKS & MATERIALS

CLASSROOM MANAGEMENT & DISCIPLINE:
1. Albert, Linda. *A Teacher's Guide to Cooperative Discipline.* AGS, 1989 .
2. Cummings, Carol. *Managing to Teach.* Teaching, Inc., 1996.
3. Ingraham, Phoebe. *Creating & Managing Learning Centers.* CSB, 1997. (Primary)
4. Viorst, Judith *Alexander and the Terrible, Horrible, No Good, Very Bad Day.* Aladdin, 1972.

CURRICULUM & ASSESSMENT:
1. Davies, Anne et al. *Together Is Better.* Peguis, 1992.
2. Feldman, Jean R. *Wonderful Classrooms Where Children Can Bloom!* CSB, 1997.
3. Fiderer, Adele. *Teaching Writing: A Workshop Approach.* Scholastic, 1993.
4. Goodman, Gretchen. *I Can Learn!* (1995) & *More I Can Learn!* (1998) CSB.
5. Pavelka, Patricia. *Learning Skills Through Literature K-2 (1995) & Learning Skills Through Literature 3-6* (1997). CSB.
6. Wittels, Harriet & Jean Greisman. *How to Spell It.* Grosset & Dunlap, 1973.

LOOPING:
1. Forsten, Char et al. *Looping Q&A: Practical Answers to Your Most Pressing Questions.* CSB, 1997.
2. Grant, Jim et al. *The Looping Handbook: Teachers & Students Progressing Together.* CSB, 1996.
3. Forsten, C & Jim Grant, *The Looping Video.* CSB, 1998. (60 m.)
4. Forsten, Char. *The Multiyear Lesson Plan Book.* CSB, 1996.
5. *Multiyear Assignment of Teachers to Students.* (A collection of articles prepared by Josephine L. Franklin) Educational Research Service, 1997.

SCHOOL CHANGE & REFORM:
1. Conner, Daryl. *Managing at the Speed of Change.* Villard, 1995.
2. Covey, Stephen R. *Principle-Centered Leadership.* Simon & Schuster, 1991.
3. Hunter, Madeline. *How to Change to a Nongraded School.* ASCD, 1992.
4. Miller, Bruce. *Children at the Center: Implementing the Multiage Classroom.* Northwest Regional Library, 1994.
5. Payne, Ruby. *Poverty: A Framework for Understanding and Working with Students and Adults from Poverty.* RFT Publishing, 1995.
6. *Prisoners of Time.* by Members of the National Education Commission on Time and Learning. 1994.

TRANSITION BOOKS:
1. de Saint-Exupery, Antoine. *The Little Prince.* 1943.
2. Fox, Mem. *Wilfrid Gordon McDonald Partridge.* 1984.
3. Penn, Audrey. *The Kissing Hand.* Child Welfare League, 1993.
4. Dr. Seuss. *Oh, The Places You'll Go!* 1990.
5. Viorst, Judith. *The Tenth Good Thing About Barney.* 1971.
6. Williams, Margery. *The Velveteen Rabbit.* 1983.

UNDERSTANDING LEARNERS & LEARNING:

1. Armstrong, T. *Multiple Intelligences in the Classroom.* ASCD, 1994.
2. Grant, Jim. *Every Parent's Owner's Manuals.*
3. Jensen, Eric. *The Learning Brain.* Turning Point, 1995.
4. ___. *Super Teaching.* Turning Point, 1995.
5. Kovalik, Susan. *Integrated Thematic Instruction (3rd ed)* 1994.
6. Parker, Steve. *Brain Surgery for Beginners.* Millbrook, 1993.
7. Sylwester, Robert. *A Celebration of Neurons: An Educator's Guide to the Human Brain.* ASCD, 1995.
8. Wolfe, Dr. Pat. *Translating Brain Research Into Classroom Practice.* (audio tapes) ASCD, 1996.
9. Wood, Chip. *Yardsticks Children in the Classroom Ages 4 - 14.* Northeast Foundation for Children, 1994.

WEB SITES:

1. http://www.socdeved.com   *National Alliance of Multiage Educators (N.A.M.E.)*
2. http://www.teachnet.com   *Teachnet*
3. http://www.classroom.net   *Classroom Connect*
4. http://www.ed.gov/pubs/pubdb.html   *US Dept. of Education*

MISC. SEMINAR BOOKS:

1. Dakos, Kalli. *Don't Read This Book, Whatever You Do!* Trumpet, 1993.
2. Grant, Jim & Irv Richardson. *What Principals Do When No One Is Looking.* CSB, 1998.
3. _____. *What Teachers Do When No One Is Looking.* CSB, 1997.
4. Heller, Ruth. *Kites Sail High* (& other books on nouns, adj., & adv.) Sandcastle Books, 1988.
5. Ohanian, Susan. *Ask Ms. Class.* Stenhouse, 1996.
6. Thaler, Mike. *The Teacher From the Black Lagoon.* Scholastic, 1989.

PUBLISHERS & DISTRIBUTORS:

Crystal Springs Books
10 Sharon Road
Peterborough, NH 03458
(800) 321-0401

Cuisenaire/Dale Seymour
PO Box 5026
White Plains, NY 10602
(800) 237-3142

Dandy Lion Publications
3563-L Sueldo
San Luis Obispo, CA 93401
(800) 776-8032

Interact (Simulation Units)
1825 Gillespie Way, #101
El Cajon, CA 92020
(800) 359-0961

Looping Requires a Two-Teacher Partnership

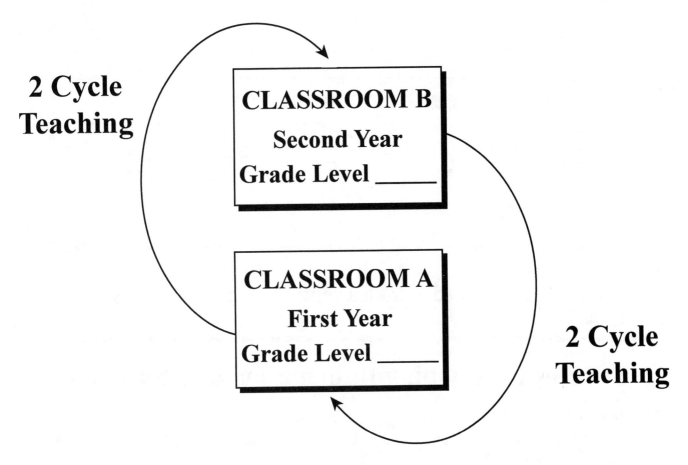

2 Cycle Teaching

CLASSROOM B
Second Year
Grade Level _____

CLASSROOM A
First Year
Grade Level _____

2 Cycle Teaching

The classroom A teacher is "promoted" to classroom B with the class and keeps students for a second year. The classroom B teacher returns to classroom A to pick up a new class and begins another two-year cycle.

Looping Facts

- Student attendance in grades 2 through 8 has increased from 92% average daily attendance (ADA) to 97.2% ADA.

- Retention rates have decreased by over 43% in those same grades.

- Discipline and suspensions, especially at the middle schools (grades 5 through 8), have declined significantly.

- Special education referrals have decreased by over 55%.

- Staff absenteeism has been reduced from an average of seven days per staff member per year, to less than three.

Provided by the Attleboro, Massachusetts School System

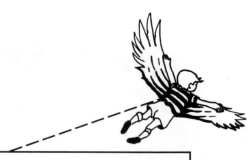

Learners' Runway

1st Grade		2nd Grade

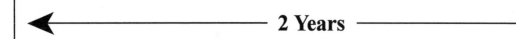

← ———————— **2 Years** ———————— →

Some students need extra learning time, not an extra year

Sources for Looping Information and Support

Publications

1. Forsten, Char; Jim Grant, Bob Johnson and Irv Richardson. *Looping Q&A: 72 Answers to Your Most Pressing Questions.* © 1996 Crystal Springs Books. 128 pp. *

2. Grant, Jim and Bob Johnson. *A Common Sense Guide to Multiage Practices.* © 1995 Teachers' Publishing Group. 128 pp. *

3. Grant, Jim; Bob Johnson and Irv Richardson. *The Looping Handbook: Teachers and Students Progressing Together.* © 1996 Crystal Springs Books. 157 pp. *

4. Grant, Jim; Bob Johnson and Irv Richardson. *The Multiage Handbook: A Comprehensive Guide to Multiage Practices.* © 1996 Crystal Springs Books. 157 pp. *

5. Jankowski, Elizabeth. *Perceptions of the Effect of Looping on Classroom Relationships and Continuity in Learning.* © 1996. A Dissertation. University of Sarasota. 97 pp. **

6. Forsten, Char, et. al. *Multiage Classrooms: An ASCD Professional Inquiry Kit.* © 1997. ASCD, Alexandria, VA. ***

7. Payne, Ruby K. *Poverty: A Framework for Understanding and Working with Students and Adults from Poverty.* © 1995. RFT Publishing. *

8. Wood, Chip. *Yardsticks: Children in the Classroom Ages 4-14, A Resource for Parents and Teachers.* © 1994, 1997. Northeast Foundation for Children.

9. *Multiyear Assignment of Teachers to Students.* © 1997. Educational Research Service, 2000 Clarendon Blvd., Arlington, VA 22201

Video

1. **The Looping Classroom** *featuring Jim Grant and Char Forsten..* © 1998. Crystal Springs Books. 60 minutes. *

* Available from Crystal Springs Books, Ten Sharon Road, Box 500, Peterborough, NH 03458 • 1-800-321-0401.

** Available from Betty Jankowski, Ed.D, Hilton Head Elementary School, Hilton Head, SC 29926.

*** Available through the Association of School Curriculum and Development, Alexandria, VA • 1-800-933-2723

Multiple Year Classroom Benefits

✔ 1. There are fewer student/teacher transitions

2. Multiyear relationships create a cohesive family atmosphere

3. There is an increased cooperative spirit between students and between students and teacher(s)

4. There is an increased sense of stability for students as a result of classroom routine and consistency

5. There is an increase in mental health benefits for the students

6. There is less pressure and stress on the classroom teacher

✔ 7. Teachers report a higher level of discipline

✔ 8. Principals report improved student attendance

✔ 9. There are fewer new parents for the classroom teacher to get to know every year

10. Principals and teachers report an increase in parent involvement

✔ 11. There are fewer new students for the teacher to get to know every other year

✔ 12. The teacher has increased student observation time

13. Teachers are not pressured to make high stakes decisions and may postpone these important decisions until they have more observation and instructional time with the students

14. There tends to be decrease in special needs referrals

15. Educators report fewer grade level retentions

✔ 16. A multiple year configuration allows for semi-seamless curriculum

17. Multiple year classrooms are more time efficient instructionally

Numbers 18-26 are classroom benefits unique to the multiage configuration

✔ 18. "Old-timers" eavesdrop and revisit concepts taught to newcomers

✔ 19. "First-timers" eavesdrop on concepts taught to the "old-timers"

20. "Old-timers" model appropriate behavior to newcomers

✔ 21. The more knowledgeable students assist the less knowledgeable

22. Extra learning time is provided without the stigma of grade level failure

23. There is a higher ceiling on the curriculum every other year

24. The classroom is more inclusionary for differently-abled students

25. There is an opportunity for students to reach "senior citizen" status every two or three years

26. There is a broader age-range of friends

✔ *Time efficient aspect of the multiyear classroom*

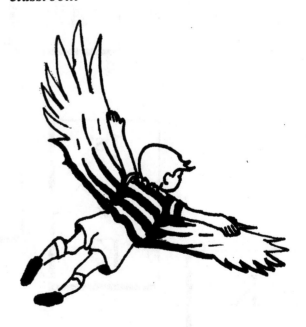

Jim Grant / Bob Johnson / Char Forsten

Caution . . . the road to the multiyear classroom has some potholes

1. Child/teacher personality clash produces no winners

2. A marginal, poor performing teacher places a student at-risk

3. The dysfunctional class from the "Black Lagoon" may be too difficult to teach

4. Too many difficult children create an unbalanced classroom

5. Long term exposure to difficult parents place teachers under too much stress

6. The multiyear classroom may mask a learning disability

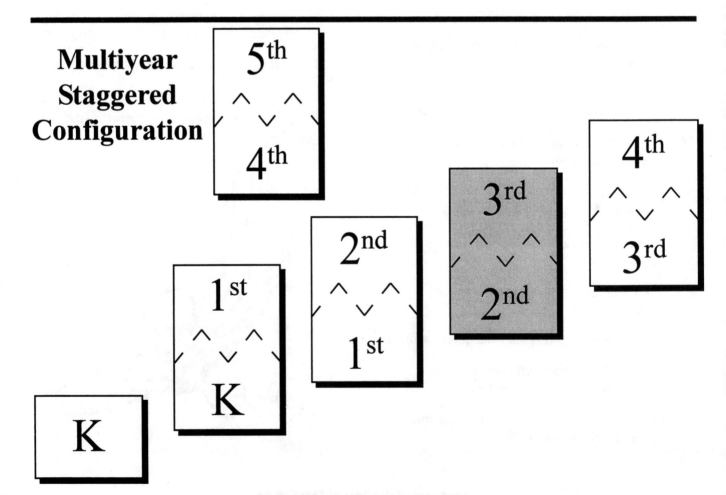

Multiyear Staggered Configuration

Jim Grant / Bob Johnson / Char Forsten

The Positive Aspects of Implementing Looping

1. Career(s) are not placed at risk

2. Short lead time is required for implementing looping

3. No extensive training is necessary to loop

4. Looping builds a teacher's confidence

5. There is a lower stress level for looping teachers

6. Curriculum changes are minimal

7. Additional physical space is not required for looping

8. Midyear decision allows the teacher who moves up to "road test" the class

9. All of the down sides of looping are totally correctable

10. Termination of looping is possible without being "noticed"

11. Looping can be the prerequisite ground work for creating a multiage configuration

12. There are minimal things to go wrong with looping

13. Looping with a partial class is permissible

14. Minimal financial resources are required to implement looping

15. The only permission necessary to secure is from the parents of the future second year students

---

The Hidden Consequences of Looping

Teachers:

1. who change grade levels may lose their teaching assistant

2. must learn the curriculum of a new grade

3. may need special training for: Health, DARE, etc.

4. must learn the ages and stages of the students at the new grade level

5. may move to a grade with mandated:
   • Testing
   • Promotional standards

6. may need to change pods (located in another wing), thus becoming separated from established teacher colleagues

7. may move up to "high pressure" grade level (i.e., 1st, 3rd or 7th grade)

8. may move to a grade level that does not embrace a child-centered philosophy (i.e. departmentalized situation)

9. may change to a grade level and be required to increase class size

10. may find a high number of pre-first graders identified as differently-abled when they move up to 1st grade

11. may find that their state requires 2 teacher certification

12. may find that some local teacher unions require posting positions before allowing a teacher to change grade levels.

Char Forsten / Jim Grant / Bob Johnson

Looping with Kindergarten (½ day) and First Grade

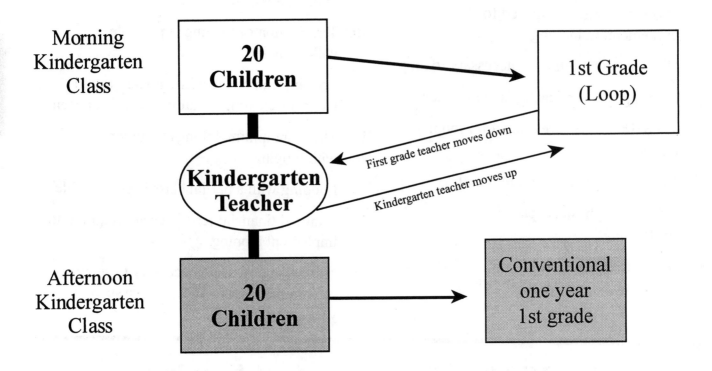

Morning Kindergarten Class — 20 Children → 1st Grade (Loop)

First grade teacher moves down

Kindergarten teacher moves up

Kindergarten Teacher

Afternoon Kindergarten Class — 20 Children → Conventional one year 1st grade

Note: Looping with a two session ½ day kindergarten program requires two first grades.

Student Selection *

- The AM class can loop

- The PM class can loop

- 10 students from the AM plus 10 students from the PM can loop

- Select 20 out of 40 AM/PM student to loop (random selection)

* Selected from a group of students whose parents have opted for a looping configuration.

A. Yes, it can be extremely effective. As a matter of fact, several parental concerns can be put to rest by creating a good teaching team.

Parents might be concerned that their child is placed with a teacher for two years in a row who isn't particularly strong in a certain subject (math, for example). With a team arrangement, a savvy principal can put together two individuals with different academic strengths, so that one team member teaches reading, writing, and social studies, for instance, while the other member teaches math and science. Teachers can also cooperatively teach some subjects and take turns assisting in other subjects.

Q.

Would team teaching be a good arrangement in a looping classroom?

Devising large group, small group and individualized instruction is much easier and more efficient with two teachers in the room. Some schools have even hired one teacher certified in special education as a member of a two-member team, or have included a special education teacher as a third member of a team. These teaming structures have been very successful at integrating special-needs students into the regular classroom without shortchanging other students.

Another concern, both of parents and teachers, is when a personality conflict develops between a teacher and a child. A good teaching team can short-circuit that; while one teacher may have a difficult time with a particular child, the other team member may not. Their instructional strategies and personal approach may be more compatible with the child's needs, which can help ameliorate any potential problems. The same theory can also work in a parent-teacher personality conflict.

The recently published book, *Team Teaching,** lists a number of benefits to students of team teaching:

- The student receives more individual attention; there is more time to tune in to individual student needs.
- Children in need of special support can be pulled aside in small groups and helped.
- Students are never left unattended.
- Interaction with students increases.

---

* Northern Nevada Writing Project Teacher-Researcher Group. *Team Teaching.* York, ME: Stenhouse Publishers, 1997.

Excerpted from *Looping: 72 Practical Answers to Your Most Pressing Questions*, by Char Forsten, Jim Grant, Bob Johnson, and Irv Richardson. Peterborough, NH: Crystal Springs Books, 1997.

- A teacher is always on hand to help with a thought or a spelling word, or to explain what is expected in the lesson.
- Someone is always available to walk around and monitor learning.
- Someone is available to answer questions.
- The curriculum moves on even if one teacher is absent.
- There is a better chance of finding out whether there is a breakdown in communication.
- Thought processes can be modeled.
- There is flexibility in paperwork and assignments.
- Students are given less busywork.
- Students can be helped to look for alternatives.
- There is more time to introduce more detailed information.
- There are more opportunities to read.
- Students learn how to ask questions.
- Students are exposed to more ideas.
- Students can relate to more than one teacher personally.
- Teachers can use different skills in different situations.
- Discipline is easier. The partners have the ability to consult with each other and to plan strategy.
- Students can be assessed informally by one teacher while the other leads the class.
- Grading and evaluation are enhanced because there are two views of the student.
- A student's social, emotional, and curricular needs can be discussed with another person who has an equal understanding of the child.
- Situations that develop without warning can be given immediate attention.
- Students can observe a good working relationship between adults and experience a positive role model for adult interaction.
- There is more flexibility to make phone calls to parents.
- Conferences are easier, and the parents get more than one view of the child.

Teaching teams are formed for a variety of reasons, some philosophical, others demographic or financial. Some teachers have a choice in the process; others are informed that they'll be doing this, and might be assigned a team member.

Whatever the reasons a teaching team is formed, the structure requires hard work, open communication, negotiating ability, and emotional maturity on the part of both team members for the arrangement to succeed. Teaming isn't for everyone. Ideally, the administration should incorporate an "opt-out" clause into the implementation plan.

© CRYSTAL SPRINGS BOOKS • PETERBOROUGH, NH • 1-800-321-0401

Q.

Are there any teaching strategies that are particularly effective in a looping classroom?

A. Yes, there are strategies you can use to make learning more effective in a multiyear classroom. Thematic planning, simulations, cooperative grouping, and strategies to help children become independent learners are all particularly suitable for the multiyear classroom. Learning centers are a valuable tool here; if you don't have a lot of space for learning centers, you can create megacenters, turning your classroom into a resource area where students take on more responsibility for locating and choosing materials that provide practice, enrichment, or extension for their learning.

Since a looping classroom is such a positive social experience for children, you might also want to explore acceptance activities (to deal with issues of special-needs kids) and themes that develop an understanding of social and cultural diversity. Conflict resolution is an effective technique that encourages self-management and responsibility for one's own behavior, rather than having the students rely on a teacher to "control" the group.

The continuity provided in a looping classroom can be enhanced by creating a "summer bridge" of activities for children at the end of the first year.

Q.

How can I blend my curriculum to make it more effective and meaningful over two years?

A. Looping provides a great opportunity to integrate your curriculum and provide meaningful, enjoyable learning experiences for your children over a two-year span, as opposed to just *covering* material in isolated bits across one school year.

A good way to start is to create a chart or a graphic organizer listing all the academic areas you will teach. Next, add the different concepts and skills that you want to teach, including any topics such as multiple intelligences and real-world connections you want to emphasize. Then, pull together:

1. any curriculum requirements from your district.
2. any state testing requirements.
3. any national testing requirements.
4. any child-driven interests, projects, and themes that your students would like to pursue.
5. any interests of your own that you would like to pursue with your students.

Dovetail all these pieces and plan your curriculum over your two-year instructional period, integrating the instruction whenever possible, making sure you plan activities for whole group, small group, and individual learning.

A. Schools are moving in the direction of using authentic, ongoing assessment tools to monitor "how we are doing" instead of "how did we do?" With looping, you have time to take better advantage of these tools. For instance:

- anecdotal notes become very important to help you make crucial decisions regarding children.
- portfolios or folders with student work help you to gauge their progress.
- rubrics are good tools to assess where children are before instruction, and to gauge their progress after instruction has taken place. Rubrics also help you, as a teacher, plan and assess your own instruction.
- projects based on multiple intelligences and connected to thematic units allow children to demonstrate what they've learned in ways other than pencil-and-paper methods.

There is a danger in a looping classroom that potential learning problems might be overlooked because of the forgiving nature of the classroom; therefore, it is doubly important to have a good reliable method of ongoing, authentic assessment in place.

Q.

How do I assess students in a looping classroom?

The Multiyear Assignment
Good for Kids, a Challenge for Teachers

I t all started about six years ago when the school administration of Attleboro, Massachusetts, decided to tackle some of the problems Attleboro kids were facing.

"We wanted to provide some stability in our students' lives. We have a lot of kids who move around a lot, and a lot of homes that aren't too stable," said Ted Thibodeau. The administration, led by Dr. Joseph Rappa, Attleboro's superintendent, decided to try two-year teaching assignments to provide some of the stability students needed. They began with small pilot programs at Coelho Middle School and Willet Elementary School, with a handful of teachers who had expressed an interest in multiyear teaching. Those teachers had very positive experiences, and "talked it up" with their colleagues; by the second year there were five or six teaching teams ready to try the concept.

By the third year, confronted with a group of enthusiastic teachers and evidence of substantial benefit to the students, the administration was faced with a decision. "We had to decide whether we were just going to go with the people who wanted to do it, or say, 'This is good for kids, so we're going to do it for everybody,' " said Thibodeau. "Dr. Rappa decided that everyone was going to do it." Now all teachers in grades one through eight throughout the Attleboro school system take part in multiyear assignments.

Today, the multiyear assignment has been accepted and is supported by the vast majority of teachers, students and parents, although "it went over better at some levels than at others," said Thibodeau. The teachers in the early grades accepted it more readily; there was more resistance at the middle school level.

"Seventh and eighth grade was the real battleground," Thibodeau said. "There were teachers who had been teaching eighth-grade science for twenty, thirty years, and they said, 'Now I've got to go back to seventh grade, and I've got to teach math and science?' We provided summer workshops in those areas where people felt they needed them, both in team building and in unfamiliar content areas."

In a survey conducted in 1994 by the school district, 70 percent of the seventh- and eighth-grade parents, students and teachers said they liked the multiyear assignment. "Today, that would be even higher," said Thibodeau.

A Reborn Math Specialist

One teacher who is described by Ted Thibodeau as "reborn" because of the multiyear assignment is twenty-five year math specialist Dave Cox of Coelho Middle School. Cox now shares a two-year seventh- and eighth-grade teaching assignment with his team member, Pam Puccio; he teaches math and science, while she teaches communications and social sciences. Cox spoke, enthusiastically and at length, about the two-year assignment and two-person teaching teams

**Excerpted from *The Looping Handbook: Teachers and Students Progressing Together*, by Jim Grant, bob Johnson, and Irv Richardson.
Peterborough, NH: Crystal Springs Books, 1996.**

Simple Concept, Complex Structure

The multiyear assignment is essentially a very simple concept; but in Attleboro it's part of a complex collection of instructional strategies and structures that include emphasis on critical thinking skills, cooperative learning, and teaming of students and teachers.

Two- and sometimes three-person teaching teams are at the heart of many of Attleboro's classrooms. Teachers are assigned to a team by district superintendent Rappa based on a number of criteria.

"We're usually trying to get a blend of someone who's strong in math/science and someone strong in the languages, or in some cases male/female, in other cases veteran and newcomer," Thibodeau said. "The superintendent has made a number of transfers to achieve a better balance in the three middle schools.

"It's not easy for the teachers."

Although the administration makes the final decision about teaming arrangements, it will consider teaming requests from teachers. "We don't let teachers just voluntarily pick their teams, but when we know there's a bond that exists, and we know it's a positive one for the kids, not just something of comfort for the adults, we go with that," Thibodeau said.

Multiyear Teaming Improves Teaching

Dr. Rappa considers teaming a powerful administrative tool for monitoring and improving the quality of teaching in Attleboro. Not only does teaming allow the administration to balance the instruction in a classroom in terms of the teachers' strengths, but it is a way to build the competency of teachers who may be new, or may be less than adequate in their performance.

"New teachers are paired with a more experienced teacher; we don't put two new teachers together on a team," reports Thibodeau. "If we have someone whose performance is marginal, we pair that person with one or two teachers who are excellent, so that the marginal teacher learns or is challenged by his or her partners. We've seen a lot of improvement."

Multiyear Quality Control

Some people have left the system because of the pressure involved in multiyear teaching. One veteran teacher resigned after having received a less than favorable response from her group of parents. "We've had about five people take career leaves," said Thibodeau.

"Dr. Rappa believes that the multiyear assignment is actually a good supervisory tool, because in the long run, the parents aren't going to settle for mediocrity with a two-year arrangement. In the past they might have said, 'Okay, for one year we'll put up with it.' And if it's only in one subject area, too, parents will say, 'Oh, all right, we'll put up with it.' But when it's concentrated like this, the principal has to be a better supervisor; and we have to be very careful about whom we give tenure or professional status to."

The teams are evaluated every year, and are reassigned as necessary at the end of the two-year assignment. "Right now, the fifth and seventh grade teachers are beginning to wonder what's going to happen next," Thibodeau said. "We may move a teacher because another school needs a strong math/science teacher, or to create a better blend in terms of

Attleboro Public School District

100 Rathbun Willard Drive
Attleboro, MA 02703

Phone: 508-222-0012
FAX: 508-222-5637

Open to Visitors: yes

Contact:　Dr. Joseph Rappa,
　　　　　Superintendent
　　　　　Theodore Thibodeau,
　　　　　Asst. Superintendent

teaching style. One very good team may not be together forever, because they're both so very strong, we may have to pair each of them with someone who needs some assistance."

Generally after teachers make a change, they're happy. "They get a new lease on life." Sometimes, when the team hasn't exactly been a comfortable match, the team members welcome the administration's initiative in making changes. "It takes the onus off them," Thibodeau said. "They don't have to ask for a team divorce."

Thibodeau provided The Society For Developmental Education with an opportunity to visit several Attleboro schools and talk with principals, teachers and students about multiyear assignments.

. . . But The Kids Like It

The day after some parents expressed opposition to the multiyear assignment at a public forum, a team of 55 to 60 eighth-grade students met with representatives from NELMS (the New England League of Middle Schools) to discuss the multiyear assignment. "The kids were there, sitting on the floor and talking, and practically everything that the parents had said the night before, the kids said the opposite," said Thibodeau. " 'We love teams; we get to know each other.' 'No, we aren't limited in the number of friends, because we see them elsewhere; and when we go to the high school we'll have stronger friends, from having known them for two years, and we'll make other friends; we're not worried about that.' One teacher from another system said, 'There must be something wrong with it; doesn't anyone have any complaints?' and one kid got up and said, 'Yeah, the teachers know us too well.' "

This group had some special-needs students in it who took part in the program put on for NELMS, and, as Thibodeau said, "You never ever would have known it; they fit right in."

Some Parent Opposition . . .

Most parents who've expressed an opinion have embraced the multiyear concept as highly beneficial for their children. Few parents — less than one percent — request that their child be transferred out of a classroom after the first year of a two-year assignment — an option that's been in place from the beginning of the program.

"That's mostly because the kids are happy with the team they're with; it may also be partly that parents are reluctant to stand out and make that choice," Thibodeau said.

"When the multiyear assignment is successful, the parents usually credit its success to the teacher; when it doesn't work well, the multiyear assignment itself is blamed." This was the case at a recent forum, where a small but vocal group of seventh- and eighth-grade parents spoke out against the multiyear assignment.

A Complicated Issue

Thibodeau believes that the opposition is about more than the two-year structure. "We have full inclusion; we have two-person teams, which means we don't have a departmental approach; we're dealing with some serious behavioral problems — kids that other towns might send away to a residential facility are included in the public school systems in Attleboro. We're a very diverse community, too, and we have kids with limited English speaking ability, and in some schools a larger Hispanic and Cambodian population, and that's part of the opposition, too.

"What some parents are really looking for is a return to a departmental, subject-specific, high-content kind of program."

Social issues get mixed in too; many more people are attempting to get their children into honors programs at the high school, partly in an effort to get them out of inclusive classrooms and away from behavioral problems; and the high school teachers are complaining, saying they're not getting the same caliber of student they're accustomed to getting.

"It's all very complicated," said Thibodeau. "A lot of different issues get mixed in."

The Harvard Education Letter

Volume XIV, Number 1   *Published by the Harvard Graduate School of Education*   January/February 1998

Multi-age Classrooms: An Age-Old Grouping Method Is Still Evolving

Despite mounting challenges, the multi-age classroom continues to be an attractive option for educators

BY NANCY WALSER

Seven years ago, when Connie Chene took over as principal of the Puesta Del Sol Elementary School in Rio Rancho, NM, she issued this challenge to her teachers: If they had any ideas about how to do things differently to benefit kids, all they had to do was talk to her.

Located just outside Albuquerque in one of the state's fastest growing cities, Puesta Del Sol had a not-so-progressive classroom arrangement. All special education students were taught outside the school in portable buildings; all regular education students were taught inside the main building. Chene was immediately besieged by proposals from regular and special education teachers who wanted to combine their students. Teachers knocked down walls between rooms, more proposals came in, and Chene now presides over a smorgasbord of classrooms: both single grades and mixed ages in both regular and inclusion classrooms, including one inclusion class that spans kindergarten through the 3rd grade.

"Teachers began to see the power of kids with different abilities and different points of view working together in the classroom," says Chene. "They began to buy into the idea that society is multi-age, families are multi-age, and we wanted the classrooms to reflect real life."

On the other side of the country, at the Graham and Parks Alternative School in Cambridge, MA, students have been combined in multi-age classrooms for 25 years. However, Graham and Parks is also home to the district's only Haitian-Creole transitional bilingual education program, and with bilingual Haitians now making up more than 30 percent of the school population, principal Len Solo is reassessing their system of combining two grades per classrooms in 1st through 8th grades. Especially in the higher grades, he contends, there are simply too many ability levels in each room for teachers to handle.

"You can have an eight- or nine-year spread in terms of levels," Solo says. "I've got a staff that kills themselves to meet kids' needs, and it's beginning to get really difficult to do that."

> "Society is multi-age, families are multi-age, and we wanted the classrooms to reflect real life."

A Long History

Since the days of the one-room schoolhouse, multi-age grouping in this country has been buffeted by changing times and shifting priorities. Largely abandoned for single grades beginning in the mid-19th century, the practice was revived in the 1960s and 1970s with the growing interest in developmentally based education. Today

Classroom Grouping Terms

Looping: Students stay with a teacher(s) for more than one year. A multi-age classroom is considered one form of looping.

Multi-age (or mixed-age): Students in two or three grade levels are mixed in one classroom based on the philosophy that this form of grouping improves learning and attitudes toward school. Multi-age grouping is practiced more often in elemenary schools than in secondary schools.

Multi-grade (also combination grades or split grades): Students from one or more grade levels are grouped due to low enrollments or uneven class sizes. Students in these different grade levels are usually taught separately although they are in the same classroom.

Multi-year: An umbrella term for any classroom where students stay with the same teacher(s) for more than one year. Includes multi-age classrooms and looping.

Non-graded (or ungraded): Students of different ages are mixed based on the mixed-age philosophy that emphasizes continuous progress by individuals rather than grade-level expectations. Since state education departments require reporting by grade level, however, this form of mixed-age classroom is more rare.

Single-grade: Students of roughly the same age are assigned to the same grade for one year. This is the most common form of grouping.

---

most multi-age classrooms mix two, or more rarely three, grade levels containing a minimum of four chronological ages, according to Jim Grant, executive director of the Society for Developmental Education of Peterborough, NH.

Supporters say the practice of mixing different ages in the same classroom still holds much promise, arguing that it improves learning by emphasizing project-based curricula, continuous progress (as opposed to an annual pass-fail system), cooperation, and the sharing of knowledge. In theory, teachers in multi-age classrooms focus on individuals rather than on grade-level expectations. They also have more time to address individual needs because children spend more than one year in their class.

Detractors focus on the difficulties of managing multi-age classrooms and some practitioners report a new threat to the viability of multi-age education: the emergence of tests tied to grade-specific curriculum frameworks, which adds to the difficulty of teaching more than one grade level at a time.

Types of Grouping

Multi-age classrooms have been used in a variety of ways for a variety of reasons. One type, multi-grade classrooms, are forced upon teachers as a way to manage low enrollments and shrinking budgets (see box). Because of this variety, simply counting the number of districts with mixed-age

classrooms has proved illusive and made it difficult to judge their effectiveness.

When comparing achievement and other kinds of success in multi-age and single-grade classrooms, research is decidedly mixed. In a study published in 1995, Simon Veenman of the University of Nijmegen of Norway examined 56 studies, including 33 in the U.S., which compared standardized test results for single-grade classrooms with multi-

---

The emergence of tests tied to grade-specific curricula adds to the difficulty of teaching multi-age classes.

---

grade and multi-age classrooms. While he concluded that multi-age classrooms "appear to be generally equivalent" to single-graded in terms of achievement, he found that tests measuring self-concept and attitudes toward school registered "a small positive effect for students in multi-age classes." Veenman excluded studies of non-graded classrooms—a more deliberate and rarer form of multi-age classroom that rejects all things labeled by grade —since non-grading is "a philosophy that permeates the entire school organization and program." In an attempt

to look at only the effects of different grouping methods, he excluded studies in which teachers had received training in multi-grades or multi-ages.

In a 1992 study comparing non-graded with single-grade classrooms, however, Temple University professor Barbara Nelson Pavan reviewed 64 studies in the U.S. and Canada and found that the majority (58 percent) of non-graded classrooms performed better on achievement tests, as well as on tests for mental health and school attitude (52 percent). All seven studies that compared students who spent their entire elementary years in a non-graded school with single-graded counterparts found "superior performance by non-graded students." According to Pavan's definition, a non-graded school "does not use grade-level designations for students or classes" and progress is reported "in terms of tasks completed and the manner of learning, not by grades or rating systems."

Given the range of types of multi-age classrooms that exist, according to these studies, duplicating these positive results is a tricky business. In Kentucky, confusion over how to set up non-graded primary classrooms resulted in changes to the state's six-year-old education reform act mandating "multi-age/multi-ability" classrooms. Now school-based councils decide how primary-grade classrooms will be structured within general goals outlined by law. At least some of Kentucky's elementary schools now use multi-age grouping for only a portion of the day, with basic skills and drills often reserved for single-age grouping, according to Pam Williams, a consultant for the Kentucky Department of Education.

Emerging Consensus

After more than 30 years of dedicated study, some areas of consensus have emerged about mixing ages within classrooms. No one argues the fact that multi-age classrooms are harder to teach and require more preparation and training. And multi-grade classrooms—the kind forced on teachers for budgetary purposes—are particularly beset by "common problems and concerns," according to Veenman. These include "lack of time for teaching the required content, a greater work load, lack of time for individual attention and remediation, lack of adequate classroom management skills, lack of adequate preparation during teacher training, inadequate materials, and parental concerns about the academic achievement of their children."

Conversely, schools that use multi-age classrooms successfully are marked by several common traits, according to Bruce Miller, a researcher with the Northwest Regional Educational Laboratory in Portland, OR, who has written extensively about multi-age education in rural America. In a 1996 review of five schools in the Northwest that have used multi-age classrooms for more than four years, Miller found these commonalities: dedicated teachers, supportive principals and parents, and solidarity and teamwork among the staff. He also identified five requirements for implementing multi-age classrooms: review the research before beginning, don't settle on a single model, avoid "bottom up or top-down" mandates, recognize that a major conceptual change is required in terms of attitudes toward teaching and children, and get prepared for "evolving long-term change" through "strategic, incremental" steps. "Too many educators are implementing multi-age classrooms and schools with insufficient forethought, planning, and participation of key stakeholders," he concludes.

Threat of Tests

But even supporters say the best multi-age classrooms are threatened by the trend toward grade-specific cur-

riculum requirements and tests. "Multi-age is a philosophy that is truly wonderful for learning, and in a perfect world where you do not have curricular barriers, it is doable," says Char Forsten, who leads seminars around the country for the Society for Developmental Education. Forsten, who taught mixed ages in New Hampshire for 18 years, says she learned these difficulties first-hand. "The minute you were asked to teach them as 4th and 5th graders instead of the blend, you were going against the multi-age philosophy to address them as one group of learners."

Other teachers, however, have gotten around these barriers by outlining

---

No one disputes the fact that multi-age classrooms are harder to teach and require more preparation and training.

---

district expectations for all the grade levels in their classroom and concentrating on the common areas; by teaching one curriculum one year and another the next; or by using sufficiently broad themes to cover all the bases. Looping—which groups a single or mixed-age class with the same teacher for more than one year—can also help bring teachers up to speed on combining curriculums, according to Forsten. "If I'd been a 3rd-grade teacher for 10 years before I took on a 3/4 class, I'd take the 3rd graders up to 4th grade so I would know what the 4th-grade curriculum is like before I taught both grades together in the same classroom," she says

It's exactly this kind of flexibility that practitioners point to as one of the most useful aspects of multi-aging: as a tool that can be used by teachers who want to use it and by schools that want to offer it to interested parents.

In Rio Rancho, principal Connie Chene has not formally compared test results of children before and after the introduction of inclusion and multi-age classrooms. But teachers have noticed a dramatic increase in writing skills and improvement on tests in areas they have identified as important. In a 1997 survey of all 200 parents whose chil-

dren were in multi-age classrooms, all but two said they wanted their children to stay in the classrooms with mixed ages. Results like these prove the concept is working, says Chene. "There are many parents who still don't like it, and I make sure I have enough single-grade classrooms to accommodate them," she says. But even these classes have banded together to do mixed-age activities once a week—an arrangement that also gives one teacher some extra planning time each week, she says. "There's no one way of doing things around here," she emphasizes.

At Graham and Parks, principal Len Solo says he will be asking his school community to look into looping by single grades as a substitute for some or all multi-age classrooms to reap the benefits of having children stay with one teacher for more than one year, while at the same time reducing teacher work load and the need for tutoring after school and at home. "The measurable benefit [of multi-aging] comes from having a child for two years," he says. "The kids might have a good first year, but they have a much better second year; the achievement goes up by more than a year."

Despite the changes he is contemplating at his school, Solo still considers himself a staunch advocate of multi-age classrooms. "I just see so many benefits," he says. "They really contribute to the sense of community that we try to build here and we'll use them as long as we can."

For Further Information

M. A. Bozzone. "Straight Talk From Multi-age Classrooms: Why Teachers Favor Nongraded Classes and How They Make Them Work." *Instructor* 104, no. 6 (March 1995): 64-70.

P. Chase and J. Doan. *Full Circle: A New Look at Multiage Education.* Portsmouth, NH: Heinemann, 1994.

B. A. Miller. "What Works in Multiage Instruction," *Education Digest* 61, no. 9 (May 1996): 4-8.

B. N. Pavan. "The Benefits of Nongraded Schools." *Educational Leadership* 50, no. 2 (October 1992): 22-25.

Society for Developmental Education. *The Multiage Resource Book, 1993.* PO Box 577, Peterborough, NH 03458; 800-462-1478.

S. Veenman. "Cognitive and Noncognitive Effects of Multigrade and Multi-Age Classes: A Best Evidence Synthesis." *Review of Educational Research* 65, no. 4 (Winter 1995): 319-381.

Nancy Walser is a freelance journalist and the author of Parent's Guide to Cambridge Schools. *She lives in Cambridge, MA.*

Growing a Multiage Classroom

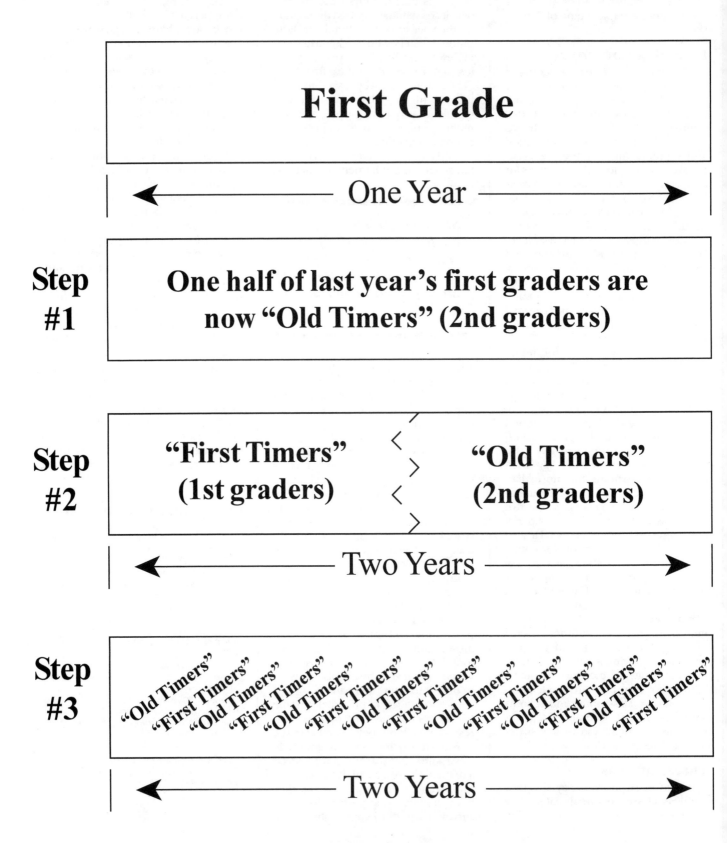

First Grade

← One Year →

Step #1

One half of last year's first graders are now "Old Timers" (2nd graders)

Step #2

"First Timers" (1st graders)   **"Old Timers" (2nd graders)**

← Two Years →

Step #3

"Old Timers" "First Timers" "Old Timers" "First Timers" "Old Timers" "First Timers" "Old Timers" "First Timers" "Old Timers" "First Timers" "Old Timers" "First Timers" "Old Timers" "First Timers"

← Two Years →

Jim Grant/Bob Johnson/Char Forsten

The Graded Classroom ("Parts List")

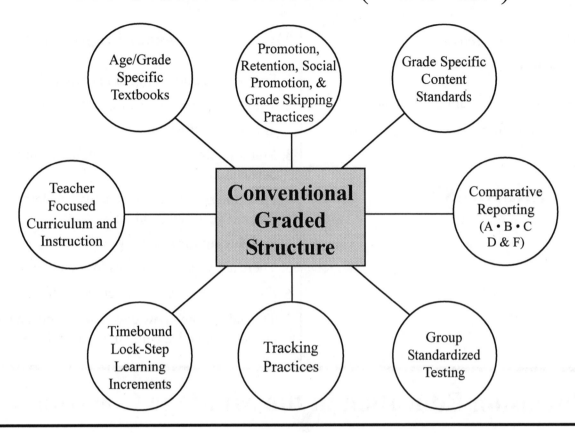

Conventional Graded Structure

- Age/Grade Specific Textbooks
- Promotion, Retention, Social Promotion, & Grade Skipping Practices
- Grade Specific Content Standards
- Teacher Focused Curriculum and Instruction
- Comparative Reporting (A • B • C D & F)
- Timebound Lock-Step Learning Increments
- Tracking Practices
- Group Standardized Testing

The Multiage Classroom ("Parts List")

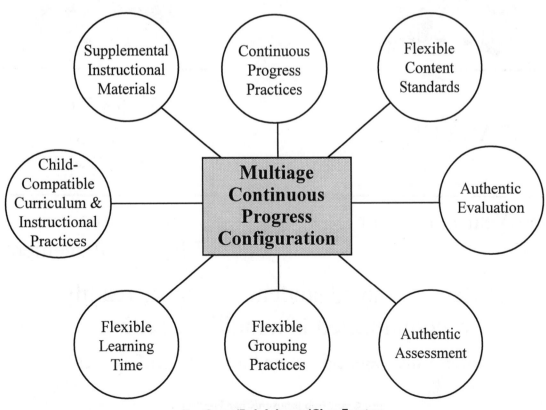

Multiage Continuous Progress Configuration

- Supplemental Instructional Materials
- Continuous Progress Practices
- Flexible Content Standards
- Child-Compatible Curriculum & Instructional Practices
- Authentic Evaluation
- Flexible Learning Time
- Flexible Grouping Practices
- Authentic Assessment

Jim Grant/Bob Johnson/Char Forsten

Gifted and Talented Students

**Conventional One Year/
Single Grade Classroom**

1. Extended learning program is available
2. Tutoring opportunities offer a "teaching role"

That's all, folks!

Multiage Continuous Progress Classroom

1. Extended learning program is available
2. Tutoring opportunities offer a "teaching role"

   and during the first year
3. Multiage classrooms have a higher ceiling on the curriculum
4. First-timers can be more readily accelerated into the next years' curriculum

   and during the second year
5. There are younger students to socialize with
6. Students can gain "senior citizen" status
7. The older more knowledgeable students have the chance to practice being in a leadership role

Inclusion Education in the Multiage Classroom

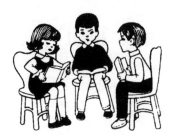

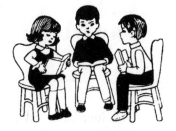

GRADE ONE

5 • 6 • 7 • 8
Year-olds
First/Second Grade Blend

One-Year Placement

Two/Three Year-
Multiage Placement

Differently-abled students are more readily accommodated in a multiage setting

Note: A multiage classroom "forgives" differences

Jim Grant/Bob Johnson/Char Forsten

Curriculum "Flip-Flop"

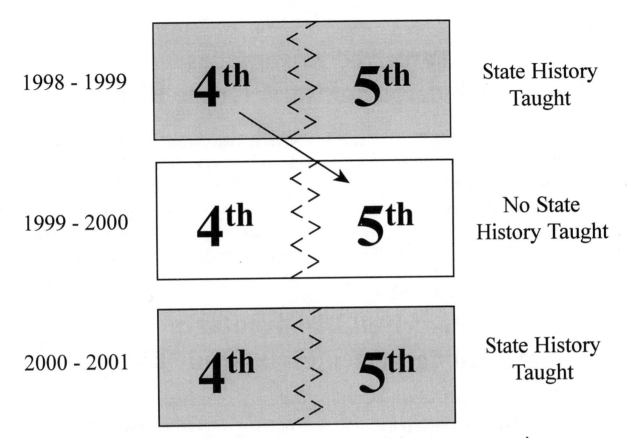

1998 - 1999	4th < > 5th	State History Taught
1999 - 2000	4th < > 5th	No State History Taught
2000 - 2001	4th < > 5th	State History Taught

Note: School officials should secure a test waiver to move testing to the end of Grade 5 as well as permission to rotate the curriculum.

Departmentalization:

1. Defeats the benefits gained by being placed with a significant adult in a consistent setting over time

2. Defeats the benefits of students being together in a school family over time

3. Is an inefficient use of instructional time

4. Creates "stop and go" teaching blocks

5. Sends the wrong message! All things in life are somehow unrelated and unconnected

6. Distorts curriculum planning

7. Creates too many transitions

8. Contributes to the harried/hurried child syndrome

9. Allows no one person to be accountable

10. Doesn't allow teachers to know children deeply

11. Is a major obstacle to integrating the curriculums

Note: Departmentalization is a sixties concept considered to be a developmentally inappropriate practice that benefits only the teachers.

Books That Give Insight into Departmentalization at the Elementary Level

The Hurried Child by David Elkind

Yardsticks by Chip Wood

ITI: The Model by Susan Kovalik

A Place Called School by John Goodlad

Jim Grant/Bob Johnson/Char Forsten

Kindergarten/First Grade Multiage Classroom

Perceived Advantages of a Kindergarten/First Grade Blend

- Mixed-age eavesdropping opportunities
- There is a higher ceiling on the curriculum
- There are peer modeling opportunities
- There are over two dozen multiyear placement benefits
- There can be an additional year of learning time without the stigma of "staying back"
- Grade one is afforded more play opportunities
- There is additional time available for "kid watching"
- In some schools kindergartners go home at noon reducing the class size for first grade in the PM
- There are real benefits to scaffolding
- There are tutoring opportunities for both groups
- There are 50% fewer new first graders to teach to read

Perceived Disadvantages of a Kindergarten/First Grade Blend

- Kindergartners may be denied play opportunities
- Many of today's kindergartners have very high needs
- Class is too diverse developmentally
- First graders may be shortchanged academically
- Some schools have four-year-olds in kindergarten due to a late entrance date and/or a year-round school schedule starting in July
- The needs of five-year-olds are very different from six-year-olds
- Kindergartners may be overwhelmed by more experienced first graders
- There may not be enough quality kid watching time
- Kindergarten is time intensive to teach
- Some entire kindergarten classes are too dysfunctional to keep together as a group for multiple years
- Kindergartners who are learning handicapped, yet unidentified, may not qualify for special needs intervention services
- If there is an AM and PM kindergarten (2 groups) there may be too much lost time transitioning

Various Factors to Consider Before Blending Kindergarten and First Grade

- Class size
- Entrance date
- Program support: Parents, teachers, administrators, school board
- Condition of the student population
- Number of non-English speaking children
- Conflicting mandates from the state, county, and local education officials
- Grade specific curriculum requirements
- Number of identified special needs children
- Number of children with "invisible" disabilities (unidentified)

Class Size Matters

Compared to large classes:

- small classes ameliorate the effects of large schools
- fewer students are held back a grade
- while small classes benefit all students, minority students benefit the most
- students receive more individual attention
- smaller classes are friendlier and more intimate
- there are fewer discipline problems in smaller classes
- students are more likely to participate in activities

Consider some potential cost savings from using small classes in grades K-2 or K-3

- There are fewer retentions
- Less need for remediation and /or special education
- Improved behavior
- Increased achievement

Center of Excellence for Research in Basic Skills • Tennessee State University
330 Tenth Avenue North, Suite J • Nashville, TN 37203 • 615-963-7231

Contact Dr. Gary Peevley for more information on the Student/Teacher Achievment Ratio Project (Project STAR). The project has studied the effect of class size on learning.

Guidelines to balancing the multiyear classroom

- Equal number of students from each grade level *
- Equal number of boys and girls
- Racially/culturally/linguistically balanced
- Socio-economically balanced
- Equal range of ability levels
- The percent of special needs students should be the same as conventional classrooms

Additional factors to consider include: Student motivation, behavior problems and emotional problems.

Note: Remember, it is not always possible to achieve the above ideal guidelines.

* Does not pertain to single grade looping classrooms

Jim Grant/Bob Johnson/Char Forsten

Times when it's appropriate to separate your multiage class by grade level for a specific purpose

- Annual environmental camping trip

- Occasionally some specific lessons require splitting your class by age/grade in music and physical education

- D.A.R.E. drug program (local police request only 5th graders receive the program)

- Sex education programs

- Mandated group standardized testing

- Occasionally some types of field trips may require separating the class by age or grade level

- Sometimes an outside sponsored activity by the 4-H club, Boy Scouts, Girl Scouts, Cub Scouts, Brownies, etc. may require dividing classes by age/grade. (This is unique to inner city schools with an unsafe neighborhood.)

Note: Splitting your multiage class on occasion by age/grade level will not undermine the integrity of your program and at times can actually be beneficial.

The Role of Administrators in a Multiyear Classroom

1. The administration should secure waiver(s):
   - to change the timeframe and sequence for teaching mandated grade specific curriculum content
   - to eliminate promotional gates
   - requiring teachers to hold dual certifications (i.e., kindergarten and elementary certification or elementary and middle school configuration)
   - to postpone group standardized testing until the end of the second year

2. Principals must permit teachers to deemphasize the conventional grade barrier at the end of the first year as well as the beginning of the second year.

3. The principal should actively participate in school board, staff and parent presentations.

4. The principal needs to be proactive and take measures to reduce/minimize/eliminate staff dissension.

5. The administration should secure adequate funding for supplemental materials, site visits, training, research, substitutes, etc.

6. The principal needs to create opportunities for teachers to:
   - visit the next grade level
   - visit model multiyear classrooms
   - attend seminars/conferences
   - have collaborative planning time

7. The principal needs to assure that multiyear classrooms have balanced, teachable student populations.

8. The principal must provide options for giving some students an additional year of learning time.

9. The school administration should "guarantee" the rights of teachers to have a "voice" in creating his/her workplace.

Multiyear Teachers' Bill of Rights

1. Teachers are not mandated to teach in a multiyear classroom against his/her will.

2. Teachers have a right to take a hiatus from teaching in a multiyear classroom if his/her life's circumstances change.

3. Teachers have the right to transfer a student to another class if a personality clash is unable to be resolved.

4. Teachers are not required to keep an unreasonable or disgruntled parent for more than <u>one</u> year.

5. Teachers are <u>not</u> required to keep a dysfunctional class for more than one year.

6. Teachers have the right to create a classroom with a balanced, teachable school population.

7. Teachers who agree to take a disproportionately higher number of high needs students should be provided additional classroom support, a reduced class size, and not receive transient students during the school year.

Q.

What exactly are the differences between multiage instructional practices and developmentally appropriate practices used in a single-grade classroom?

A. None. The needs of individual children still must be met through a quality program of instruction, regardless of the span of abilities and age ranges of their classmates.

Both multiage and developmentally appropriate single-grade classrooms should have a literacy program that helps children develop a love for reading through exposure to quality literature, while improving their ability to decode and comprehend text. A math program appropriate for young children would incorporate the National Council of Teachers of Mathematics (NCTM) standards and would focus on using manipulatives and a variety of other activities to help children build a sound foundation of mathematical concepts. Programs for science should involve children exploring their world while using appropriate scientific materials and processes. Curricula for other subjects should also be taught in ways that are congruent with how young children learn.

For information about what activities are developmentally appropriate for children at different ages, read *Developmentally Appropriate Practice in Early Childhood Programs Serving Children From Birth Through Age 8* (Sue Bredekamp, ed.) and other books published by the National Association for the Education of Young Children (NAEYC). Other good books on developmentally appropriate practices include *Yardsticks*, by Chip Wood, and *A Notebook for Teachers: Making Changes in the Elementary Curriculum*, both of which are published by the Northeast Foundation for Children; and *Developmental Education in the 1990's* by Jim Grant, published by Modern Learning Press.

Excerpted from *Multiage Q&A: 101 Practical Anwers to Your Most Pressing Questions*, by Jim Grant, Bob Johnson, and Irv Richardson. Peterborough, NH: Crystal Springs Books, 1996.

A. No. The need for two-year kindergartens and transitional first grades may be reduced when a district has an effective multiage program in place. It is not eliminated, especially in larger-enrollment districts.

It is vital that multiage programs be widely available and commonly used. This assumes much more than just a grouping of different ages together. It requires methods, materials, time schedules, and curriculum which support such a program. Multiage is not just multigrade!

When integrated curriculum, hands-on and activity-based learning, strong literature-based instruction, and cooperative learning are integral to the program, then the multiage program is likely to be an effective one. When pupils experience an effective multiage program, fewer of them may need an extra year of learning time within their primary program.

If either the availability or quality of multiage programs is restricted, the need for readiness kindergartens and transitional first grades will continue to exist. These programs have been very productive and positive for children, and can continue to meet a real need for some pupils (Uphoff 1995).

Multiage programs are a major step toward providing children with the quality of instruction that, too often, only the extra-year programs provided previously.

Q. Does a multiage classroom eliminate the need for a transitional kindergarten for young fives or a transitional first for young sixes?

Q.

Are there potential drawbacks to a multiage classroom?

 Yes! Every reform has its drawbacks, and multiage classrooms are no exception.

Paying attention to the following potential pitfalls will help assure a smooth transition to a multiage classroom.

· *Neglecting Gifted and Talented Students.* This is a major parental concern. Every effort needs to be made to challenge advanced learners, while making sure these students are not taken advantage of as free teachers' aides to tutor less knowledgeable students.

· *Assigning a Marginal Teacher to a Multiage Classroom.* Students should never be subjected to a poor teacher for one year, let alone two or three. (Fortunately, marginal teachers usually don't offer to teach in such a demanding classroom environment.) The principal can quiet parental fears by ensuring that only the highest energy, most qualified teachers will be assigned to teach in multiage classrooms.

· *Perpetuating a Dysfunctional Class.* It seems every few years a school ends up with a class with an unusually difficult combination of students. It is unfair to everyone involved to keep this group together in a multiple-year placement. This class is overwhelming to teach, and is unfair to the students, parents, and teacher.

· *Concentrating Too Many Problem Students in One Class.* Keeping too many high-impact students together in a multiple year placement is a form of tracking. The effect these students have on each another as well as on the teacher often produces negative results.

· *Placing Too Many Handicapped Students in One Class.* There may be a tendency to overload a multiage classroom with special-needs students due to the accommodating nature of the program. Steps must be taken to assure that the multiage classroom does not turn into a special education room or a dumping ground.

· *Masking a Learning Disability.* When grade lines are deemphasized, it is not unusual for a student with disabilities to be inadvertently overlooked during the first year in a multiage classroom. The oversight may delay much needed special education intervention.

· *Keeping Difficult Parents More Than One Year.* Having unreasonable, difficult parents for even one year can be very trying for the teacher. It is in everyone's interest not to force parents and teachers together against their will.

· *Creating Too Much Diversity Among Students.* Too much is too much! When the range of ages and abilities is too great it becomes nearly impossible to meet the wide variety of needs. This environment becomes unworkable and too stressful for the teacher. Too much student diversity is the reason most often attributed to the failure of a multiage program.

· *Clashing Student/Teacher Personalities.* In rare cases an unresolvable personality clash develops between a teacher and student. Moving the student to another classroom seems to be the best way to extricate the child from this unpleasant situation. Schools would be wise to have a policy in force to handle this dilemma should the occasion arise.

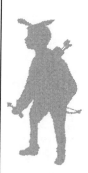

Select Students for a Multiage Classroom With Careful Thought

The key to a successful multiage classroom is balance — providing enough diversity among classmates so that children may learn from each other and support each other, but not so much diversity that the classroom becomes unmanageable, and thus unteachable. It is crucial to balance the natures and needs of all the students, including the differently-abled and developmentally different.

The first rule for selection is to draw from a pool of students whose parents have indicated an interest in their child being placed in a multiage classroom. Nothing will jeopardize a well-planned, thoughtfully implemented multiage program more quickly than parents who have been forced to place their child in a program which they believe is not suited to meet their or their child's needs.

A classroom should also be balanced, whenever possible, in terms of age, number of students from each grade, racial and cultural diversity, linguistic diversity, a broad range of ability levels, and gender.

Much care must be taken when including differently-abled and developmentally different students in the multiage venue. Some communities are being told by well-intentioned staff and administrators that multiage, nongraded continuous grouping can replace or eliminate the need for special education programs. Wrong!

A developmentally appropriate multiage classroom may minimize the need for some students' placement in special education classrooms, but developmentally appropriate practices alone will not necessarily adequately meet the needs of high-impact children. These children typically may be behaviorally disordered, emotionally unstable, learning-disabled, economically disadvantaged, severely developmentally delayed or difficult children. To meet success, these students will need additional support and attention, requiring more of the multiage classroom teacher's time than her other students.

Realistically, these same students may need the additional services in the multiage classroom of the special educator, speech and language therapist/pathologist, occupational or physical therapist, school counselor, bilingual teacher, instructional aide or a parent volunteer. Too many hard-to-teach students create an imbalance that makes it harder for the teacher to provide good instruction to all of the students in the room.

Excerpted from *Our Best Advice: The Multiage Problem Solving Handbook*, by Jim Grant, Bob Johnson, and Irv Richardson. Peterborough, NH: Crystal Springs Books, 1996.

Parents should also know, and we must help them understand, that placement in a multiage program is an annual choice involving the student, the parents, and the teacher. All must concur for the placement to work.

It is important to remember that not all communities will reflect the diversity necessary to create an ideally balanced, culturally diverse multiage classroom.

Our Best Advice ✓

Assuring a balanced, teachable student population is critical to the success of quality teaching in the multiage classroom. This is one very important aspect that must not be left to chance.

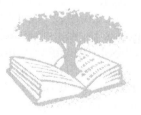

Don't Start With Too Many Grades

Have you recently awakened in the middle of the night with cold sweats and nightmares from the lack of sufficient challenges? or worst yet, from too little stress and misery in your life?

If the answer to this question is yes, then you may well be a candidate to teach a three- or four-grade multiage blend. As with all decisions about the number of grades to include when creating a multiage classroom, common sense must prevail.

Some experts suggest you need three grades blended together to be a true multiage classroom, while others fear that if they don't create a three-grade or greater blend, a teacher may continue to group students using the tracking-by-ability practices of the past. The rationale for this rests in the notion that creating ability groups for three or more grades would be too difficult, thus forcing a teacher to look for other ways of grouping. Neither concept makes sense.

Our advice is to start where you feel comfortable and build from that base. Sometimes our initial zeal and excitement for a new experience causes us to make choices that hindsight may later abhor.

Consider these simple facts: A three-grade blend typically will include a five- to six-year chronological age span, a three- to eight-year developmental range, and an ability range that can span 70 points (70–140 IQ). Although it's true that diversity is an asset when considering the potential for inclusion of differently-abled and developmentally different students, too much diversity will likely undermine the potential opportunities for all the students placed in the classroom.

While many states are encouraging exploration of different grouping configurations, including multiage grouping, they may still insist on continuing rigid grade-level expectations in their curriculum. As an example, many states require state history to be taught in fourth grade, U.S. history in fifth grade, and world cultures/civilization in sixth grade. The more grades included in the multiage class, the more difficult it will be to reconcile the demands of the grade level curricula.

Some teachers choose to handle broad multiage groupings — three grades or more — by instituting cross-grade team teaching. In this configuration, the team plans together, often centering instruction around broad thematic units integrating social studies and the sciences. The teaching team and all the students come together to share during the thematic unit, but otherwise remain in one of several multiage classrooms for the remainder of the class time.

Another challenge is how to effectively use specialists teaching music, art, physical education, computer, foreign language, and library skills within a more-than-two-grade multiage classroom. One of the most common reasons cited for discontinuing multiage grouping is the difficulty of accommodating the diverse range of developmental levels, ability ranges, learning styles, and personalities in these specialties.

Add to this the high number of students who come to school with learning disabilities, from families in crisis, with health and nutrition problems, with emotional problems, and poverty, and the diversity becomes staggering for some and just plain overwhelming for others.

Our Best Advice ✔

When implementing multiage education, start with a two-grade blend and let your own common sense dictate when or if to expand to three or more grades. Success breeds success; start at your comfort level, and grow in confidence. Think big, start small!

MANY FACTORS INFLUENCE
Developmental Diversity

BY JAMES K. UPHOFF, ED.D.

The school bells ring in mid- to late summer and thousands of children march through the schoolhouse doors without anyone giving any thought as to whether these children are ready — physically, socially, emotionally, academically — for the curriculum awaiting them.

This article aims to provide parents and teachers with information about a number of major factors which need to be considered in making the decision about a child's readiness for school. These same considerations are relevant when parents are thinking about giving their child the *gift of time,* another year in the current grade in order to grow and mature, or a year in a readiness/K or transition K-1 program.

Too often parents and school officials confuse verbal brightness with readiness for school. *Being bright* and being *ready for school* are not the same thing! An inappropriate start in school too often tarnishes that brightness.

Today's K-3 curriculum has been pushed down by our American "faster is better" culture to the point that what is often found in today's kindergarten was found in late first or early second grade just three decades ago. Many schools are trying to change from the "sit-still, paper-pencil" approach of the present to a more active, involved, manipulative curriculum which enables young children to learn best. However, until this latter learning environment is available for every child, parents and teachers must decide whether each child is ready.

Each of the following factors indicates a potential for problems. The more factors which apply to an individual child, the more likely he or she is to encounter difficulty — academically, socially, emotionally, and/or physically — and each of these areas is crucial to a well-rounded human being. *No one factor should be the only basis for making a decision.* Look at all of the factors, then decide.

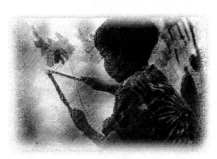

The more factors which apply to an individual child, the more likely he or she is to encounter difficulty— academically, socially, emotionally, and/or physically— and each of these areas is crucial to a well-rounded human being. *No one factor should be the only basis for making a decision.* Look at all of the factors, then decide.

Readiness Factors

Chronological Age at School Entrance: My own research and that of many others indicates that children who are less than five-and-a-half years of age at entrance into kindergarten are much more likely to encounter problems than children who are older. This would put the cutoff for birthdate at about March 25 for many schools. The younger the child is, the more likely it is that the current academic paper/pencil kindergarten curriculum is inappropriate.

Problems at Birth: When labor lasts a long time or is less than four hours, or when labor is unusually difficult, the child is more likely to experience problems in school. Long labor too often results in reduced oxygen and/or nourishment for the child just before birth. Some studies have found birth trauma to be associated with later emotional problems including, in the extreme, suicidal tendencies.

Early General Health and Nutrition: Many factors involving general health and nutrition:

- Poor nutrition in the preschool years puts the child at greater risk in terms of school success.
- The child who experiences many serious ear infections has been found to have more difficulty in learning to read.
- Allergies, asthma, and other similar problems can also inhibit learning. Any type of illness or problem which results in a passive child — either confined to bed or just forced to "be very quiet" day after day — is likely to result in physically delayed development. Lack of body and muscle control can be a major problem for learners.

Family Status: Any act which lessens the stability of the child's family security is a problem; the closer such acts/events occur to the start of school, the more likely that start is to be a negative one. The following destabilizing factors should be considered:

- Death of anyone close to the child. This includes family, friends, neighbors, or even pets.
- A move from one house or apartment to another; even though the adults may see it as a positive relocation — more space, own bedroom for child, etc. — the child may miss friends, neighbors, or the dog next door.
- Separation from parents or close family members whether by jobs, military duty, divorce, prison, remarriage, or moves can create problems for a child in early school experiences.
- The birth of a sibling or the addition of new step-family members can be very upsetting.

Birth Order: If the gap between child number one and child number two is less than three years, then child two is more likely to have problems in school. When there are more than three children in a family, the baby of the family (last born) often experiences less independence and initiative. There are exceptions to these factors as with the others, but they remain as predictors, nevertheless.

Low Birth Weight: A premature child with low birthweight often experiences significant delays in many aspects of his or her development.

Gender: Boys are about one month behind girls in physiological development at birth, about six months behind at age five, and about twenty-four months behind girls at ages eleven and twelve. (Some contend that we males never catch up!)

Boys need extra time more than girls, but research shows that girls actually benefit from it more. Their eyes, motor skills, etc., are ahead by nature, and when given time, become even "aheader"! Boys fail far more often than do girls and have many more school problems than do girls.

Vision: Being able to see clearly does *not* mean that a child's vision is ready for schoolwork. It is not until age eight that 90 percent of children have suffi-

cient eye-muscle development to do *with ease* what reading demands of the eyes. The younger the child is, the more likely he or she does *not* have all of the vision development required.

For example, many children have problems with focusing. Their eyes work like a zoom lens on a projector, zooming in and out until a sharp focus is obtained. Much time can be spent in this process and much is missed while focusing is taking place. Other eye problems include the muscle's inability to maintain focus and smooth movement from left to right; lazy eye; and mid-line problems.

Memory Level: If a child has difficulty remembering such common items as prayers, commercials, his or her home address or telephone number, the child may well experience problems with the typical primary grade curriculum. Many times memory success is associated with one's ability to concentrate; thus this factor is related to the next one.

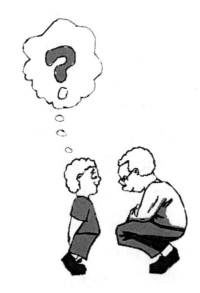

Attention Span: Research has clearly shown a strong connection between the amount of time a child spends working on skill content (the three Rs) and the achievement level reached. The child who is easily distracted and finds it difficult to focus attention for ten to fifteen minutes at a time on a single activity is probably going to experience much frustration in school. Discipline problems are likely, as are academic ones. Sitting still is very difficult for the typical 5½- to 6½-year-old child and this normal physiological condition is at great odds with the

typical sit still/paper-pencil curriculum which still exists in many schools.

Social Skills: The child with delayed social development is often reluctant to leave the security of a known situation (home/sitter/preschool/etc.). This child is very hesitant about mixing with other children, is passive, and slow to become involved. Noninvolvement is often associated with lower learning levels. Tears, urinary "accidents," morning tummyaches, a return to thumb sucking, etc., are all signals of such a delay. Some research has found correlations between short labor deliveries and such problems.

Speaking Skills: A child's ability to communicate clearly is closely related to maturation. In order to pronounce sounds distinctly and correctly, muscle control is essential. Hearing must also be of good quality; this is often reduced by early ear infections, allergies, etc. Inappropriate speech patterns (baby talk) and/or incorrect articulation (an "r" sounds like a "w") are major concern signals.

Reading Interest: If a child does not like to be read to, has little desire to watch a TV story all the way through, or rarely picks up a book to read to him- or herself, the odds are high that the child is not ready for the curriculum of the typical kindergarten. Few of us do well those things in which we are not yet interested, and our children are no different!

Small Motor Skills: The ability to cut, draw, paste, and manipulate pencils, colors, etc., is very important in today's pushed-down kindergarten. The child who has some difficulty with these, uses an awkward grip on the pencil (ice-pick, one or no fingertips on the pencil, etc.), and/or has trouble holding small cards in the hand during a game is a candidate for frustrations. Eye/hand coordination is vital for a high degree of success.

Large Motor Skills: It is typical for a five- to six-year-old child to "trip over a piece of string," yet the typical curriculum assumes major control over one's body movements. Ability to skip, jump on one foot at a time, walk a balance beam, hop, jump from a standing position, etc., is a set of skills which research has found to be related to overall school success. For example, some testing of such skills just before the start of school has been found to predict reading success levels at grades five and eight!

Summary

A child's self-concept needs to be positive. He or she should see school as a good place to be. Giving a child the best start in school demands that the parents and school work together to be sure that the curriculum will allow him or her to find success and positive experiences.

Parents can also provide support for the school in its efforts to reduce the amount of paperwork in the early grades. Working together, the home and the school can help each child establish a firm foundation for a lifetime of learning.

"Is this child ready for school?" is a major question for parents and teachers to answer. This article merely highlights some of the key factors one should consider when making such a decision. I urge all schools to adopt a thorough assessment procedure which considers all of these factors so as to provide parents and teachers with as much information as possible on which to base their decisions.

For more information on transition and readiness programs, see Dr. Uphoff's book, Real Facts from Real Schools, *published by Programs for Education, 1995.*

The book provides a historical perspective on the development of readiness and transition programs, presents an in-depth look at the major issues raised by attacks on such programs, and summarizes more than four dozen research studies.

To contact Dr. Uphoff, you may write him at the College of Education and Human Services, Wright State University, Dayton, Ohio 45435, or email him at JKUphoff@aol.com.

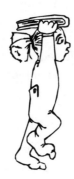

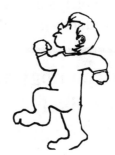

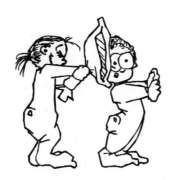

Factors and Circumstances That Create Developmental Diversity

1. Chronological age at entrance
2. Gender
3. Low birth weight
4. Prematurity
5. Mother's level of education *
6. Living below the poverty level *
7. Non-English speaking mother *
8. Mother unmarried at time of the child's birth *
9. Single parent family *
10. Homelessness
11. Transiency (resulting in excessive absences)
12. Difficult/traumatic birth/forcep birth
13. Lack of health care, i.e., untreated ear infections, untreated asthma, lack of dental and vision care
14. Lack of prenatal care
15. Traumatized, i.e., divorce, violence, death of a family member, abuse/neglect
16. Damage resulting from smoking/alcohol/drugs prenatally
17. Lack of pre-school experience
18. Family in crisis, i.e., unemployment, parent incarcerated, etc.
19. Malnutrition
20. Chemical injury, i.e., lead, pesticides, etc.

* **Major Family Risk Factors** (One half of today's preschoolers are affected by at least one of these risk factors and fifteen percent are affected by three or more of them. Children with one or more of these characteristics may be educationally disadvantaged or "at-risk" of school failure. — *National Center for Educational Statistics*)

Note: Some factors are not considered to be a root cause of unreadiness in children, however they may exacerbate the condition.

The chronologically younger children in any grade are far more likely than the older children in that grade to:

1. have failed a grade
2. become dropouts
3. be referred for testing for special services and special education
4. be diagnosed as Learning Disabled
5. be sent to the principal's office for discipline problems even when in high school
6. be receiving various types of counseling services
7. be receiving lower grades than their ability scores would indicate as reasonable
8. be behind their grade peers in athletic skill level
9. be chosen less frequently for leadership roles by peers or adults
10. be in special service programs such as Title I
11. be in speech therapy programs
12. be slower in social development
13. rank lower in their graduating class
14. be a suicide victim
15. be more of a follower than a leader
16. be less attentive in class
17. earn lower grades
18. score lower on achievement tests

School Readiness and Transition Programs: Real Facts From Real Schools

by James K. Uphoff, Ed.D

Jim Grant

Children Progress Through School on a Broken Front

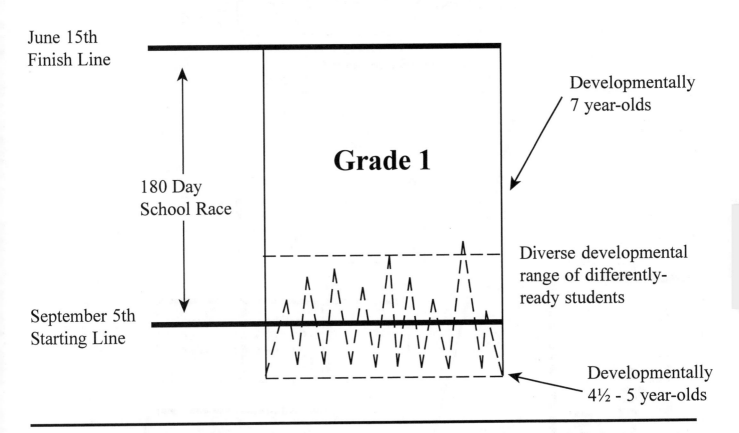

June 15th
Finish Line

180 Day
School Race

September 5th
Starting Line

Grade 1

Developmentally
7 year-olds

Diverse developmental
range of differently-
ready students

Developmentally
4½ - 5 year-olds

Children Enter Kindergarten on a Broken Front

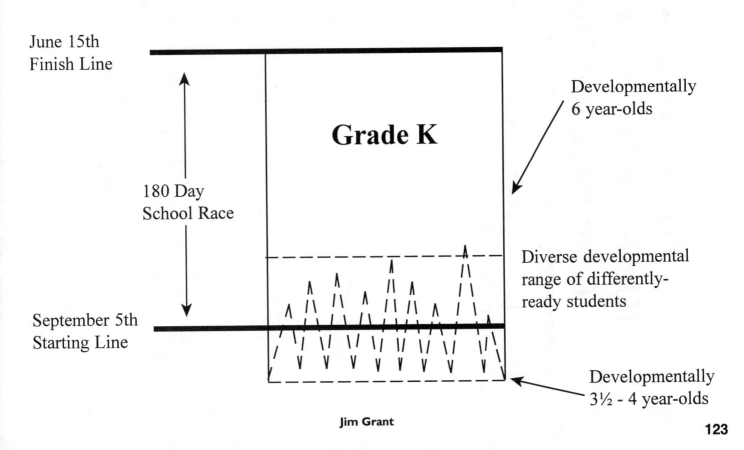

June 15th
Finish Line

180 Day
School Race

September 5th
Starting Line

Grade K

Developmentally
6 year-olds

Diverse developmental
range of differently-
ready students

Developmentally
3½ - 4 year-olds

Jim Grant

Pre-Kindergarten/
Kindergarten/First Grade
Configuration Options

Caution: The special needs population tends
to be overrepresented in transition classes.

Jim Grant

Block	Description
2nd (optional) / 1st / K	K/1 or K/1/2 Multiage classroom (one teacher or team teachers)
1st / K (loop)	K/1 Loop
1st / Pre-1st	Pre-first/first grade Multiage classroom
1st, Pre-1st, K	Self-contained classroom for Kindergarten, pre-first and first grade
Pre-1st / K	K/Pre-1st Multiage classroom
K / Pre-K	Pre-K/K Multiage classroom
Pre-K	Pre-K for "Young Fives"
Universal Preschool	Pre-K for 4 year-olds

When Compared to Boys . . .

Girls entering kindergarten are more likely to:

- Hold a pencil correctly

- Button their clothes

- Write or draw rather than scribble

- Be able to identify more colors

- Count to 20 or beyond

- Write their own name

- Recognize more letters of the alphabet

- Have a longer attention span

- Fidget less

- Show an interest in reading

- Have speech understandable to a stranger

- Not stutter or stammer

On-Time Bloomers Have More Assets

They:

- Seem to cope better emotionally

- Often are older and more mature

- Seem better able to focus and attend

- Seem to have the physical stamina to sustain a demanding school experience

- Often have a greater general knowledge base

- Seem better able to complete tasks

- Seem to have higher social abilities

- Have more school related accomplishments

- Tend to have fewer school related difficulties

Babies Born at Low Birth Weight (weighing 5.5 pounds or less) are more likely to:

1. Have learning disabilities

2. Be retained in grade

3. Fail school

4. Have a short attention span

5. Have health related problems

6. Have developmental delays

7. Have overall low academic performance

"As decisions about preschool, kindergarten and first grade arise, the following reasons to give children extra time should be considered.

Family patterns of slow development — "late bloomers"

Prematurity or physical problems in early life

Immature motor development — awkwardness, poor motor skills such as in catching or throwing a ball, drawing or cutting

Easy distractibility and short attention span

Difficulty with right/left hand or eye/hand coordination, such as in copying a circle or diamond

Lagging social development — difficulty taking turns, sharing or playing. If the child is shunned by children her own age, take it seriously.

Each of these might be a reason to allow a child to mature another year before starting preschool, or to stay in preschool or kindergarten a year longer."

— T. Berry Brazelton, M.D., *Touchpoints*

Recalibrate Your Curriculum & Instruction

- Bring vertical handwriting back to K/1

- Eliminate/reduce board and chart copying

- Eliminate greater than and less than (> <) before 4th grade

- Eliminate the missing addend/subtrahend $3 + \square = 7$, $7 - \square = 4$ before 4th grade

- Do not require left to right eye tracking until children are developmentally ready

- Eliminate workbooks in K/1 for most children

- Reduce the volume of drill sheets in the early grades

- Provide more play-based experiences throughout the elementary years

- Reduce seat time for young learners

- Eliminate all group standardized testing before grade four

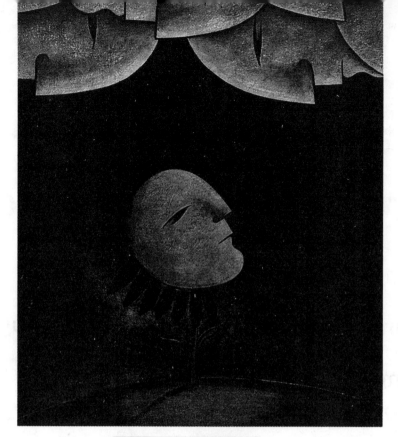

RESEARCH REPORT

HOW DO YOUR CHILDREN GROW?

By Susan Black

The best preschool programs allow children to
invent, experiment, and play

THE RESEARCH ON EARLY-CHILDHOOD EDUCATION LEAVES NO ROOM FOR DOUBT: Preschoolers learn best—and they become better students in later grades—when they follow their natural dispositions. They need to explore, wonder, question, create, and—most importantly—play.

In a compelling study of early-childhood programs in the District of Columbia Public Schools, Rebecca Marcon, a developmental psychologist and professor of psychology at the University of North Florida in Jacksonville, found that educators cannot assume that "just any

Susan Black is a research consultant in Hammondsport, N.Y.

preschool curriculum will achieve positive results." As Marcon discovered when she was called in to investigate high rates of retention in the district's first grades, many youngsters weren't getting smarter with each year they spent in school. In fact, Marcon soon determined, many kids were failing even though they'd been enrolled in readiness programs such as Head Start, prekindergarten, and kindergarten.

As Marcon says, she and others involved in her study were "filled with surprises" at how little consistency they found when they investigated preschool programs serving 4-year-olds in the D.C. schools. Based on information collected from teacher surveys and classroom visits, Marcon sorted the district's preschool programs into three categories: (1) the child-initiated model, in which teachers encourage children to choose and develop their own learning and in which a child's social and emotional needs are considered more important than academic learning; (2) the academically directed model, in which teachers stress academic learning and readiness for the upcoming grades; and (3) the "middle-of-the-road" model, which borrows features from the other two.

Which of these programs works best for kids? As Marcon's data conclusively show, only the children in the child-initiated preschools benefited (in both the short-term and the long-term) from their early experience in school. (Each time Marcon replicated her study, in fact, only the children in the child-initiated model continued to master basic skills and to excel in upper grades.) In contrast, children from the academically directed preschools lost ground, especially in first-grade reading and math. In addition, children in the academic preschools lagged in social development, and boys, especially, fell behind in their overall academic achievement and development. (Girls, Marcon notes, were more ready than boys for academic experiences, but girls did better in classrooms that valued social-emotional development instead of academic preparation.)

RESOURCES

Bettelheim, Bruno. "The Importance of Play." *The Atlantic Monthly*, March 1987, 35-46.

Elkind, David, ed. *Perspectives on Early Childhood Education.* Washington D.C.: National Education Association Professional Library, 1991.

Glascott, Kathleen. "A Problem of Theory for Early Childhood Professionals." *Childhood Education*, Spring 1994, 70, 131-132.

Marcon, Rebecca A. "Doing the Right Thing for Children: Linking Research and Policy Reform in the District of Columbia Public Schools." *Young Children*, November 1994, 8-20.

"NAEYC [National Association for the Education of Young Children] Position Statement: A Conceptual Framework for Early Childhood Professional Development." *Young Children*, March 1994, 68-73.

Standards for Quality School-Age Child Care. Alexandria, Va.: National Association of Elementary School Principals, 1993.

Trepanier-Street, Mary. "What's So New About the Project Approach?" *Childhood Education*, Fall 1993, 70, 25-28.

The middle-of-the-road preschools offered no discernible benefits: Children in these programs were found to have significantly lower mastery of basic skills, especially language skills, and they were slower to develop their social and motor skills.

When she followed the 4-year-olds through the upper grades, Marcon found that by age 9 the effects of a child's preschool experience were clearly apparent. For instance, by fourth grade, children in the academic programs were earning lower grades and passing fewer reading and math objectives. By fourth and fifth grades, these same children were behind their peers developmentally, and they displayed more maladaptive behavior, such as hyperactivity, depression, anxiety, and defiance. According to Marcon's research, these children had more difficulties adjusting and learning than children whose first school experience is in a supportive social-emotional setting. (For Marcon's recommendations for early-childhood programs, see the sidebar on page 19.)

Smarter each year?

If your school has an early-childhood program—or if your district is contemplating adding a program for preschoolers—that research means you need to lay down the law for both teachers and parents: In the early-childhood program at your school, you need to say, preschoolers are not going to be thought of and treated simply as smaller versions of older kids. And they won't be filling out workbook pages and ditto sheets or studying so-called academic subjects (such as math and science) the way older students do. (The National Association of Elementary School Principals, or NAESP, criticizes such an approach, saying preschoolers don't need "bite-sized nibbles" of what older children are getting.) Children in your early-childhood program, you should insist, will be doing what they do best—playing.

You'll also want to make NAESP's two priorities for preschool programs clear to staff members and parents: One goal is that, through play, your 3 and 4-year-olds (as well as younger children if they're also being cared for in your school) will develop a genuine pleasure in learning; the second is that your young charges will develop self-confidence in their ability to learn and to accomplish challenging tasks.

"I try to show—not just tell—parents and teachers what an early-childhood program should look like, sound like, and feel like," says a curriculum specialist who coordinates preschool programs in her school district. "In our classrooms, we provide children with all sorts of interesting toys and supplies, such as water tables, sandboxes, interlocking blocks, and dollhouses. We also give the children lots of time and encouragement to invent and experiment as they play. And we offer constant social and emotional security by making our centers happy and secure places where kids feel respected and loved."

But, as Kathleen Glascott, an assistant professor at Middle Tennessee State University at Murfreesboro, claims, there's more to running a high-quality early-childhood center than making sure you have the right equipment and that you focus on kids' social and emotional development. Far too many teachers "don't completely understand the theory behind their classroom practice," says Glascott. If teachers can't describe the research on early-childhood education—especially the research that says kids learn as they play—it's likely their efforts won't be taken seriously, Glascott maintains. Teachers ought to be able to link their methods—such as providing uninterrupted playtime and having children select their own play activities—with research findings for two reasons, Glascott contends: For one thing, most parents and educators unfamiliar with early-childhood education need to be persuaded—with sound research evidence—that for very young children, play *is* learning; for another, teachers need to demonstrate that play during early childhood pays off in terms of increased academic achievement in later years.

But even those teachers and school executives who have a handle on the research that supports a more relaxed and playful approach to learning for young children have their frustrations. As they tell it, convincing parents that time spent playing is better for their children than studying can be difficult. "I spend countless hours explaining to parents that the best programs concentrate on 'kid stuff,'" says an early-childhood consultant. "Teachers and parents sometimes get impatient with letting kids play freely. They want to force kids to do more grown-up 'school stuff' even though the kids aren't ready to read, print, or listen to a teacher's instructions."

Playing up play

Although approximately 50 percent of 3 and 4-year-olds are in some form of preschool today—and predictions show more school districts plan to adopt early-childhood programs—there's still a "muddled understanding" of what constitutes learning for children this age, says Gary Salyers, former president of NAESP, in his essay "The Critical Preschool Years." Somehow, educators keep missing the boat when it comes to the youngest learners, according to Salyers. Instead of promoting learning that is "developmentally appropriate"—that is, the way a child learns at each stage of growth—schools too often push the kindergarten and first-grade curriculum down into preschool. Unfortunately, the tendency to start preschoolers off with more controlled learning is wrong, Salyers notes, and so is the idea that kids are learning only when they're seated quietly and studying school subjects.

In "The Importance of Play," an essay published in the *Atlantic Monthly,* Bruno Bettelheim, the noted child psychologist and researcher, describes the role of play in a young child's life. Drawing from observations first recorded by Freud, Bettelheim says that children work through and master "complex psychological difficulties of their past and present" as they play. For children, play—especially when it's freewheeling, without rules or goals, and chosen for pure enjoyment—is a "royal road" to their conscious and unconscious inner worlds, says Bettelheim.

Play is actually an intellectual activity, Bettelheim maintains. Through play, children learn cognitive skills

(such as numbering and sorting), motor skills (such as balancing), and personal habits (such as perseverance). But it's important, Bettelheim cautions, for adults to allow young children to "own their own struggles" as they play. Teachers and parents who interfere—by suggesting a "right" way to use a toy, for instance—actually rob children of their chance to solve their own problems, resolve anxieties, and experience the joy of learn-

AN EARLY-CHILDHOOD CHECKLIST

Rebecca Marcon presented the following recommendations for early-childhood education to the administrators and school board members of the District of Columbia Public Schools. The recommendations are based upon her study, "Early Learning and Early Identification Follow-Up Study: Transition from the Early to the Later Childhood Grades":

1. Preschool programs should be individualized to match children's levels of development and natural approaches to learning. Activities in preschool programs should be child-initiated (rather than teacher or subject-initiated).

2. Early-childhood education should focus on children's social and emotional development instead of academic learning. Children who are pushed into academic learning too soon are likely to develop social and scholastic problems by fourth grade. It might take time to see the benefit of a developmentally appropriate early childhood program, but it is worth the wait.

3. Kindergarten should be an extension of preschool rather than a jump start on first grade. Kindergarten should not rush children into academic learning.

4. Schools should concentrate on identifying and assisting children in early-childhood programs who have problems with social, emotional, behavioral, and learning problems. Early intervention—rather than retaining students in kindergarten or first grade—is a better policy and one that is more likely to help students overcome school problems.

5. Schools should encourage and welcome parent involvement in their children's early-childhood education. Parents can positively affect children's scholastic achievement, classroom behavior, and later school success.

6. Schools should plan smooth transitions between early-childhood and later-childhood grades. School personnel should communicate the changes in curriculum and instruction, expectations for students, and information about classrooms and facilities to students and parents.

7. Schools should provide comprehensive counseling and psychological services to all young children. Services should include screenings and evaluations for maladaptive behaviors; staff training on developmentally appropriate teaching and learning; help for students who are anxious and depressed; and community-based outreach programs to help families help their children succeed in school.—S.B.

ing. And, Bettelheim and others note, children invariably lose interest and abandon their activity as soon as adults intrude on their play.

What's more, Bettelheim reminds us, a child's play often doesn't make much sense to an adult, but a child's decisions while playing—such as pushing around a cardboard box or climbing into a wagon and pretending to sleep—fulfill needs that can't always be seen. Remember, researchers say: Play is a constructive activity that allows children to act out problems and dilemmas in their lives, recreate enjoyable moments, and discover their own interests and personalities.

"It's hard to stand back and watch toddlers try over and over to build a tower out of blocks," says a teacher with a roomful of 3-year-olds. "But I've learned not to underestimate these little ones. Instead of rushing to their rescue, I realize now that it's a wonderful moment—one worth waiting for—when they finally get that top block in place and the tower sways but doesn't tumble." Learning that some tasks take considerable time and effort is a valuable lesson kids can get from their play, Bettelheim states. Kids as young as 3 can learn not to give up when things don't go right the first time.

According to the research, schools are on the right track when they give children plenty of time and plenty of room to move, play, and try out ideas. As Bettelheim puts it, teachers should provide ample play opportunities to help kids develop their own "inner life of creativity and imagination."

Howard Gardner, the cognitive psychologist who studies how children and adults learn, urges teachers to take note of what kids choose to play and how they go about playing. According to Gardner, teachers should use the data they collect from observing kids at play to encourage a state of "happy concentration" in their regular studies, such as music and history.

In Indianapolis's Key School (which is organized according to Gardner's theories) youngsters attend a "flow room" each week where they go about the serious business of playing board games, making models, and participating in other activities of their own choosing. According to Gardner and other researchers, play helps put kids into a "state of flow"—a psychological term that describes a point at which learning is neither too easy nor too hard, and solving problems and meeting challenges are extremely satisfying. (For more information on Howard Gardner's research, see the Research Report in the January 1994 issue.)

Ready to receive

According to Rebecca Marcon and many other early-childhood researchers, schools also should be wary of the national education goal that insists: "By the year 2000, all children in America will start school ready to learn." (That school-readiness goal is the first of six goals drafted by the National Governors' Association,

supported by Presidents George Bush and Bill Clinton, and passed legislatively as Goals 2000.)

As Frank Newman, president of the Denver-based Education Commission of the States (ECS), notes in his essay "School Readiness and State Action," schools across the country are trying to figure out what readiness means and how they should go about getting young children ready to learn. As an elementary principal in Maine puts it, "We talk about getting kids ready to learn in our school, but, the truth be told, we don't have a systematic plan to get every child ready for kindergarten or first grade. So far, our best effort involves sending calendars home to parents with suggestions for daily activities they can do with their preschoolers—such as going to a library story hour and touring a local sailing museum. It's a nice touch, but it isn't exactly a readiness plan."

But, researchers such as Lorrie Shepard of the University of Colorado and Mary Lee Smith of Arizona State University say the goal of school readiness should be turned around. Instead of "shoehorning children into programs that don't fit them," Shepard and Smith say, schools ought to concentrate on helping teachers design ways to teach kids as they come. The last thing a school should do is prepare a "readiness checkoff," these researchers say: Thinking that all children can be lumped into a "mythical homogeneous group" in which everyone learns the same way at the same time denies children's natural racial, ethnic, and cultural diversity, Shepard and Smith say.

As for the national goal for school readiness, Frank Newman says school administrators and teachers need to ask a fundamental question: "Readiness for what?" In Newman's view, getting preschoolers ready to do kindergarten work and kindergartners ready for first-grade reading and other subjects, is a "hollow reform." Reflecting on the findings from her research in Washington, D.C., Rebecca Marcon notes that politicians and educators need to shift their thinking from getting kids "ready to learn" to getting schools "ready to receive" eager young learners. "I've had a serious turnabout in my thinking," says a veteran preschool teacher who agrees with Marcon's position. "I now welcome all my little ones with open arms—just as they are—instead of mentally sorting them into groups of learners and non-learners during the first week of school."

A kindergarten teacher in an inner-city school offers this observation: "My teaching partner and I used to moan and groan about kids coming to school not knowing how to hold a book and not ever having counted out buttons or blocks. But now we use this information as a starting point for their learning. We've learned to backtrack when we have to. So, for some kids, we hold them on our lap and show them a book—right side up—and we point out the cover, the title, the print, and the pictures. There's a big difference in where we start with our kids now. I guess you could say we, the teachers, have to be ready to learn." ⬛

TRANSITIONAL
Classrooms

BY ANTHONY COLETTA

Transitional classrooms are designed for normal children who need more time to acquire the maturity, learning habits, motivation, and attention span needed to succeed in school. For such children, the extra year of time and stimulation promotes success and supports positive self-esteem. These children, according to language consultant Katrina deHirsch, develop slowly despite excellent intelligence, and fare better if their school entrance is deferred, "since one more year would make the difference between success and failure."

Participants are placed either in a readiness class prior to kindergarten, or a transitional first between kindergarten and first grade. After completing the readiness class, students enter kindergarten. The transitional first grade is for students who have finished kindergarten but who have been identified as needing extra time before entering first grade.

The additional year is provided within a child-centered environment. In many schools, transitional classrooms provide a model for primary-grade teachers interested in creating a "developmentally appropriate curriculum." Susan Sweitzer, Director of Education and Training for

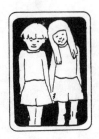

Clearly, children do not languish or "mark time" in these programs. A well-planned transition class is intellectually stimulating. Moreover, the curriculum does not repeat what the students have experienced the year before. Instead, the concepts are extended and elaborated upon.

the Gesell Institute in New Haven, Connecticut, recommends the use of traditional classrooms as a "transition" to developmentally appropriate practice. She states: "Until we get to the point where these practices are extended up to the early grades, there have to be some options."

Clearly, children do not languish or "mark time" in these programs. A well-planned transition class is intellectually stimulating. Moreover, the curriculum does not repeat what the students have experienced the year before. Instead, the concepts are extended and elaborated upon. The additional year allows the children to mature in all areas of development while they are exposed to stimulating learning experiences. As Harvard University Professor Jerome Bruner, author of ***Towards a Theory of Instruction***, says about readiness, the teacher "provides opportunities for its nurture."

As early as 1958, Gordon Liddle and Dale Long reported in the ***Elementary School Journal*** that transitional classrooms were valuable in improving academic performance. During the 1970s and 1980s, students in New Hampshire's public schools consistently achieved the highest scores on the Scholastic Aptitude Test (SAT), even though New

Hampshire ranks 50th in state aid to public schools. In **All Grown Up & No Place to Go**, David Elkind writes that "In New Hampshire children are not hurried. It is one of the few states in the nation that provides 'readiness' classes for children who have completed kindergarten but who are not yet ready for first grade."

Research on Transitional Classrooms

The extent to which extra-year programs yield academic gains is subject to controversy, but their beneficial effect on social growth and self-esteem seems clear. As Robert Lichtenstein states in a paper entitled, "Reanalysis of Research on Early Retention and Extra Year Programs," transitional classrooms "offer significant advantages in non-academic areas (e.g., self-concept, adjustment, attitude toward school)."

Jonathan Sandoval, Professor of Education at the University of California, published research in which he studied high school students who years ago had completed the transitional (junior) first grade. The results showed beneficial outcomes. The children placed in the transitional class were superior to the control group on three out of four indicators of academic progress. The students also had favorable attitudes about the transitional program, indicating that the experiences helped them do better socially and emotionally, as well as academically. Sandoval speculated that without the transitional program, they might not have done as well.

A much publicized 1985 study, conducted by Professors Lorrie Shepard and Mary Lee Smith, concluded that transitional classrooms, though not harmful, do not boost academic performance in schools as had been expected. They conducted a study of 80 children in Boulder, Colorado, which led them to state there were no clear advantages to having an extra year of school prior to first grade. However, even they found a slight difference in achievement test scores in favor of the extra-year students. And, Shepard and Smith's published conclusions omitted the positive social-emotional effects of giving children more time to grow. Their original study includes figures showing that in every area of "Teacher Ratings" (reading, math, social maturity, learner self-concept, and attention), the group receiving the extra year (the "retained" group) scored higher. Most important, the figures were especially higher in the areas of social maturity and learner self-concept. The Shepard and Smith study also does not separate those children who repeated kindergarten from those who were placed in transition programs. All were part of the "retained" group.

Shepard and Smith contend in their book, **Flunking Grades**, that the study of extra-year programs is "limited by the lack of systematic investigation of long-term effects." However, they do not mention Betty McCarty's eight-year study of the effect of kindergarten non-promotion on developmentally immature children. McCarty's results indicated that non-promotion of developmentally young kindergarten children had a positive effect on subsequent levels of peer acceptance, academic attitude, classroom adjustment, and academic achievement.

In general, studies which have reported negative effects of transitional classrooms, such as those described in Gilbert Gredler's article, "Transitional Classes," studied children who were academically at risk. It must, however, be remembered that a transitional program is not intended for remediation. It is developmental, and therefore is based on the premise that children have not yet acquired academic skills.

More than 25 studies of transitional classroom programs are summarized in Dr. James K. Uphoff's **School Readiness and Transition Programs: Real Facts From Real Schools**. According to Uphoff, these studies show that students in transitional classes have at least done as well as fellow students in regard to academic achievement in later years, and in many cases they have surpassed the national averages. The classes have also produced very positive benefits in regard to student self-concept, and emotional and social maturity. Further, there has been overwhelmingly strong satisfaction and support for transitional classes among parents whose children participated in such classes.

The Transitional Class Debate

Transitional classrooms have become a controversial issue. Supporters view them favorably because they help children who might do poorly in a rigid, academic curriculum, by providing instead the opportunity to be successful in a more relaxed, developmentally appropriate environment. Extra-year programs are therefore seen as a clear alternative to grade retention.

Critics, however, argue that such classrooms often become a "dumping ground" for children with low abilities and emotional problems. There may be merit to this argument if schools use transitional classrooms for children who have handicaps or learning problems, or if they inaccurately identify children using techniques and instruments which are insensitive to maturational factors.

Critics also argue that transitional classrooms are a form of retention in which children are stigmatized because they do not progress directly to the next grade. However, as Dr. James Uphoff writes in the article "Proving Your Program Works," "Clearly there is a tremendous difference between a child whose school experience has been one of failure, and a child in a success-oriented program providing time to grow."

The National Association for the Education of Young Children (NAEYC) opposes transitional classrooms because it believes lack of school readiness is most often due to rigid, inappropriate curriculums. NAEYC argues the schools should change so children do not need extra time in order to succeed. They have proposed a shift toward more developmentally appropriate practices in kindergarten and in the primary grades as a way of reducing the large number of children deemed to be unready for school. In an NAEYC publication titled, **Kindergarten Policies: What Is Best for Children,** co-author Johanne Peck states that instead of increasing the age of school entry, "resources and energy should instead be redirected to offering a good program." Many supporters of this position feel that transitional programs impede progress toward the goal of creating appropriate curriculums for all students.

There may be some truth to this, but I am not aware of any hard data which supports this position. And, eliminating readiness and transition classes does not mean that a school will quickly or even eventually implement a developmental curriculum. Many schools will have great difficulty changing to a system that requires additional teacher training and smaller class sizes.

Robert Wood, director of the Northeast Foundation for Children and co-author of **A Notebook for Teachers**, believes that kindergarten teachers are hard-pressed to create a curriculum that meets the individual needs of children, when the developmental age range in a typical class may vary as much as three years. In an average kindergarten, where some children behave like 4 year-olds and others like 5 or 6 year-olds, responding to individual student needs requires high levels of diagnostic teaching skills and more specialized preparation than teachers normally receive.

School personnel interested in providing a developmentally appropriate curriculum for all students realize it is a worthwhile goal that may take time to achieve. In the meantime, many of these schools have established, or are considering, transitional classrooms. To be effective, such programs must be carefully implemented. A series of guidelines that can help parents and educators prepare for success are included in my book, **What's Best for Kids.**

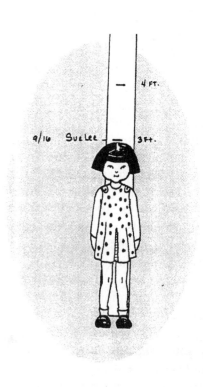

PROPER PLACEMENT

in the beginning

Assures Success
AT THE END

BY JIM GRANT

When I graduated from Keene State College in 1967, I found a job teaching 5th grade in a small, rural community in New Hampshire. My first year as a teacher was a tremendous experience, and I felt I had achieved a lot of success. When I went back for my second year, the Assistant Superintendent of Schools came to see me. He said, "Jim, we're pleased with you, and we want to give you a chance to experience upward mobility. We're going to make you Principal of the Temple Elementary School."

"Well," I said, "I may not look very bright, but I am gifted in math, and I know that would make me Temple's fifth principal in twenty-four months. I'm not sure I can stand that kind of upward mobility." In spite of my reservations, when I woke up the following Monday, I was the principal of an elementary school.

The teacher of the first/second multiage classroom presented me with my first challenge. "I don't know what I'm going to do with my twenty-five children," she said. "They're all over the place. I have trouble getting them to slow down long enough for me to teach them."

I went to her classroom, opened the door, and quickly

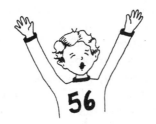

"A child who is eager and ready for kindergarten and first grade is likely to become a lifelong learner.

A child who is pushed to do too much too soon will never really like school and is likely to have problems all the way through.

These are your child's formative years, and starting school should be a positive, rewarding experience."

— Judy Keshner,
Starting School

closed it. Nothing in my teacher education classes or one year of actual teaching experience had prepared me to deal with what I saw.

It was then that I brought in my former teacher, Nancy Richard, as an early childhood consultant who could advise me on the children's development. She observed the class and said, "You have second graders doing third grade work, second graders doing second grade work, second graders doing first grade work, first graders doing second grade work, first graders doing first grade work, first graders doing no work at all, and then there are two boys in the corner who aren't toilet trained after lunch."

"Some of these children," she continued, "aren't yet ready to do first grade work. Chronologically, they are 6, but developmentally they are still too young to succeed in that class." She then suggested I take a course on "developmental readiness."

In that course, I was surprised to learn that up to twenty-five percent of the children in American schools repeat a grade, and as many as another twenty-five percent are often struggling and not succeeding in their current grade. I checked the registers covering a six-year period at my school and proved those statistics were flawed. In my school, thirty-three percent of the kids had repeated! This informal survey also showed that most of the children who repeated were boys, and the grade most children repeated was first grade.

Being a bright, young, "overplaced" principal, I immediately made two brilliant deductions: boys are stupid, and first grade teachers are incompetent. Further reflection, observation, and discussion led me to some different conclusions, however. I began to consider the possibility that girls tended to develop more rapidly in certain respects than boys, and that these differences reached the crisis point in first grade, when all the children were expected to learn how to read and write.

One September in the late 1960's, we began to screen children to help determine their developmental readiness for a first grade experience. We discovered that many of the children eligible for first grade on the basis of their age that year were at risk for a traditional first grade program. When I shared that news with their parents and recommended that the developmentally young children remain in kindergarten for another year, the parents were very unhappy. They decided to send all of those late-blooming children into first grade together, thinking that the children being together would somehow make a difference in their developmental readiness for the demands of first grade.

Of course, it did not. By the middle of October, several of the children had been withdrawn from first grade at their parents' request and moved back to kindergarten. The problems that were surfacing at home and at school made the parents realize that these children really did need more time to grow and prepare for first grade. The rest of the developmentally young children ended up taking two years to complete first grade.

The next year, when we assessed the entering children's developmental levels, we did more to inform the parents — at PTA meetings, in one-on-one meetings, through literature. That year, many children who were developmentally young stayed in kindergarten for an extra year, and then entered first grade when most were 7-years-old. That first group of children, who had the advantage of an extra year to grow, graduated from high school in 1982, and many went on to graduate from college in 1986. We've been using this developmental approach in schools across New Hampshire for well over two decades — with success.

Nationwide, thousands of schools also began providing developmentally young children with extra-time options during the 1960's, helping tens of thousands of students master the curriculum and achieve success in school. This concept, which was formulated in 1911 and formalized as a Title III government program in New Hampshire in 1966, spread rapidly as teachers and parents recognized firsthand how much some children benefited from having an extra year to develop, which then gave them a much greater chance to succeed in school.

Now, when many parents and politicians are demanding stricter standards and measurements of progress, at the same time that many young children are feeling the effects of the disintegration of families and communities, there is a greater need than ever to provide extra-time options for children who are developmentally too young to succeed in a particular grade or program.

Time-flexibility Options

Programs that provide children with an extra year of growing time have many different names, but they share a number of common features. A good time-flexibility program offers reasonable class sizes, an environment rich in materials, and a room with space for movement. Here children can develop their physical and motor capabilities, learn social skills, work with hands-on math and science materials, practice listening and speaking, gain experience with different types of literature, explore the creative arts, and develop problem-solving abilities. As a result, children in these programs can develop the habits of success and a positive attitude toward school.

These programs emphasize an interest-based approach to learning rather than a curriculum based on text books and "time-on-task," access to a wide variety of literature instead of just basal readers and workbooks, and the use of authentic assessments rather than standardized achievement tests. All of these characteristics should be found in any of the time-flexibility options described below:

Readiness Classes for "Young 5's"

Many schools continue to find that a large number of entering students are developmentally too young to learn and succeed in kindergarten. This may be due to a child's innate but still normal rate of development, or environmental factors which have left a child unprepared to work well in a kindergarten class. Readiness classes provide the time needed to grow and make the transition to the school environment in a supportive setting, which then makes kindergarten a much more positive and educational experience. This is particularly important because, as kindergarten teacher Judy Keshner explains in her booklet, *Starting School*, kindergarten "is not a preview of what is to come — it is the foundation on which the following years will grow. Each grade builds on the one that came before, and kindergarten sets the pattern and the tone."

Developmental "Two-tier" Kindergarten

In this type of program, all 5-year-olds enter kindergarten at the same time, based on the legal entrance age, but some stay for one year and some stay for two. After enrollment, each child is developmentally assessed and continues to be observed throughout the year, so that detailed information about children's rate and stage of development is available. At the end of the school year, those children who are developmentally ready move on to first grade. Children who need more time to develop in order to enhance their experience in first grade can remain in kindergarten for a second year, or move into the sort of pre-first or transition class described below.

Pre-first Grade, Transition Grade, Bridge Classes

Call it what you will, this sort of extra-year option has been adopted by concerned parents, teachers, and administrators across America. It provides developmentally young 6-year-olds with a continuous-progress, full-day program in which they have extra time to grow and learn. This helps them make the very difficult and important transition from the play-oriented learning of kindergarten to the more formal "academic tasks" which become increasingly important in first grade. Developmentally young children who have had this extra-year experience are then much better prepared to enter first grade with confidence and a reasonable expectation of success.

Readiness/First Grade (R/1) Configuration

This approach acknowledges the reality that continues to exist in most first grade classes: children who need extra time to grow are blended with those who are developmentally ready for first grade. What makes the R/1 configuration different is that the parents of children who need extra time know from the very beginning that their children can have two years to complete this blended first grade, if needed. This takes the pressure off everyone — students, teachers, and mom and dad. There are no high-stakes campaigns to pass "or else," and no end-of-the-year trauma for children who just need more time to grow and develop.

Some schools chose the R/1 configuration to save money — by not having a separate readiness class, they save on classroom space, staffing, and materials. Other schools choose this option because it is the one the educators prefer and the community accepts. It also provides many benefits of the multi-age classes described below, such as allowing developmentally young students to work closely with and learn from more experienced students during their first year, and then to become the models for new students during their second year.

Multi-age Primary Classes

An increasing number of schools now offer multi-age primary classrooms, in which children of different ages work and learn together, staying together with the teacher for a multi-year placement. These classrooms eliminate the artificial time constraints created by having separate grades from kindergarten through third grade.

One important result is that more time is available for teaching and learning, especially at the start of the year, as teachers and students don't have to spend time getting to know one another and learning to work well together. This approach also eliminates worries about "running out of time" to complete the curriculum by the end of each year, and it eliminates many high-stakes decisions which otherwise have to be made each year. In addition, if a child needs extra time to develop and complete the curriculum before moving on, a multi-age class works particularly well because it already contains a wide range of age levels and a flexible timetable, rather than a rigid, lock-step grade structure.

Multi-age classrooms decrease the risk of failure for all children, because these classes allow students to develop and learn at their own rate in a much less hurried environment. Staying in the same class with the same teacher and classmates for more than one year also provides a sense of consistency and belonging, which can be particularly helpful for the many children who now grow up in fast-changing families and communities. And, the developmental diversity that naturally occurs in a multi-age classroom makes it easier for transfer and special-needs students to be included in them.

An Extra Year of Preschool

Unfortunately, too many parents have to cope with schools which do not offer viable extra-time options for children who are developmentally too young to succeed in kindergarten. Under these circumstances, allowing developmentally young children to spend an extra year in preschool can be a very positive alternative to sending them off to kindergarten and waiting to find out if they "sink or swim." Having an extra year to grow and learn in a supportive preschool environment greatly decreases the odds that such children will flounder and need rescuing in the primary grades.

High-quality preschools provide children with a range of developmentally appropriate activities that foster continued growth and learning. And, the mixed age levels found in most preschools makes it easy for developmentally young children to fit in, just as in a multi-age class. This sort of environment also tends to make preschool teachers aware of the importance of readiness and adept at working with children who are at various developmental levels. Unfortunately, in most cases this option is only available to financially advantaged parents.

An Extra Year at Home

Some parents may prefer to provide their late bloomer with day care and learning experiences at home for an extra year. In situations where there is a parent at home every day who has the time, inclination, and understanding to work with a child in this way, it can be a viable alternative, especially now that more materials and support networks have been developed for the small but growing number of parents who opt to provide their children's entire education at home.

In many cases, parents can simply notify the local school of their intent and send children to kindergarten when they are 6-years-old. However, young children need opportunities to grow and learn with their peers, which contribute in many ways to a child's overall development. And, well-trained preschool and elementary school teachers can often provide a wider range of supportive and educational learning experiences for a developmentally young child than a parent.

Dropping Out and "Stopping Out"

When developmentally young children do not take extra time early in their educational career, they tend to take the time later on. They may repeat a grade in middle school or high school, or flunk out or drop out altogether. They may also obtain their high school diploma but feel the need to take time off before going to college. Some "stop out" — a phrase used to describe students who take a leave of absence while at college. Statistics show that a large number of students do take time off during college, and interestingly enough, the percentage is about the same as the percentage of children found to need extra time when they start school!

Some young people may be ready to put the extra time to better use when they are older, but too many end up with negative attitudes, low self-esteem, and poor skills that interfere with their ability to create productive and fulfilling lives. Early intervention in a positive and supportive way can be far more effective than a wait-and-see approach.

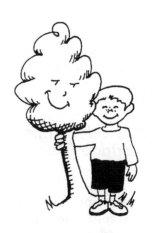

Look at the **Quality** of the Materials

1. **Supportive, repetitive language patterns** (emergent)

2. **Direct correlation between text and illustration** (emergent readers)

3. **Illustrations clear and simplistic** (for emergent readers)

4. **Supportive language patterns** (emergent)

5. **Illustrations supportive enough of difficult words and concepts** (early & fluent)

6. **Illustrations "comfortable" and inviting**

7. **Layout of the page**
    - **size of print**
    - **spaces between words**
    - **amount of "white air space"**
    - **number of words on a line**
    - **number of lines on a page**

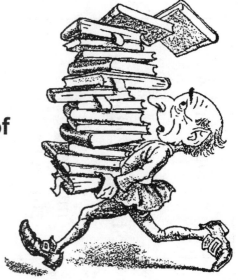

8. **Labeling and organization at back of book discreet yet helpful to teacher**

Day One

Strategy Coaching

- integrating strategies

- cross checking

- articulating strategies used

Day Two

Retelling

- summarizing
- comprehension

Revisiting

- challenging pages

Reread

Mini-lesson

Writing responses/ innovations

Day Three

Writing/ "publishing" innovations

Mini-lesson

Reread

Guided Reading Materials Publishers

The Wright Group
19201 120th Ave. NE
Bothell, Washington
98011-95612
1-800-648-2970

• Story Box
• Sunshine
• New Sunshine
• Visions
• TWIG

Rigby
P.O. Box 797
Crystal Lake, IL 60014
1-800-822-8661

• Literacy 2000
• Satellites
• Literacy Tree

Sundance Publishing
234 Taylor Street
Littleton, MA 01460
1-800-343-8204

• Little Red Readers
• Little Blue Readers

Scholastic, Inc.
P.O. Box 7502
Jefferson City, MO 65102
1-800-325-6149

• Shoebox Library

Richard C. Owen Publishers
P.O. Box 585
Katonah, NY 10536
1-800-336-5588

• Books for Young Learners

SRA
Macmillan/McGraw-Hill
250 Old Wilson Road
Suite 310
Worthington, OH 43085

• Voyages

Literature Circle Directors

for

_____

1. "Discussion Director"
   1.
   2.
   3.
   4.
   5.
   6.

2. "Selection Director"
   1.
   2.
   3.
   4.
   5.
   6.

3. "Art Director"
   1.
   2.
   3.
   4.
   5.
   6.

4. "Wild & Crazy Word Finder"
   1.
   2.
   3.
   4.
   5.
   6.

5. "Connector Director"
   1.
   2.
   3.
   4.
   5.
   6.

6. "Summary Director"
   1.
   2.
   3.
   4.
   5.
   6.

Kathryn L. Cloonan

Group Overview

Title/ Level	Name	m s v	skills /	needs
	1.			
	2.			
	3.			
	4.			
	5.			

Title/ Level	Name	m s v	skills /	needs
	1.			
	2.			
	3.			
	4.			
	5.			

Guided Reading

Recently a great deal of attention has been focused on the importance of grouping children according to their instructional needs. At the same time, we want to be careful not to repeat the errors of the past — that is, placing children in static groups that remain the same year after year. Individual children make progress at different rates; thus we need to group (and regroup) them for guided reading based on careful observations of how they are applying their skills, knowledge, and strategies while they are reading and writing. In their excellent book on learning how to conduct guided reading groups within the context of a balanced literacy program, Fountas and Pinnell (1996) also emphasize flexible grouping based on children's developing control of the reading process. A wise time management expert once said of time, "We have all there is and there isn't enough." If there were an extra day in the week or an extra month in the year, somebody would have undoubtedly discovered it by now. Since there won't be any extra hours to get it all done, you need to look at the time you do have and make some different decisions about how to spend that time.

In guided reading, the teacher works with a small group of children with similar instructional needs. The teacher's role is to predict the type and amount of support the group needs in order to be able to read and understand the book or story. She prompts them to apply reading strategies, regulating her assistance according to the developing control of the individual children in the group. She intervenes only when a student is unlikely to problem-solve independently, is frustrated, or is in jeopardy of losing meaning and does so by asking questions that relate to the reading process. She also provides specific feedback that praises an appropriate processing behavior: for example, "That's good that you went back to the beginning and reread that part. That helped you figure it out."

Guided reading helps children develop an appreciation and understanding of the story and at the same time stimulates problem-solving conversations about how to apply reading strategies in context. Competence as well as independence is encouraged as the teacher models ways of responding when one encounters difficulty in text.

When Do I Begin Guided Reading in My Classroom?

Although there isn't a pat answer to this question, there are observable characteristics that indicate children are ready to participate in these more formal groupings:

- Do they have many of the early concepts of print almost under control (i.e., can they distinguish between text and illustration)?
- Do they have some knowledge of one-to-one matching?
- Do they know the difference between letters and words?
- Do they know the letters of the alphabet and a few frequently encountered words (e.g., *I, the, a*)?
- Do they actively participate in shared reading by predicting events and language structures that show an awareness of comprehension, rhythm, and rhyme?
- Do they spend time reading and noticing a few details of print?
- Do they explore the print on the classroom's walls?
- Do they notice that the same words appear in many different contexts?
- Do they link sounds with symbols when they write?
- Do they articulate words slowly as they write?

If the answer to some of these questions is yes, chances are children are ready to learn more about how printed language works, Some children are ready to begin guided reading in kindergarten, while others need many more opportunities and experiences with print before reading a book in a small group.

Elements of a Guided Reading Lesson

Book Selection

Book selection is critical. Books need to be chosen based on children's interests, prior knowledge, and competency. When selecting books for young readers, teachers should consider important factors such as text layout, specialized vocabulary or concepts, the child's oral language facility, and his potential to apply problem-solving strategies to figure out the words he is unlikely to know. A carefully selected book enables a child to learn more about reading each time he reads.

The book selected needs to be able to be read at 90 percent accuracy or better. Analyzing running records of previously read texts (see Clay 1993) will help you with this judgment call. When reading accuracy falls below 90 percent, the child may be unable to retain the meaning of the story.

Many books that might be considered easy for some children can be too difficult for others. Reading is a problem-solving process by which the reader creates meaning through interacting with the text. Meaning is created as the reader brings prior knowledge and personal experience to the page. The physical design of books and the way their stories are constructed are critical elements in the process. Children begin school with varied literacy backgrounds — some have so little experience that they may not even understand that the print conveys the message. Limited experiences in a child's environment may hinder his or her understanding of the content (e.g., if a child has never been to a zoo, he may be unfamiliar with some of the animals in a zoo book). Therefore, teachers must be very careful to select books for beginning readers that not only meet the goal of instruction but also support the children's level of knowledge and experience: are the picture cues clear? is the type large enough? is the layout of the text easy to follow? does it re-

•Ch. 4 "Guided Reading." Excerpted from *Apprenticeship in Literacy: Transitions Across Reading and Writing*, by Linda J. Dorn, Cathy French and Tammy Jones. York, ME: Stenhouse Publishers, 1998.

quire knowing about certain concepts?

For a child to be able to read a book effectively, the book needs to contain more supportive features than challenging ones. Answering the following questions should help you select an appropriate book for guided reading:

1. Does the book allow the child to construct meaning?
2. Does the book contain structural patterns that are within the child's language control?
3. Does the book include letters and some words that the child can use to monitor his or her reading?
4. Does the book allow the child to use his or her current strategies and skills to problem-solve?
5. Does the book promote fluency?
6. What are the supportive features of the book?
7. What are the challenging features of the book?

Setting the Focus

In cognitive apprenticeship, the teacher is the more capable person. Through sensitive observation, she is always aware of the cutting edge of her children's development. The focus of a guided reading lesson is determined by the strengths and needs of the children in the group. The teacher can use the following questions (Clay 1991; Fountas and Pinnell 1996) to help her set the proper focus for instruction:

1. Can the child match one-to-one?
2. What strategies is the child using (e.g., rereading, searching pictures, using first-letter cues, noticing chunks in words)?
3. What strategies does the child not use?
4. What does the child do at point of difficulty (e.g., appeal to the teacher, sound out the word, reread, correct himself)?

As children become competent readers, the focus of instruction may shift to deepening their understanding of the story. For example, the teacher may ask questions about the characters and the plot, the author's writing style, characteristics of the genre, or literary devices used by the writer to express meaning.

Book Introduction

Before a group reads a new book, the teacher introduces the book. The introduction prepares children to read the story by creating a supportive context for building meaning. The teacher relates the story to the children's personal experiences, invites them to make predictions about the book based on its cover, and identifies the title, author, and illustrator. In her orientation, the teacher prompts the children to integrate meaning, structural, and visual cues. She helps the children build *meaning* by giving a brief overview of the story and prompting them to discuss the pictures. She exposes them to *structure* by identifying recurring language phrases and patterns, being careful to use the precise vocabulary of the story as she and the children talk about it. She introduces the children to visual or *graphophonetic* cues by having them find a frequently encountered word they know or predict a letter at the beginning of an unknown word. As the children gain more control, she can ask them to predict letters in ending and medial positions as well. As the children become more competent readers, the introductory discussion can include a conversation about the content, characters, setting, plot, and writing style.

The book orientation provides a framework for children to use as they explore the written text. The teacher sets the purpose for reading and quickly discusses with the group how to overcome possible challenges within the text. This gentle reminder encourages the children to consider alternatives and to make informed decisions in order to gain meaning.

Their attention is freed so they can concentrate more closely on the visual details of words and letters when they need to.

The level of support in the introduction diminishes as the children move toward self-regulated reading. During the emergent reading stage, the teacher provides a rich introduction with active discussions around the pictures and the story line. As the children move into subsequent stages, the introduction may be reduced to a summary statement and a few selective questions about the story. When the children have become fluent, self-regulated readers, they introduce the books themselves, with only a little help from the teacher. Figure 4.1 illustrates how the teacher adjusts her degree of support as children develop control of the reading process. As the children become more competent readers, they are able to introduce new books to themselves, a necessary skill for independent reading.

First Reading

Once the story has been introduced, the children have the background for constructing meaning. The first reading is an opportunity for them to use the skills and strategies they know with the assistance of a supportive and responsive teacher. Each child begins reading at his or her own pace. Instructional interactions with the children are varied and are determined by individual strengths and needs. Many times the teacher helps children apply problem-solving strategies to visual information in context, such as letters, chunks, rhyming patterns, whole words, affixes, roots, or

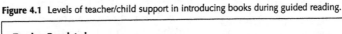

Figure 4.1 Levels of teacher/child support in introducing books during guided reading.

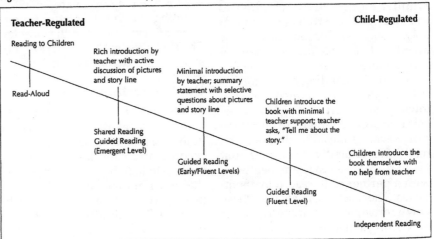

sound sequences.

After everyone has read the book, the teacher selects one or two important teaching points that will boost the children's learning to a higher level. These points are based on careful observation of the children's processing behavior during the first reading.

As children become more competent readers, they are asked to do the first reading silently. The teacher's questions focus on enhancing the children's comprehension and initiating thoughtful discussions. She can ask them to respond personally to specific events in the story: "What would you do if you were all alone during a storm?" She can ask them to locate specific information: "Read and find the part in the story that describes how the girl felt when the storm hit the island." She can use the text to initiate learning opportunities: "Where can we go to find out more information about storms?"

In second and third grades, partner prompting can be a useful technique. At this level, children are usually competent readers who know flexible ways to help themselves read. in this approach, after the book is briefly introduced by the teacher, each child selects a reading partner and the two of them find a quiet corner where they can read the text together silently. Afterwards they discuss the story together. They can also help each other problem-solve tricky words, but a general rule is that one partner can't simply give the word to another.

Subsequent Readings

Subsequent readings of a story give children opportunities to strengthen newly made connections, thus fostering higher-level thinking. Rereading familiar stories allows children to practice reading strategies comfortably, promotes reflection, and frees the attention to be able to notice new information. All these things promote a deeper understanding of the story.

During the days immediately following the guided reading lesson, the children are encouraged to reread the story several times. The children who read independently during the first reading are ready to share their book with a partner or to read it by themselves. The teacher can also use these now-familiar texts for mini-lessons or for writing activities.

Levels of Guided Reading

Below we provide examples of guided reading interactions at the emergent, early, and fluent levels. Remember: successful guided reading interactions depend on the teacher's ability to (a) observe the children's processing behavior and respond accordingly, (b) use language prompts that focus on cue integration and effective processing strategies, and (c) select appropriate materials that support reading development.

Emergent Guided Reading

Children in kindergarten and the first half of first grade are typically emergent readers. They are used to "making sense." Their oral language provides additional cues, and the things they remember about the story guide their interactions with the text. The observant teacher uses information from the *Observation Survey* (Clay 1993) and ongoing documentation of children's processing behavior (as recorded during shared reading, interactive writing, and journal writing and on running records) to determine the aspects of print to which children are attending and thus come up with an appropriate focus for small-group instruction. Although at this level the pictures provide major cues to reading books, the teacher wants the children to realize that the story resides in the text. So she directs their attention to the print by asking them to point to the words, locate known words, and search for unknown words based on their knowledge of a beginning-letter/sound relationship. The children's behavior is observable evidence that they are learning about the processes of reading: they send signals that they are aware something is wrong and they begin to search for alternatives to resolve the problem. The sensitive teacher is alert to these signals and responds accordingly.

Book Selection

For a guided reading group at the emergent level, the teacher uses ongoing assessments such as running records and samples of children's writing to help her select a new book that is within the children's zone of proximal development. As the teacher analyzes the children's processing behavior in both reading and writing,

Figure 4.2 Reading and writing behavior at the emergent level.

Reading Behavior	Writing Behavior
Relies on pictures	Writes one or two letters to represent one word or phrase
Attempts at one-to-one word matching are inconsistent	Can retell a story after hearing it, but does not consistently use one-to-one matching with print
Enjoys the rhythm and rhyme of language	Knows how to form most letters and knows that letters represent language
Can read one-line text with strong picture support	Can writes a simple sentence with supportive drawing

she is collecting data that will drive her instructional focus during guided reading, assisted writing, and word-building activities. Figure 4.2 lists the typical reading and writing behavior of a child at the emergent level.

Let's look at a typical emergent guided reading group. Lynn, the teacher, realizes the importance of selecting books that will help the children gain control of early reading behavior. She is aware that the children are still relying primarily on the picture. Looking through the books that have been identified as being at the emergent level, Lynn notices that most of them have only one sentence or line per page. The sentence usually matches what is seen in the picture. She also observes that most of the texts have a picture on both the left-hand and right-hand pages, with a single line of print positioned at the bottom of the page. Lynn knows that the position of the text is critical for emergent readers: when they open a book, the first thing they should notice is the print on the left-hand page. Therefore, she searches through the books for ones with the print on the left-hand page and the picture on the right-hand page. She wants the children to discover that the message is in the print, not the picture.

Continuing to analyze the books, Lynn looks for those in which the spacing of the letters and words on the page will give the children room to move their finger from word to word as they read. In some emergent-level books the spacing between words is so small that the children cannot practice the speech-to-print match successfully. Lynn believes this supportive feature will serve as a conceptual model the children can apply to other reading and writing contexts.

Narrowing her choice still further, she looks carefully at specific words and letters. She has observed that the children are becoming more aware of particular letter forms as they write and read daily. She wants to select a text that will give them the opportunity to use their limited knowledge of print to check on their own reading. Finally, Lynn selects a book that contains the following features:

- Print begins in the upper-left corner. This directs children's attention to an appropriate starting point.
- Pictures are placed on the right-hand pages. Children will look at the print first, then at the picture.
- Print is large and spaces are bold. The children will be able to pay attention to one-to-one matching.
- A simple repetitive language pattern occurs on each page. The one-word change is supported by the picture.
- One or two frequently encountered words are repeated throughout the text.
- Several known letters are used in the context of the repetitive pattern.

Setting the Focus

After carefully analyzing the children's reading and writing behavior, Lynn sets an overall focus for the group that will take them to a higher level of cognitive development. She knows that the children must learn how to use what they know to check on their own reading progress. She realizes the children are inconsistent with their one-to-one matching. For instance, instead of using known words in texts to monitor their responses, the children rely on their oral language and their memory. Lynn wants the children to use their finger to guide their speech-to-print matches. With these goals in mind, Lynn is ready to introduce the new book to the emergent reading group.

Book Introduction

During the book orientation, Lynn introduces the children to specific concepts they will encounter in the story. Her aim is to create anticipation and to construct a meaningful framework for the story. First she shares the cover of the book, *Me* (Randell 1996), and gives a brief summary of the story: "Today we are going to read a story called *Me*. The little girl in this story tells us about the things that she can do." By encouraging the children to share some things they can do, Lynn activates their background knowledge. Next, she gets them to discuss the pictures in the book, simultaneously planting the language of the text in their minds: "Let's look at the pictures and see what the little girl can do." Several children exclaim, "She can eat!" Lynn validates these responses and at the same time adjusts the language to accommodate the words in the text. "Yes," she comments, pointing to the words as she says them, "I am eating."

Finally Lynn passes out individual copies of the book to the children and prompts them to apply phonological skills for predicting a first-letter cue in an unknown word:

Lynn: *(Stressing the initial sound of the word* sleeping *during pronunciation)* Who can tell me what letter *sleeping* begins with?
Children: *S!*
Lynn: Yes. Can you find the word *sleeping* in your book?

As the children locate the word and frame it with their fingers, Lynn watches to see whether they are successful. When Sarah experiences dif-

ficulty, Lynn increases her level of support: "Find the word that starts with an *s*." She is prepared to pull out a magnetic letter *s* if Sarah needs additional support. After all the children have located the word, Lynn prompts them to confirm their response: "Check it with your finger to be sure it is the word *sleeping*." Confirmation is a critical part of the reading process.

To promote further attention to visual information, Lynn puts magnetic letters on the overhead projector and shows the children the word *am* (see Figure 4.3). Then she instructs them to locate the word *am* in the story. She selects *am*, a partially known word, for two important reasons. First, the word is encountered frequently and she wants the children to notice it. Second, she believes the structural position of the word (it falls in the middle of a three-word repeated pattern) will give the children a strong anchor for one-to-one matching. The children already have control of the word *I*, which is the first word on each page of the story, and they can use a strong picture cue to get the last word of the repeated pattern.

After the children locate the word *am*, Lynn says, "This is an important word in your story. I want you to use it to help yourself when you are reading." With this prompt, Lynn is sending a critical message: the children must use known words as anchors in the text to monitor and guide their reading.

First Reading

Before asking the children to read the text, Lynn tells them, "Use your pointing finger to help you as you read."

Figure 4.3 Lynn uses the overhead projector and magnetic letters to show the children an important word from the text.

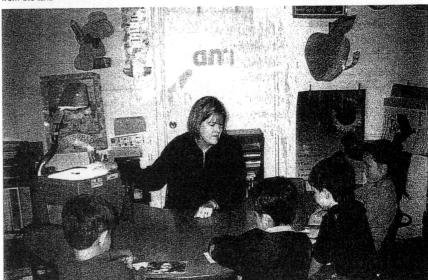

Then she circulates among them while they read. She observes their behavior and prompts them toward constructive activity: "What is happening in the picture?" "Can you find a word that you know?" When the reading is completed, Lynn uses her observations of the children's reading behavior to emphasize three carefully selected teaching points:

- *Teaching point 1 (validating a previously learned response):* "That's good that you used your finger to point to the words while you were reading. That helped you to match your words, didn't it?" Here Lynn acknowledges the children's attempts at one-to-one matching.
- *Teaching point 2 (activating a new response):* "Also, I noticed that when several of you came to the word *laughing* on page 3, you started to say *smiling*. How did you know the word was not *smiling*?" Here and in the next teaching point, Lynn illustrates the importance of using first-letter cues to monitor one's reading.
- *Teaching point 3 (activating a new response):* "You all know that the word *smiling* starts with an s, don't you? Like *sleeping*. Let's take a look at some other words that start with s."

Subsequent Readings

The books are now placed in the children's "familiar reading" baskets, and over the next few days they are encouraged to reread the story several times. The children who read independently during the first reading are ready to share their book with a partner or to read it by themselves.

Early Guided Reading

As children develop and refine their reading skills, they integrate cues and apply flexible strategies for solving new words. They exhibit behavior that indicates they are using visual information to check on the printed message (e.g., they rely less on the pictures). They are less dependent on the finger for matching speech to print, and the teacher encourages this greater control, prompting them to "read it with your eyes." Precise and deliberate matching is replaced by more fluent reading. The breaks between the words disappear, and

groups of words are read with correct phrasing and intonation. The stories are read more naturally and sound more like the language that children use every day. Let's look at a group of first graders who are participating in an early guided reading group.

Book Selection

Sandy, the teacher, selects *The Seed* (Cowley 1996) as an appropriate text for a guided reading group at the early level. Her choice is based on a careful analysis of the children's processing behavior as documented on previous running records, her observations of their reading strategies during independent and guided reading, and her observations of their problem-solving strategies during assisted and independent writing.

Figure 4.4 lists reading and writing behavior typical of children in this group. These characteristics are important criteria for selecting an appropriate text.

Figure 4.4 Reading and writing behavior at the early level.

Reading Behavior	Writing Behavior
Displays knowledge of several frequently encountered words and uses them to monitor reading	Writes several frequently encountered words with fluency and ease
Uses first-letter cues to cross-check against meaning and structure cues	Articulates words slowly when writing
Initiates some problem-solving actions on unknown words	Hears and records beginning, ending, and some medial consonant sounds in sequence; also some vowels
Displays understanding of one-to-one matching and does not need to use the finger during most reading	Shows consistent control of spacing between words
Rereads to confirm meaning and pick up new information for solving problems	Rereads to confirm meaning and expand the message
Corrects errors by matching sources of information	Applies early revision strategies, such as crossing out words and making new attempts

Setting the Focus

Based on her analysis of their reading and writing behavior, Sandy concludes that the children need more opportunities to apply problem-solving strategies for examining words during reading. She knows that it is critical for the children to have flexible ways to analyze unknown words at points of difficulty. This same focus will be emphasized during writing activities and word-building activities.

Book Introduction

Sandy introduces the book to the children by engaging them in a discussion that draws on their background knowledge:

Sandy: What do you think our story is going to be about?
Child: Planting seeds.
Sandy: Yes, we can tell from the picture on the cover that the man is going to plant some seeds. Have any of you ever planted seeds?

Several children share personal experiences with planting seeds. Sandy acknowledges their contributions and gently guides them back to the story.

Sandy: When you planted your seeds, what are some things that your seeds needed in order for them to grow?
Child: Water!
Another child: Sunshine.
Sandy: Yes, water and sunshine are very important for seeds to grow. When you planted your seeds, did you wait and watch for them to grow?
Children: Yes!
Sandy: Well, in this story Bobbie and Annie planted some seeds, but they were afraid their seeds wouldn't grow.

At this point Sandy invites Leigh to read the title of the story, giving the group an opportunity to think about the importance of using things they know about words to solve new words.

Sandy: Leigh, read the title for us.
Leigh: *Seeds . . . Seeds.*
Sandy: What helped you with that word *seeds*?
Leigh: *See.*
Sandy: Right, the word *see* helped you with the word *seeds*. Now, let's go inside the story and see what Bobbie

and Annie are going to do with seeds.

Here Sandy and the children have a short conversation about the story, making predictions based on the pictures and the story line. When Jason predicts the word *hoe* for *rake*, the teacher accepts the response because it will give the group an opportunity to cross-check meaning and visual cues when they read the text.

Next, Sandy directs the children's attention to a visual feature of the text and models how to use a known word to get to an unknown word:

Sandy: If you were going to read the word *away*, what chunk would you see at the end of the word?
All: *Way.*
Sandy: (*Makes the word* way *with magnetic letters on the overhead, then puts the letter* a *in front of it*) That's right. If I put the letter *a* in from of *way*, what new word did I make?
Children: *Away.*
Sandy: Yes, there are other words that start like *away* — *about, around, across.* Now I need everybody to look on page 7 and find the word *away.* (*Placing the word in the context of the story*) What did Bobbie and Annie do? They went where?
Children: They went away.
Sandy: That's right. They went away!

First Reading

As the children read the story independently, Sandy moves among them and listens. Willis comes the word *forgot* in his story and hesitates. First, Sandy prompts him to use meaning cues: "What did Bobbie and Annie do after they planted the seed?" Willis responds, "They went away." Since this prompt has not helped Willis with the problem word, Sandy tries a visual cue. When she frames the two parts of the word with a masking card, Willis is able to produce the correct response. Last, Sandy asks Willis to reread the line and check to see if the word makes sense.

After the children finish reading the story, Sandy praises them for specific strategies they used. She leads them in a quick review of things to do to help themselves when they are reading.

Sandy: What are some things that you can do when you get stuck on a word?

Child: Go back and reread.
Another child: Think about the story and look all the way through the word.
Another child: See if there is a part of the word you know.
Sandy: Yes, it helps you to do those things as you read. Now, I want you to take your book and read your story with a partner. When you have both read the book, please put it in your familiar-reading basket.

Subsequent Readings

During subsequent readings, the children might reread the book with a partner or read it alone. The important thing is that children be give the opportunity to practice fluent rereading behavior.

Fluent Guided Reading

At this level, children are competent readers and can apply strategies to help themselves read text within their instructional range. Reading becomes more silent, which enables children to increase their speed. Children need lots of time to read independently, because they continue to improve with each book they read. Reading now takes on a new focus: reading to learn. As children read a much wider range of material, they use their knowledge of *how* to read nonfiction and fiction material anywhere they find it. Children respond emotionally and read with increasingly deeper understanding of the author's intended message.

In order to examine the children's processing behavior and determine reading group placements, the teacher may occasionally ask the children to read aloud for a running record. It is expected that fluent readers' processing will be more refined and automatic. When they encounter difficulty, children use the text as the main source for solving the difficulty. Errors tend to be single, isolated words, and substitutions are often visually similar words. Self-corrections diminish as the children apply preprocessing strategies to solve words before errors occur.

Book Selection

Selecting books for the fluent reader is based on a much wider range of criteria: interest, content, thematic units, and story genre. Books at this

level have complex structures, which are generally characterized as (a) repetitive, (b) cumulative, (c) cultural, (d) chronological, (e) problem-centered, and (f) rhythm and rhyme. At this level, readers must be able to deal with diverse material that includes various organizational structures, multiple writing styles, and specialized vocabulary. Figure 4.5 lists reading and writing behavior typical of children at this level.

Figure 4.5 Reading and writing behavior at the fluent level.

Reading Behavior	Writing Behavior
Acquires rapidly expanding vocabulary and concept knowledge through reading	Writes complex sentence structures about varied topics with ease
Applies flexible strategies with good control of visual patterns	Shows good control of visual patterns; spelling is generally at the conventional and transitional stages
	Applies a range of editing and revising techniques
Adjusts reading to accommodate author's message and intended purpose	Knows how to write for different audiences and different purposes
Selects books independently and enjoys reading	Chooses to write often and enjoys writing
Reads with expression and fluency	Incorporates various punctuation and literary devices
Preprocesses information before making errors (self-corrections are less obvious)	Understands the writing process and the purpose of first drafts, revising, editing, and final drafts

Setting the Focus

The fluent reader can already integrate cues and flexibly adapt reading strategies to fulfill a range of purposes. Therefore, the focus of instruction varies according to the topic or subject matter. The focus may include (but is not limited to) learning how information is presented in a variety of ways (maps, drawings, charts, tables of contents, indexes, glossaries, headings, subtopics, diagrams, and labels); making comparisons and contrasting information between texts; exploring the author's style of writing; developing an increasing range of comprehension skills (oral and written retellings) or increasing mastery of story elements (setting, main characters, plot, problem, resolution). The range of possibilities in setting a focus for a fluent guided reading group is immense, as are the opportunities for moving children forward to a higher level of competency. Let's look at two examples of how to conduct a guided reading group with fluent readers.

The Tale of Peter Rabbit:
Book Introduction

Judy, the teacher, introduces *The Tale of Peter Rabbit* (Potter 1993) by building on background experience: "Have any of you ever done something your mother or father told you not to do?" Several children relate their personal experiences. Next, Judy presents a brief overview of what the story is about: "Well, in this story, Mother Rabbit warns Flopsy, Mopsy, Cottontail and Peter not to go into Mr. Mcgregor's garden, or something terrible might happen to them, like it did to their father." Then she encourages the children to make predictions:

Judy: What do you think might happen if the rabbits go into the garden?
Ryan: The scarecrow might scare them.
Lisa: They might get poisoned from bug spray or fertilizer.
Jarred: No! I think another animal will eat them, like a dog or a cat.
Judy: (*Praising the children's predictions*) Those are all terrible things that might happen to the little rabbits if they don't mind their mother.

Next Judy provides the children with enough detail to stimulate their interest and leave them wondering about what will happen to the rabbit: "Well, unfortunately, one of the rabbits disobeyed Mother Rabbit and went into Mr. Mcgregor's garden anyway. Needless to say, he ran into a lot of trouble. Several things happened to him that really frightened him and

made him wish he had listened to his mother."

The Tale of Peter Rabbit:
First Reading

Now that the children are familiar with the overall theme of the story, they are eager to begin, and Judy prepares them for a silent reading. First, she sets a purpose for reading: "I want you to read pages 2 and 3 with your eyes and find out why Mother Rabbit didn't want the young rabbits to go into Mr. Mcgregor's garden." After the children silently read the pages, Judy asks, "Who can find the part that tells why Mother Rabbit didn't want her bunnies to go into Mr. Mcgregor's garden?" Lisa reads, "Your father had an accident there; he was put in a pie by Mrs. Mcgregor." Judy responds: "Well, no wonder Mother Rabbit didn't want her babies to go in there."

Next Judy prompts the children to read pages 4 through 7 to find out what happened to one of the rabbits as he squeezed under the gate of Mr. Mcgregor's garden. After they've read these pages silently, Judy starts a discussion:

Judy: On page 4, what did Peter do when he entered the garden?
Children: He ate the vegetables in the garden.
Judy: Read the part that describes what happened to Peter in the garden.
Ryan: "First he ate some lettuce and some French beans; and then he ate some radishes. And then, feeling rather sick, he went to look for some parsley."
Judy: (*Coaching the children to think beyond the story*) Why do you think that Peter went to look for some parsley?
Lisa: He ate so much that he got a tummy ache.
Nicholas: Yeah, and the parsley will make him feel better.

The children continue to predict their way through the text and use rereading to confirm or discount their predictions. At appropriate places, Judy guides the children to make further inferences: for example "How do you think Peter felt when he had to face his mother?" She prompts them to relate these textual events to life: "Have you ever disobeyed like Peter and had to face your actions? What

happened to you? How did you feel? What lesson did you learn?" These questions are selective and are naturally interspersed with extended stretches of reading.

The discussion during the first reading does not deter the children from comprehension or the sheer enjoyment of reading. It simply engages them in the reading process as they learn to read for the author's intended meaning. As children gain experience and expertise in silent reading, they are encouraged to read increasingly longer passages at one time, until a whole book can be managed.

After the first reading, the teacher may focus on some problem-solving strategies if the children have encountered any troublesome spots. For instance, she might select one or two appropriate words from the story for extending the children's knowledge about words and use magnetic letters or a white board to illustrate appropriate problem-solving techniques. This is in direct contrast to introducing vocabulary words or potentially difficult words before reading the story. Waiting until after the first reading before discussing the tricky parts gives the children the opportunity to meet and overcome the challenges independently.

Frog and Toad Are Friends:
Book Introduction

Mrs. Vest introduces the book *Frog and Toad Are Friends* (Lobel 1970) to a guided reading group. Together, they read the title and the name of the author and illustrator on the cover. Mrs. Vest explains that the book is an anthology of adventures about two very good friends named Frog and Toad. She turns to the table of contents and briefly notes the different stories in the book. Then she informs the children that today they will be reading the first story, "Spring."

Next Mrs. Vest taps into the children's prior knowledge by initiating a discussion about hibernation. The children talk about animals who sleep during the winter months and awaken in the springtime from their long winter naps. This provides a nice framework to introduce the story. Mrs.. Vest says, "In today's story, Frog tricks Toad into waking up too soon from his long winter nap." Then she coaches the children to think of ways

Frog might trick Toad to do this. Mrs. Vest records the children's predictions on a chart and comments, "After you read the story, we will check to see if you were right."

Next Mrs. Vest sets a purpose for reading the story: "I want you to read the story silently and find out how Frog convinced Toad to believe it was about half past May and time to get up." She is careful to plant the language chunk "half past May" in the introduction, so that the children can hear this unfamiliar phrase. "What do you think is so important about 'half past May'?" Several children exclaim, "That's when it's time for Toad to get up from hibernation."

Before the children begin reading, Mrs. Vest also initiates a brief conversation about ways the children can problem-solve independently: "When you come to a hard word, what are some things you can do to help yourself?" The children's responses indicate their understanding of problem-solving strategies: "Search for chunks in words." "Notice how the word starts and check to see if the word makes sense and looks right." Mrs. Vest reminds the children to try various ways to solve the problem but tells them that if they are unsuccessful in their attempts, they can mark the word with a sticky note: "We will help you figure the word out after you finish reading the story."

Frog and Toad Are Friends:
First Reading

To set the scene and establish a fluent pace, Mrs. Vest reads the first two pages of the story. Then she says, "Now, I want you to read the next six pages to yourself." Next she guides the children to view the characters from different perspectives: she asks some children to focus on the feelings of Frog and others to focus on the feelings of Toad. After the reading, Mrs. Vest guides the children in a short discussion around the emotions of Frog and Toad. She accepts all responses, occasionally inviting children to read passage that support their interpretations of the characters' feelings. As the first reading comes to an end, Mrs. Vest says, "Now, finish reading the story to yourself to find out how Frog finally got Toad out of bed."

After the children finish the story, Mrs. Vest directs them back to their original predictions from the chart. They confirm or discount their initial predictions with supportive passages from the text. Next, she asks them to locate any word that they had difficulty with during the first reading. She selects one or two words for group problem-solving. Mrs. Vest coaches the children to apply strategies for solving the problem. When appropriate, she uses magnetic letters or the chalkboard to illustrate strategies for

analyzing words. Afterward, the children are encouraged to return to the text and read the problematic part within the context of the story. Then, taking the textual experience to a new level, Mrs. Vest asks the children to debate whether they feel the trick was fair and to predict what they think will happen if Toad ever finds out it really was not "half past May." These lively discussions lead to writing connections that allows the children to explore feelings and story elements.

Closing Thoughts

In the apprenticeship approach to guided reading, the following characteristics need to be emphasized:

- The teacher designs instructional interactions that build on the knowledge children bring to the reading task.
- The teacher provides adjustable scaffolds that reflect ongoing observations of the children's skills, strategies, and knowledge of the story.
- The teacher moves the children into higher-level guided reading groups as they become more competent readers.
- The teacher uses language techniques such as modeling, coaching, scaffolding, articulating, and reflecting to enable the children to experience successful interactions with the text.

Patricia M. Cunningham
Dorothy P. Hall
Margaret Defee

Nonability-grouped, multilevel instruction: Eight years later

This article reports on the long-term development, implementation, and assessment of a framework for beginning reading instruction, best known as the Four Blocks approach.

Eight years ago, the three of us embarked on a journey. We wanted to figure out how to provide reading instruction to children with a wide range of entering levels without putting them in fixed ability groups. The results of our first year were published in this journal (Cunningham, Hall, & Defee, 1991). Since that first year we have extended our efforts across grade levels, schools, and states. In this article, we will share an updated model of multilevel, multimethod instruction that has come to be called the Four Blocks.

Teachers usually try to meet the needs of struggling readers by putting them in a "bottom" reading group and pacing their instruction more slowly. The data on this method does not hold out much hope that it will ultimately solve the problem. Children who are placed in the bottom group in first grade generally remain there throughout their elementary school careers and almost never learn to read and write up to grade-level standards (Allington, 1983, 1991).

Another variable that concerned us was the phenomenon of the "pendulum swing." Especially in the U.S., various approaches to reading come in and out of fashion. Eight years ago when we began this endeavor, literature-based reading instruction (commonly referred to as "whole language") was the recommended approach. Today, this approach is losing favor, and school boards are mandating phonics. The search for the "best way to teach reading" denies the reality or possibility of individual differences. Children do not all learn in the same way and consequently, approaches with particular emphases are apt to result in some children learning to read, and others not. When the pendulum swings to another approach, we may pick up some of those who weren't faring too well under the previous emphasis but lose some who were. Thirty years ago, the First-Grade Studies, which were carried out to determine the best approach for reading instruction, concluded that the teacher was more important than the method but that, in general, combination approaches worked better than any single approach (Bond & Dykstra, 1967, 1997).

This article describes the development of a framework for beginning reading instruction that had two goals. The first goal was to meet the needs of children with a wide range of entering literacy levels without putting them in ability groups. The second goal was to avoid the pendulum swing and find a way to combine the major approaches to reading instruction. Since our first year in which we developed the instructional framework in one first-grade classroom, the model has been refined and implemented in numerous primary classrooms.

The instructional framework

The instructional framework is the heart of our program. The basic notions underlying this framework are quite simple, but its implementation is complex. There is considerable variation depending on the grade level and how early or late in the year it is, individual teaching styles, and the particular makeup of the class. In this section we will describe the instruction and provide some sense of the variety that allows its implementation in a wide range of classrooms.

In order to meet the goal of providing children with a variety of avenues to becoming literate, language arts instructional time is divided fairly evenly between four major historical approaches to reading instruction. The 2¼–2½ hours allotted to language arts is divided among four blocks—Guided Reading, Self-Selected Reading, Writing, and Working With Words—each of which gets 30–40 minutes.

To meet our second goal of providing for a wide range of literacy levels without grouping the children by ability, we make the instruction within each block as multilevel as possible. For each block, we will briefly describe some of the formats, materials, cooperative arrangements, etc., we use to achieve this goal of multilevel instruction.

Guided reading. In our first several years, we called this the basal block because this was the time when the basal reader drove our instruction. In recent years, teachers have branched out to use other materials in addition to or instead of the adopted basal reader. Depending on the time of year, the needs of the class, the personality of the teacher, and the dictates of the school or school system, guided reading lessons are carried out with the adopted basal, basal readers from previously adopted series, multiple copies of trade books, Big Books, and various combinations of the above. The purposes of this block are to expose children to a wide range of literature, teach comprehension strategies, and teach children how to read in materials that become increasingly more difficult.

Early in first grade, most of our guided reading time is spent in shared reading of predictable books, read together in a variety of choral, echo, and other shared-reading formats. Comprehension activities often include "doing the book" in which children are given roles and become the characters as the rest of the children read the book. Little books based on the Big Books are read and reread with partners, then individually or in small groups.

The first goal was to meet the needs of children with a wide range of entering literacy levels without putting them in ability groups.

As the year goes on, the shared reading of Big Books continues to be a part of guided reading. Other books, not big and not predictable, are added. These books might be part of a basal series or multiple copies of trade books. The emphasis shifts from reading together to reading with partners or alone. Instead of reading the selection first to the children, teachers often take children on a "picture walk" through the book, leading the children to name things in the pictures and make predictions, and pointing out a few critical and potentially difficult vocabulary words students might encounter as they read the selection. Children then read the selection individually, with a partner, or in a small flexible group with the teacher. The class reconvenes, discusses the selection, and then sometimes reads it chorally or in some other whole-class format (not round-robin reading, however). Comprehension strategies are taught and practiced. Predictions made before reading are checked. Story maps and webs are completed.

The next reading of the selection might include a writing activity done by some children individually, some with partners, and others in a group guided by an adult. Often the next reading is an acting out of the selection, with

Nonability-grouped multilevel instruction

various children playing different parts as the rest of the class reads or tells the story.

Guided reading is the most difficult block to make multilevel. Any selection is going to be too hard for some children and too easy for others. We don't worry anymore about those children for whom grade-level guided reading material is too easy because the other three blocks provide many beyond-grade-level opportunities. In addition, our results have consistently indicated that students who begin first grade with high literacy levels continued to read well above grade level at the end of the year.

Children do not all learn in the same way and consequently, approaches with particular emphases are apt to result in some children learning to read, and others not.

We do, however, worry about those students for whom grade-level selections are too challenging. To make this block meet the needs of children who read below grade level, teachers make a variety of adaptations. Guided reading time is not spent in grade-level material all week. Rather, teachers choose two selections—one grade level and one easier—to read each week. Each selection is read several times, each time for a different purpose in a different format. Rereading enables almost all children to achieve fluency by the last reading. Children who need help are not left to read by themselves but are supported in a variety of ways. Most teachers use reading partners and teach children how to help their partners rather than do all their reading for them. While some children read the selection by themselves and others read with partners, teachers usually meet with small groups of children. These teacher-supported groups change daily and do not include only the low readers.

Self-selected reading. Although historically it has been called individualized reading or personalized reading (Veatch, 1959), many teachers now label their self-selected reading time Readers' Workshop (Routman, 1995). Regardless of what it is called, self-selected reading is that part of a balanced literacy program when children choose what they want to read and what parts of their reading they want to respond to. Opportunities are provided for children to share and respond to what is read. Teachers hold individual conferences with children about their books.

In our classrooms, the self-selected reading block includes a teacher read-aloud. The teacher reads to the children from a wide range of literature. Next, children read "on their own level" from a variety of books the teacher has gathered and keeps on a bookshelf or, more popularly, in dishpans or buckets. The teacher selects books for the classroom library on themes the class is studying, easy and difficult library books, old favorites, new easy predictable books, etc. Every effort is made to have the widest possible range of genre and levels available. While the children read, the teacher holds conferences with and takes anecdotal records on several children each day. The block usually ends with one or two children sharing their books with the class in a "Reader's Chair" format.

Self-selected reading is, by definition, multilevel, because children choose what they want to read. These choices, however, can be limited by the reading materials available and how willing and able children are to read from the available resources. Fielding and Roller (1992) sum up the problem many struggling readers have with self-selected reading:

> While most of the children are quiet, engaged, and reading during independent reading times, there are always a few children who are not. They are picking up spilled crayons, sweeping up shavings from the pencil sharpener, making trips to the water fountain, walking back and forth alongside bookcases, opening and closing books, and gazing at pictures. (p. 678)

Many of the children who "wander round" during self-selected reading time are the ones whose reading ability is limited. Fielding and Roller conclude that:

> Either they do not know how to find a book that they can read, or there is no book available that they can read or they do not want to read the books they can read. These children remind us of Groucho Marx: They refuse to become a member of any club that will accept them. In book terms, they cannot read the books they want to read and they do not want to read the books they can read. (p. 679)

Fielding and Roller go on to make excellent and practical suggestions about how to support children in reading books they want to read that, without support, would be too difficult and about how to make the reading of easy books both enjoyable and socially acceptable. These suggestions include helping children determine when a book is just right, encouraging children to read books that the teacher has read aloud, encouraging children to read with a friend and to do repeated readings of books they enjoy, teacher modeling of the enjoyment to be found in easier books, setting up programs in which children read to younger children and thus have a real purpose for reading and practicing easy books, and making lots of informational picture books available. Following these suggestions makes the self-selected reading time more multilevel. We have incorporated many of these ideas in our self-selected reading block.

In addition, we steer our more advanced readers toward books that challenge them. We also teach our early first graders that there are three ways to read. You can "pretend read" by telling the story of a familiar story book. You can "picture read" by looking at a book about real things with lots of pictures and talking about all the things you see in the pictures. And you can read by reading all the words. Early in the year, we model all types of reading and discuss how children at their age would probably read different books.

> *The Three Billy Goats Gruff* is a book you could pretend read because you know the story so well. Let's practice how you might pretend read it if you chose it for self-selected reading time.
>
> How would you read this book about dinosaurs? It's got lots and lots of words in little print, but you could read it by picture reading. Let's practice picture reading.
>
> Now, here is an alphabet book. You see just one word and it goes with the picture. You can probably read this book by reading the words.

Once children know that there are three ways to read books, no child ever says, "I can't read yet!"

Writing. The writing block is carried out in Writers' Workshop fashion (Calkins, 1994; Graves, 1995; Routman, 1995). It begins with a 10-minute minilesson. The teacher sits at the overhead projector or with a large piece of chart paper. The teacher writes and models all the things writers do (although not all on any one day). The teacher thinks aloud—deciding what to write about—and then writes. While writing, the teacher models looking at the Word Wall for troublesome words and inventing the spelling of a few big words. The teacher also makes a few mistakes relating to the items currently on the editor's checklist. When the piece is finished or during the following day's minilesson, the children help the teacher edit the piece for the items on the checklist.

Next the children go to their own writing. They are all at different stages of the writing process—finishing a piece, starting a new piece, editing, illustrating, etc. While the children write, the teacher confers with individuals, helping them get pieces ready to publish. In most classrooms, teachers allow children to publish a piece when they have completed three to five good first drafts. The child chooses the one to publish and then confers with the teacher. At this point, we fix all spelling errors and tidy it up mechanically, because we want a published piece that the other children can read easily—and of which the author will be proud. This block ends with Author's Chair in which several students each day share first drafts or published books.

Writing is the most multilevel block because it is not limited by the availability or acceptability of appropriate books. If teachers allow children to choose their own topics, accept whatever level of first-draft writing each child can accomplish, and allow them to work on their pieces as many days as needed, all children can succeed in writing. One of the major tenets of process writing is that children should choose their own topics. When children decide what they will write about, they write about something of particular interest to them and consequently something that they know about. Now this may seem like belaboring the obvious, but it is a crucial component in making process writing meet the needs and interests of all children. When everyone writes about the same topic, the different levels of children's knowledge and writing ability become painfully obvious.

In addition to teacher acceptance of student work, children choosing their own topics, and not expecting finished pieces each day, Writers' Workshops include two teaching opportunities that promote the multilevel nature of process writing—minilessons and publishing conferences. In minilessons, the teacher writes and thinks aloud. The children get to see how writers think. In these daily short lessons, teachers show all aspects of the writing process. They model topic selection, planning, writing, revising, and editing; they write on a variety of topics in a variety of forms. Some days they write short pieces. Other days, they begin a piece that takes several days to complete. When doing a longer piece, teachers model how to reread what was written previously in order to reestablish the train of thought and continue writing. The minilesson contributes to making process writing multilevel when the teacher includes different facets of the writing process, writes on a variety of topics in a variety of forms, and intentionally composes shorter easier pieces as well as more involved longer pieces.

Another opportunity for meeting the various needs and levels of children comes in the publishing conference. In some classrooms children do some peer revising and editing and then come to the teacher "editor-in-chief" for some final revision and editing before publishing. As teachers help children publish the pieces they have chosen, they have the opportunity to individualize their teaching. Looking at a child's writing usually reveals both what the child needs to move forward and what the child is ready to understand. The publishing conference provides the "teachable moment" in which both advanced and struggling writers can be nudged forward in their literacy development.

Finally, writing is multilevel because for some children writing is their best avenue to becoming readers. When children who are struggling with reading write about their own experiences and then read it back (even if no one else can read it), they are using their own language and experiences to become readers. Often these children who struggle with even the simplest material during guided reading can read everything in their writing notebook or folder. When children are writing, some children are really working on becoming better writers; others are engaging in the same activity, but for them, writing helps them figure out reading.

Working with words. In the working with words block, children learn to read and spell high-frequency words and learn the patterns that allow them to decode and spell lots of words.

The first 10 minutes of this block are usually given to reviewing the *Word Wall* words. Word Wall is a display of high-frequency words categorized alphabetically by first letter only. The words are written with thick black marker on colored paper. The teacher adds 5 words a week until there are 110–120 words on the wall. Students practice new and old words daily by looking at them, saying them, clapping or snapping the letters, writing the words on paper, and self-correcting the words with the teacher.

Practice with the high-frequency words on the wall takes the first 10 minutes of the words block every day. The remaining 15–25 minutes is given to activities that help children learn to decode and spell. Three of the most popular activities are described next.

Rounding up the rhymes follows the guided reading of a selection or a book the teacher has read aloud at the beginning of the self-selected reading time. Here is an example using *Ten Little Dinosaurs* (Schnetzler, 1996).

The first (and often second) reading of anything should be focused on meaning and enjoyment. *Ten Little Dinosaurs* describes in rhyme the antics of 10 different dinosaurs.

> Five little dinosaurs playing in the street.
> Ankylosaurus yelled, "A car to beat!"
> He charged into the street: squeal, screech, bleet, spleet.
> No more dinotanks playing in the street.

Revisiting the book during the words block, we draw the children's attention to the rhyming words. As we read each page, we encourage the children to chime in and to listen to the rhymes they are saying. As children tell us the rhyming words, we write them on index cards and put them in a pocket chart. Here are the rhyming words "rounded up" from the first several pages:

bed	bike	mooth	river	peak	street
head	spike	tooth	aquiver	beak	beat
said	trike	booth	shiver	shriek	spleet

Next, we remind children that words that rhyme usually have the same spelling pattern. Children then underline the spelling patterns in each set of rhymes and decide whether or not they are the same. Because we want rhymes with the same spelling pattern, we discard *bed*, *head*, and *said*; *shriek* and *beat*. We now have five sets of words that rhyme and have the same spelling pattern in our pocket chart:

b*ike*	m*ooth*	*river*	*peak*	str*eet*
sp*ike*	*tooth*	aqu*iver*	b*eak*	spl*eet*
tr*ike*	*booth*	sh*iver*		

In the final part of this activity children use these words to read and write some other words. This is the transfer step and is critical to the success of this activity for children who learn only what we teach. We begin the transfer part of this activity by telling children something like,

> You know that when you are reading books and writing stories, there are many words you have never seen before. You have to figure them out. One way many people figure out how to read and spell new words is to see if they already know any rhyming words or words that have the same spelling pattern. I am going to write some words, and you can see which words with the same spelling pattern will help you read them. Then, we are going to try to spell some words by deciding if they rhyme with any of the words in our pocket chart.

Here are the new words the children read and spelled based on their new understanding of rhymes and spelling patterns at the conclusion of this activity.

h*ike*   *liver*   *leak*   sw*eet*

Making words (Cunningham & Cunningham, 1992; Cunningham & Hall, 1997) is an active, hands-on, manipulative activity in which children learn how to look for patterns in words and how changing just one letter or letter order changes the whole word. The children are given the six to eight letters that will form the final word. The lesson begins with two-letter words, then builds to three-, four- and five-letter words until the word that can be made with all the letters is made. Students then sort the words according to a variety of patterns including beginning sounds, endings, and rhymes; they read the sorted words and use them to spell words with similar patterns.

In one lesson, the children had the letters *a, i, g, n, s, t.* They made these words:

> *it, in, an, ant, tan, sit, sat, sag, snag, sang, gain, stain, giants*

(The word *giants* was chosen because the children had read a story about a giant during the guided reading block. The last word made is "the secret word" because it always uses all the letters, and children delight in trying to figure out what the secret word can be.)

When all the words were made, the teacher led the children to sort them for rhymes:

it	*an*	*ag*	*ain*
it	an	sag	gain
sit	tan	snag	stain

Following the same procedure used in the transfer step of rounding up the rhymes, the teacher helped students use these rhyming words to read and spell other rhyming words they might meet in their reading or need to spell while writing. In this particular lesson, the transfer words were *brain*, *flag*, *plan*, and *hit*.

Guess the covered word is another popular working with words block activity. Its purpose is to help children practice the important strategy of cross-checking meaning with letter-sound information. For this activity, the teacher writes four or five sentences on the chalkboard, covering a word in each sentence with two sticky notes. Children read each sentence and then make several guesses for the word. There are generally many possibilities for a word that will fit the context, and the teacher points this out. Next, the teacher takes off the first sticky note, which always covers all the letters up to the vowel. Guesses that don't begin with these letters are erased, and new guesses that both fit the meaning and start with all the right beginning letters are made. When all the guesses that fit both meaning and beginning sounds have been written, the entire word is revealed. Most teachers adjust the length of their sticky notes so that children also become sensitive to word length.

Watching children doing the daily Word Wall practice, you would assume that they are all learning the same thing—how to spell words. But what they are doing externally may not reveal what they are processing internally. Imagine that the five new words added to the wall one week were *come, where, they, boy, friend.* During the daily Word Wall practice, children who have already learned to read them are learning to spell them. Other children, however, who require lots of practice with words, are learning to read them.

While rounding up the rhymes, some children are still developing their phonemic awareness as they decide which words rhyme and are learning that rhyming words usually—but not always—have the same spelling pattern. As they use the words rounded up to read and spell new words, some children are practicing beginning letter substitution. Children who already have well-developed phonemic awareness and beginning letter knowledge are practicing the important strategy of using known words to decode and spell unknown rhyming words.

Making words lessons are multilevel in a number of ways. Each lesson begins with short easy words and progresses to longer, more challenging words. Every making words lesson ends by the teacher asking, "Has anyone figured out the word we can make if we use all our letters?" Figuring out the secret word in the limited time available is a challenge to even our most advanced readers. Making words includes even children with very limited literacy who enjoy manipulating the letters and making the words even if they don't complete them until the word is made by the teacher with the big pocket chart letters. By ending each lesson by sorting the words into patterns and then using those patterns to read and spell new words, we help children of all levels learn to use the word patterns to read and spell other words.

Guess the covered word lessons provide review for beginning letter sounds for those who still need it. The more sophisticated readers consolidate the important strategy of using meaning, all the beginning letters, and word length as cues to the identification of an unknown word.

Connections across the blocks

So far, we have described the blocks as separate entities. In most classrooms, they each have their allotted times, and an observer can tell which block the teacher and children are in. As much as possible, teachers try to make connections from one block to another. Many teachers take a theme approach to teaching. These teachers often select books for guided reading that correlate with their theme. During the writing minilesson when the teacher models writing, he or she often writes something connected to the theme. Some of the books teachers read aloud at the beginning of self-selected reading and some of the books children can choose from are connected to the theme.

Theme words are not put on the Word Wall, which is reserved for high-frequency words. But most teachers have a theme board

in addition to the Word Wall. This board changes with each theme and, in addition to pictures, includes theme-related words that children will need as they pursue that theme. Often the secret word in a making words lesson is connected to the theme. Sometimes, the sentences a teacher writes for a guess the covered word lesson relate to the theme.

In addition to theme connections, there are other connections across the blocks. We practice Word Wall words during the words block, but children know that when they are writing, they spell words as best they can unless the word is on the Word Wall. Word Wall words must be spelled correctly.

Rounding up the rhymes occurs during the words block, but the book used usually has been read by the children during guided reading or read aloud by the teacher to begin the self-selected reading block. Sometimes, we do guess the covered word activities by using sticky notes to cover one word on each page of a Big Book. We often introduce vocabulary during guided reading through picture walks, and while reading with small groups, we coach children on how to decode words using picture, context, and letter-sound strategies taught during the words block.

In our minilesson at the beginning of each day's writing time, we model how to find words on the Word Wall and how to stretch out words and listen for the sounds in more challenging words not available in the room. When we are helping children edit, we praise them for their good attempts and spelling and coach them to use strategies and skills they are learning during the words block.

Support for struggling students

Along with the four blocks, schools and teachers use a variety of formats for providing the extra support needed by children who find learning to read unusually difficult. Some schools have Reading Recovery. Classroom teachers and Reading Recovery teachers report that the Four Blocks classroom instruction and Reading Recovery are very compatible.

Other schools in which the majority of the children need additional support use a program called FROG—Facilitating Reading for Optimum Growth (Hall, Prevatte, & Cunningham, 1995). Special teachers and the classroom teacher form FROG teams. All children receive

45 minutes of small-group FROG instruction each day. Each small group consists of four or five children and includes one of the strongest readers in the classroom, one of the weakest readers, and two or three other children. Each group is taught by one of the teachers.

The 45 minutes of daily FROG instruction includes four activities. For the first 10 minutes, children talk about and read a little from the self-selected book they have been reading during classroom self-selected time. Next, they participate in the shared reading of a big book, which is read and worked with for 1 week. The third daily activity is a word study activity such as making words, rounding up the rhymes, or guess the covered word. Each FROG session ends with each child writing a sentence related to the big book.

In addition to the four blocks, many teachers schedule a 10-minute easy reading support group in which very easy books are read and reread. This group of four or five children changes daily. Children who need easy reading are included more often, but not every day. The group is not composed of only struggling readers. Teachers include better readers as models and assure that all children are included across several weeks.

Assessment and evaluation

In the last several years, several schools and districts have evaluated the effectiveness of the Four Blocks framework. We will report some data from three different sites.

Data from the original Four Blocks school. Clemmons Elementary School in Winston-Salem, North Carolina, the school in which the framework was originally implemented, is a large suburban U.S. school with a diverse student population. Some children come from homes surrounding the school, and others are bused from the inner city. In any year, 20–25% of children qualify for free or reduced-priced lunches. Approximately 25–30% of the children are African American, Hispanic, or Asian-Pacific Island. Since the program began, the student population has remained relatively stable, with approximately 10% of the children moving in and out each year. There have been three different administrators. Approximately half of the current first- and second-grade teachers have been there for all 8 years of our work with Four Blocks. The other half, including some beginning teachers, have more recently joined the staff. All classes are heterogeneously grouped and contain an average of 23 children. No children are retained, and children are not referred for special classes until second grade. Thus, the population of this study includes all children who are in the school at the end of first and second grade. The majority of the children have had 2 years of four blocks instruction, but some children who are new to the school have had a year or less.

Throughout the year, teachers conduct assessment by observing and conferring with children, taking running records, and looking at writing samples. At the end of the year, children are given the Basic Reading Inventory (BRI) by an assessment team headed by the curriculum coordinator. Instructional levels are computed using the standard procedures and include measures of oral reading accuracy and comprehension. Because the BRI is administered at the end of the year, an instructional level of first or second grade is considered grade level at the end of first grade, and an instructional level of second or third grade is considered grade level at the end of second grade.

BRI data are reported starting with our second year, in which all first-grade teachers were involved, and continues through 6 years of first graders and second graders (see Table). Approximately 100–140 children in each grade are included in each year's data.

Across 6 years, instructional level results have remained remarkably consistent. At the end of first grade, 58–64% of the children read above grade level (third grade or above); 22–28% read on grade level; 10–17% read below grade level (preprimer or primer). On average, one child each year is unable to meet the instructional level criteria on the preprimer passage. At the end of second grade, the number at grade level is 14–25%; the number above grade level (fourth grade level or above) increases to 68–76%; the number reading below grade level drops to 2–9%, half what it was in first grade.

While we have no control group to which we can compare our results, our data were collected across 7 years and were consistent across 6 groups of 100–140 children. The data look remarkably similar, even with new teachers and several changes in school administra-

Eight years of multimethod, multilevel instruction

Year 1 (Pilot study in *one* first-grade classroom) 1989–1990

Year 2 (Grade 1)	1991		Year 3 (Grade 2)	1992	
Reading levels:	No.	Percentage	Reading levels:	No.	Percentage
Above (Grades 3–6)	64	63%	Above (Grades 4–6)	77	75%
At (Grades 1–2)	28	27%	At (Grades 2–3)	24	23%
Below (PP, P)	10	10%	Below (PP, P, Grade 1)	2	2%

Year 3 (Grade 1)	1992		Year 4 (Grade 2)	1993	
Reading levels:	No.	Percentage	Reading levels:	No.	Percentage
Above (Grades 3–6)	65	62%	Above (Grades 4–6)	74	71%
At (Grades 1–2)	26	25%	At (Grades 2–3)	21	20%
Below (PP, P)	14	13%	Below (PP, P, Grade 1)	9	9%

Year 4 (Grade 1)	1993		Year 5 (Grade 2)	1994	
Reading levels:	No.	Percentage	Reading levels:	No.	Percentage
Above (Grades 3–6)	76	61%	Above (Grades 4–6)	87	68%
At (Grades 1–2)	28	22%	At (Grades 2–3)	32	25%
Below (PP, P)	21	17%	Below (PP, P, Grade 1)	9	7%

Year 5 (Grade 1)	1994		Year 6 (Grade 2)	1995	
Reading levels:	No.	Percentage	Reading levels:	No.	Percentage
Above (Grades 3–6)	59	58%	Above (Grades 4–6)	76	78%
At (Grades 1–2)	25	25%	At (Grades 2–3)	16	16%
Below (PP, P)	17	17%	Below (PP, P, Grade 1)	6	6%

Year 6 (Grade 1)	1995		Year 7 (Grade 2)	1996	
Reading levels:	No.	Percentage	Reading levels:	No.	Percentage
Above (Grades 3–6)	87	64%	Above (Grades 4–6)	97	70%
At (Grades 1–2)	29	22%	At (Grades 2–3)	31	22%
Below (PP, P)	19	14%	Below (PP, P, Grade 1)	10	8%

Year 7 (Grade 1)	1996		Year 8 (Grade 2)	1997	
Reading levels:	No.	Percentage	Reading levels:	No.	Percentage
Above (Grades 3–6)	85	64%	Above (Grades 4–6)	118	74%
At (Grades 1–2)	32	24%	At (Grades 2–3)	26	20%
Below (PP, P)	15	11%	Below (PP, P, Grade 1)	8	6%

tion. Looking at these data across 6 years reveals that the most startling (and encouraging) results relate to those children who do not read at grade level at the end of first grade. Of the 10–15% of children who do not read at grade level at the end of first grade, half are reading on or, in some cases, above grade level at the end of second grade. Standardized test data on these children collected in third, fourth and fifth grades each year indicate that 90% of the children are in the top two quartiles. Most years, no children's scores fall in the bottom quartile.

Data from a suburban school district. The original school in which the framework was implemented does not use standardized testing until the end of third grade. Other districts, however, do administer standardized reading tests in the primary grades. One district devised an evaluation model, the results of which will be reported here. Lexington One in Lexington, South Carolina, is a suburban school district with eight elementary schools, in which 25% of the children qualify for free or reduced-price lunches. During the 1995–1996 school year, first-grade teachers in the district were given information about the Four Blocks framework and allowed to choose whether they wanted to implement the model in their classrooms. Approximately half of the teachers chose to implement the framework and were provided with several workshops, professional books, and collegial support throughout the year in their classrooms.

In January 1996, 100 first graders in classrooms using the Four Blocks and 100 first graders in classrooms not using the framework were randomly selected and were given the Word Recognition in Isolation and Word Recognition in Context sections of the BRI. Adjusted mean (average) scores for both measures favored students in the Four Blocks classrooms. For the Word Recognition in Context scores, the differences were statistically significant. Students in the Four Blocks classrooms were, on average, reading at the beginning of second-grade level. Students in the other first grades were on average at the first-grade, second-month level.

Although these results were encouraging, district officials were concerned about lack of reliability of the BRI and about teacher bias, fearing that the enthusiasm of the teachers who chose to implement the model may have created artificially high scores. They then devised an experiment using cohort analysis and standardized test results. In May of 1996, all 557 first graders in Four Blocks classrooms were administered the Metropolitan Achievement Test. Each child was matched with a first grader from the previous year (1994–1995) on the basis of his or her scores on the Cognitive Skills Assessment Battery (CSAB), a test of readiness given each year during the first week of school. The total reading mean score for the Four Blocks first graders was significantly better (.0001 level) than that of matched students from previous years. In grade equivalent terms, the average Four Blocks first grader's reading level was 2.0 while the 1994–1995 student's average reading level was 1.6.

On the basis of the standardized test data, school officials concluded that the Four Blocks framework had been much more effective than their previous ability-grouped traditional basal instruction. They hypothesized that since students selected for the basal cohort group had been taught by all the first-grade teachers in the system, teacher bias could not have accounted for the results. Furthermore, classroom observations suggested that teachers who implemented the Four Blocks framework had not all implemented it fully or equally well. In spite of the uneven implementation, children in the Four Blocks classrooms scored on average almost half a year better than the previous group.

The district then analyzed its data by dividing both groups of students into thirds according to their CSAB scores. The Figure demonstrates graphically that children of all ability levels (as defined by their CSAB performance) profited from the multilevel Four Blocks instruction. There was a 15-point difference in total reading scores for the lower third, a 23-point difference for the middle third, and a 28-point difference for the upper third. The district concluded that organizing in this nonability-group manner had profited the struggling students and had been even more successful for students who would traditionally have been placed in the top groups.

Data from one rural school. During the same year, a nearby school adopted the Four Blocks framework and mandated its use in all first- and second-grade classrooms. Brockington Elementary School in Florence School District Four in Timmonsville, South Carolina, is a small rural district in which 84% of students qualify for free or reduced-price lunches. Based on low achievement test scores, the elementary school had been placed on the list of the state's worst schools and had tried a variety of approaches to improving reading and math test scores. During the 1991–1992 school year, the school was mandated by a new superintendent to "teach the basics." A state-developed basic skills curriculum focused on "skill and drill" was implemented along with a computer lab basic skills remediation program for Chapter 1 students. End of the year achievement test scores showed no improvement. During the 1992–1993 school year, teachers took a yearlong graduate course on whole language. Again, the end-of-year test results failed to show improvement.

During the 1993–1994 school year, another new superintendent arrived. The district continued to emphasize whole language, and teachers were trained in cooperative learning. This year's test scores showed some improvement at Grades 2 and 3, though none at Grade 1. During the 1994–1995 school year, teachers were urged to continue to use whole language and cooperative learning; they were also trained in the learning styles approach of Rita Dunn. On the Metropolitan Achievement Test (MAT) only 20% of first-grade students scored at or above the 50th percentile on total reading. At the second-grade level, only 9% scored at or above the 50th percentile.

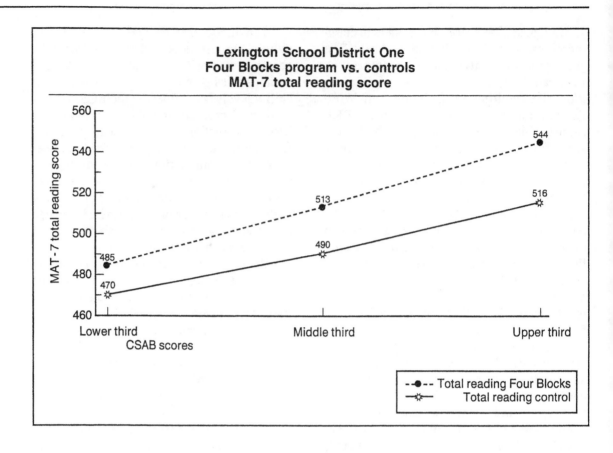

Lexington School District One
Four Blocks program vs. controls
MAT-7 total reading score

During the 1995–1996 school year, all 10 teachers—6 at first grade and 4 at second grade—were trained in and mandated to try the Four Blocks framework. The teachers were given workshops and books, as well as state department and central office support, etc. In the opinion of those central office and state department facilitators who visited classrooms weekly, 4 of the 6 first-grade teachers and 3 of the 4 second-grade teachers implemented the framework.

MAT total reading scores for all first and second graders in the school (including the three classes that did not implement the framework) indicated that 30% of the first graders and 38% of the second graders had total reading scores at or above the 50th percentile. Results for the 1996–1997 school year show 46% of first graders and 40% of second graders at or above the 50th percentile on the MAT total reading.

The results from this school system are, of course, open to speculation. Since different children were tested in the 1994–1995 group and we have no pretest data on these children, we cannot be sure that the huge jump in the number of children reading at or above grade level is due to the implementation of the Four Blocks framework. Nevertheless, officials in this school district, having tried so many programs in the previous 5 years, are convinced that the differences are real and attributable to the balanced multilevel instruction that most of the first and second graders received.

Conclusions

The last 8 years have been exciting and satisfying for us. We have seen the Four Blocks framework implemented in hundreds of classrooms in diverse settings, with varied populations of children. We have learned a great deal about teachers and about children.

Teachers who are widely criticized for not being willing to try anything new will change when the innovation has lots of familiar elements, is doable within the time frame and materials they currently have, and results in observably better readers and writers. Teachers, too, have individual differences. Most teachers like some blocks better than others. They continue teaching each block each day, however, because they see children for whom each block is critical and are convinced that if they left any block out, some children would not learn to read as well. Finally, we have learned that teachers can take this framework and put their own "stamp" or style on it. What is the same in all classrooms, however, is that we give each block its allotted time each day and we work to make each block as multilevel as possible. Beyond that, there is wide latitude for teachers to carry out the instruction in ways they and the children find most satisfying and effective.

We have also learned more about how children learn. We began with the notion that children do not all learn in the same way, and this notion has become a conviction. Some children seem equally engaged and successful in each block, but others have clearly observable preferences. If you watch closely, you can almost see them "click in" during the block that matches their learning personality.

We are even more convinced now about the dangers of fixed reading groups. Although we use many grouping formats for our instruction, the children have no notion of being in a top, middle, or bottom group. First graders who come with little print experience but much eagerness to learn maintain that eagerness and their "I can do anything" attitude. Many of our inexperienced first graders become grade-level or better readers and writers.

We realize that when we used to put children in the bottom group, we were combining two types of learners—slow learners and inexperienced learners. When slow learners and inexperienced learners are combined in a bottom group, the pace is slowed and the opportunity to learn is limited. When inexperienced but fast learners have multiple opportunities to read and write and don't become discouraged by low-group placement, they make up for lost time. We began with the theoretical abstract idea that grouping children was not the best solution to the many entering levels of children. Our abstract idea has now been replaced with "real kid" readers and writers.

Perhaps the most surprising thing we have learned from our work came not from the children with the lowest entering levels but from those children already reading when they came to first grade, the ones who would have been placed in the top reading groups. In all honesty, we didn't initially expect our model to make things much better for these children. We just hoped that not being in a top group wouldn't hurt them. As year after year of data have indicated, these children read consistently and significantly above grade level. We have come to realize that the Four Blocks framework is probably as important for the highest achievers in each class as it is for the lowest. When our children were in reading groups, the top group in first grade read in the second-grade book at the end of first grade. But this upwards modification had clearly not been enough to accelerate the achievement of the very best readers. In the Four Blocks framework, children spend half their time in the self-selected and writing blocks in which there is no limit to the level at which they can read and write. When there is no limit on how fast they can learn, our best readers will astonish us. It is clear to us now that being placed in static reading groups defined by ability levels and with a prescribed curriculum was as limiting for those in the top half of the top group as it was for those in the bottom half of the bottom group.

Previously a public school teacher and administrator, Cunningham now teaches courses in literacy education at Wake Forest University. Hall is the curriculum coordinator at Clemmons Elementary School in Winston-Salem, North Carolina, USA. Defee was the first-grade teacher at Clemmons Elementary who initially collaborated with Cunningham and Hall in developing the Four Blocks framework. She is now the curriculum coordinator for Easton Elementary School in Winston-Salem, North Carolina, USA. Cunningham can be contacted at Wake Forest University, PO Box 7266, Winston-Salem, NC 27109, USA.

References

Allington, R.L. (1983). The reading instruction provided readers of differing reading ability. *The Elementary School Journal, 83,* 549 – 559.

Allington, R.L. (1991). Effective literacy instruction for at-risk children. In M. Knapp & P. Shields (Eds.), *Better schooling for the children of poverty: Alternatives to conventional wisdom* (pp. 9 – 30). Berkeley, CA: McCutchan.

Bond, G.L., & Dykstra, R. (1967). The cooperative research program in first grade reading instruction. *Reading Research Quarterly, 2,* 5 – 142.

Nonability-grouped multilevel instruction

Bond, G.L., & Dykstra, R. (1997). The cooperative research program in first grade reading instruction. *Reading Research Quarterly, 32,* 345–427.

Calkins, L.M. (1994). *The art of teaching writing* (2nd ed.). Portsmouth, NH: Heinemann.

Cunningham, P.M., & Cunningham, J.W. (1992). Making Words: Enhancing the invented spelling-decoding connection. *The Reading Teacher, 46,* 106–115.

Cunningham, P.M., & Hall, D.P. (1997) *Making more words.* Parsippany, NJ: Good Apple.

Cunningham, P.M., Hall, D.P., & Defee, M. (1991). Nonability grouped, multilevel instruction: A year in a first grade classroom. *The Reading Teacher, 44,* 566–571.

Fielding, L., & Roller, C. (1992). Making difficult books accessible and easy books acceptable. *The Reading Teacher, 45,* 678–685.

Graves, D.H. (1995). *A fresh look at writing.* Portsmouth, NH: Heinemann.

Hall, D.P., Prevatte, C., & Cunningham, P.M. (1995). Eliminating ability grouping and reducing failure in the primary grades. In R.L. Allington & S. Walmsley (Eds.), *No quick fix* (pp. 137–158). New York: Teachers College Press.

Routman, R. (1995). *Invitations.* Portsmouth, NH: Heinemann.

Schnetzler, P.L. (1996). *Ten little dinosaurs.* Denver, CO: Accord.

Veatch, J. (1959). *Individualizing your reading program.* New York: Putnam.

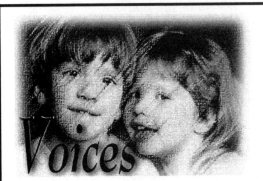

*T*he best teacher is not necessarily the one who possesses the most knowledge, but the one who most effectively enables his students to believe in their ability to learn.

— *Norman Cousins*

From *The Heart and Wisdom of Teaching: A collection of thought-provoking quotations for teachers.* Compiled by Esther Wright, M.A. TEACHING FROM THE HEART © 1997 by Esther Wright.

READING CLINIC • BY PATRICIA CUNNINGHAM

Use students' names to build basic reading skills

The school year is about to begin, which means a roomful of new students and a slew of names to learn. These activities will help you all get acquainted *and* teach some important concepts about reading.

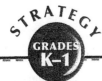

STRATEGY GRADES K–1

Develop Phonemic Awareness

PURPOSE
Phonemic awareness is not just another term for *phonics*. It is the ability to take words apart, put them back together, and change them.

■ **The following activities will help students develop phonemic awareness. They should be done orally, calling attention to the sounds in words.**

CLAP SYLLABLES
Say a student's name. Have students repeat the name with you, clapping the "beats" (syllables). Help them see, for example, that Eve and Matt are one-beat names, Manuel and Keisha, two beats, and so on.
    Determine which names have the same number of beats, then have students with those names stand up. Together, say and clap the beats in their names.

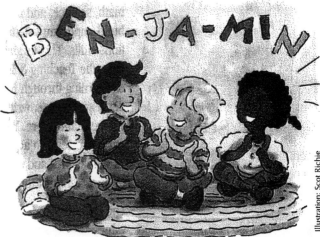

Illustration: Scot Richie

MATCH BEGINNING SOUNDS
Say a sound—not a letter—and assemble all students whose names begin with that sound. For *sssss,* for example, Samantha, Steve, and Cynthia would come forward. Be sure to always stretch out the sound. Have the whole class say the names, stretching out the initial sound.

HEAR RHYMING WORDS
Call on students whose names have lots of rhyming words, such as Pat and Nick. Say a word that rhymes with one of the names. Have students repeat the word, along with the name that rhymes with it, for example, *"sat, Pat."*

Patricia Cunningham teaches at Wake Forest University in Winston Salem, North Carolina. Her public-school teaching includes first grade, fourth grade, and remedial reading. She has published articles and books, including *Phonics They Use; Making Words* (with Dorothy Hall); and *Classrooms that Work* and *Schools that Work* (with Richard Allington), which are all available from IESS by calling (800) 644-5280.

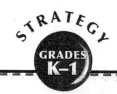

STRATEGY GRADES K–1

Promote Concepts About Words and Letters

PURPOSE
Names can also be used to develop critical word and letter concepts. For these activities, children look closely at classmates' names and sort them according to various features.

MATERIALS
strips of blank paper, preprinted letter cards or stiff paper for making letter cards

LONG WORDS/SHORT WORDS
Write each student's name on a large strip of paper. As a class, count the letters in each name and group the names with the same number of letters. After the names are sorted, read all of the names with students, helping them understand the concept of short and long words.

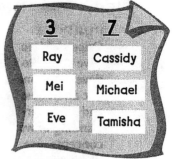

FIRST-LETTER SORT
Sort the names by first letter. Count how many names begin with each letter. Sing the alphabet song and decide which letters don't begin any of the names.

BEING THE NAMES
Distribute cards with individual letters printed on them (one letter per student, including duplicates as needed). Hold up a child's name strip. Have students compare their letter cards with letters in the name. If their letter matches any of the letters on the strip, have them line up to spell the name. This activity helps children understand left-right orientation, as well as the fact that the *order* of letters in words matters.

● READING CLINIC

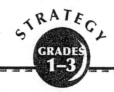

STRATEGY GRADES 1–3

Teach Letter Names and Sounds

PURPOSE
Once children have begun to develop phonemic awareness and an understanding of word concepts, use this activity to help them make connections between letters, letter combinations, and sounds.

MATERIALS
stiff paper for name cards

REVIEW BEGINNING SOUNDS IN FIRST AND LAST NAMES
With very young children I generally use only first names to teach concepts about words; for slightly older children, I include last names as well. This activity will help children understand that letters have predictable sounds, which may include more than one sound.

1 Using large name cards, sort students' first and last names according to the beginning letters, up to the first vowel. Have students say the names and divide them by the different *sounds* in the beginning letters.

2 Once the names are sorted, help students see that sometimes we "blend" the beginning letters together to figure out the words, as in Craig, Clark, and Clover. Other times combinations have a special sound, as the *Ch* in Chad and Charlene. The most common *c* sound can be found at the start of Catherine and Cari—but *c* can also have the *s* sound, as in Cynthia.

| Cynthia | Craig | Chad | Charlene | Clover | Catherine |
| Cyrus | Creighton | Chelsea | Charlotte | Clark | Cari |

Janiel M. Wagstaff

Building practical knowledge of letter-sound correspondences: A beginner's Word Wall and beyond

This article discusses the development of self-monitoring and searching behaviors in beginning readers.

"Teacher, I can't do it." Ezzie's wide eyes were eager to learn, yet teary with frustration, as the pencil wobbled awkwardly in her little fingers. I looked around the room on that first day of kindergarten to see others struggling to steady their pencils too. Before the week was over, I realized the challenge that lay ahead: Few of my students could identify letters or numbers, most had little book knowledge, none could write their names, and, like Ezzie, some had rarely had opportunities to put pencil to paper. They were beginning literacy learners in the truest sense. Where would I start teaching them what they needed to know?

My school district had an answer: Letter of the Week. I could introduce a letter and sound on Monday for my students to practice throughout the week. Bulletin boards, science, social studies, and other curricula would revolve around that letter. Using this curriculum, I might have the alphabet covered three fourths of the way through the school year. Not only did this seem painfully slow, but the approach focuses on letters and sounds in isolation. Would my students be able to understand and apply this letter-sound knowledge?

Wagstaff, Janiel M. (Dec. 1997/Jan. 1998). "Building practical knowledge of letter-sound correspondences: A beginners Word Wall and beyond." *The Reading Teacher*, 51 (4), 298-304.

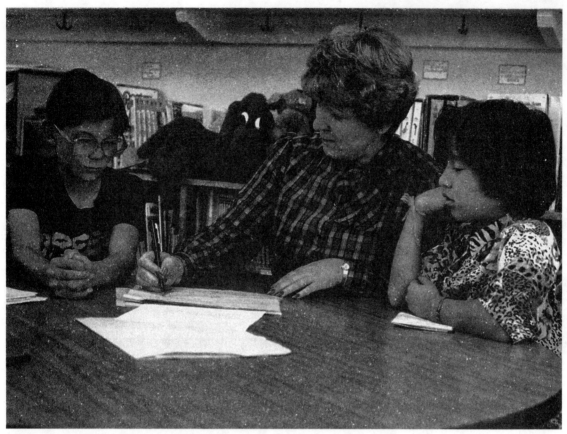

We read chorally, working on concepts of print and fluency. Photo by Robert Finken

The case against Letter of the Week

I had read *Becoming A Nation of Readers* (Anderson, Hiebert, Scott, & Wilkinson, 1985), where the Commission on Reading characterizes exemplary reading instruction as varied and fast-paced. In *No Quick Fix: Rethinking Literacy Programs in America's Elementary Schools* (1995), Richard Allington makes a case for picking up the pace of instruction: "designing schools that offer instruction that accelerates development early, in kindergarten and first grade, must become our priority" (p. 8). For Ezzie and her classmates, who enter school with few literacy experiences, the slow pace of programs like Letter of the Week is a serious disadvantage.

In addition to the problem of pacing, Letter of the Week instruction allows letters and sounds to be introduced without connection to meaningful reading and writing. Too often, reading time is spent practicing letters and

sounds in isolation or completing paper-and-pencil tasks related to the latest letter. Activities like these may leave learners with no understanding of how to apply letter-sound knowledge. Stahl (1992) relates this deficit to baseball.

> For a person learning to play baseball, batting practice is an important part of learning how to play the game. However, imagine a person who has never seen a baseball game. Making that person do nothing but batting practice may lead to the misconception that baseball is about standing at the plate and repeatedly swinging at the ball. That person would miss the purpose of baseball and would think it a boring way to spend an afternoon. (p. 620)

Yes, knowledge of letters and sounds, along with phonemic awareness, has been shown to be of utmost importance in learning to read (Adams, 1990). But a decontextualized, Letter of the Week curriculum is not the best way to help students develop that knowledge.

Yet, in some classrooms, Letter of the Week is the only reading instruction children receive. Although some educators still argue that kindergarten should serve solely a social

Building practical knowledge of letter-sound correspondences

purpose and that formal reading instruction should start in Grade 1, there is much support for kindergarten curricula that include phonemic awareness activities, the development of letter-sound correspondence knowledge, and purposeful reading and writing (Adams, 1990; Button, Johnson, & Furgerson, 1996; Clay, 1991; Fountas & Pinnell, 1996; McGill-Franzen, 1992; Richgels, Poremba, & McGee, 1996). Such activities are certainly promoted by findings from emergent literacy research that children begin learning literacy very early as they interact in a literate environment. In

---

Through shared reading of simple predictable books, I began modeling what readers do.

---

accord with this principle, Teale and Sulzby (1989) suggest daily reading and writing as a natural part of the early childhood curriculum. In New Zealand, where the literacy rate is the highest in the world, there is no debate about when literacy instruction should begin. Time is not wasted on "reading readiness"; rather, it is filled with rich literacy instruction and balanced with a variety of reading and writing activities, beginning on every child's 5th birthday (Smith & Elley, 1994).

If not Letter of the Week, what?

Even though Ezzie entered school with little book experience, she did have life experiences she could talk about. So did her classmates. It was logical to start with these stories as the basis for communicating on paper. I began writing workshop with a minilesson emphasizing that I would accept anything from scribble marks to drawings and letter-like forms, as long as students "got something down on paper." It worked. My children began writing in journals daily. They put down scribbles, drawings, and letter-like forms. Following writing time, they shared their stories with one another, and a community began to develop.

Through shared reading of simple predictable books, I began modeling what readers do: where to begin reading; left to right

progression; the difference between letters, words, and spaces; and one-to-one correspondence. I thought aloud about using initial letters and other cues to read words, and I read aloud frequently. Students began independent emergent storybook readings as they reread familiar stories based on our shared reading (Holdaway, 1979). They often checked these books out to read at home, and Ezzie led in number of checkouts.

Feeling we were off to a successful start, I thought of how I might extend these foundational lessons. My students were beginning to get a sense of letters, sounds, and their purposes as I gave them feedback on their writing and called attention to print during reading. Next, I wanted to keep track of our known and developing letter-sound correspondences. I immediately thought of building a Word Wall (Cunningham, 1995), so students would have a permanent reference to use while reading and writing.

In my years of teaching second grade, the Word Wall was an important classroom feature. I learned the technique from Pat Cunningham's book, *Phonics They Use: Words for Reading and Writing* (1995). In second grade, we built the Word Wall with key words containing useful chunks or rimes. These chunks, such as *ake* in *cake* and *art* in *dart*, help students read and write unknown words by analogy to words they already know rather than sounding out letter-by-letter or using phonetic rules. For example, using the key words *cake* and *dart*, students may more easily read or write words like *rake*, *cart*, *snowflake*, and *starting*. For a full description of building and using a Word Wall with chunks to facilitate students' reading and writing, see Wagstaff (1994; in preparation), Brown, Sinatra, and Wagstaff (1996), Cunningham (1995), Downer and Gaskins (1991), and Gaskins, Gaskins, and Gaskins (1991).

Given the needs of my kindergartners, it did not make sense developmentally to begin building a Word Wall with chunks. These students needed work in phonemic awareness and recognizing letters, letter names, and beginning consonant sounds. In second grade, we selected our Word Wall words from the context of humorous poetry. Since I had experienced great success with this method, I immersed my kindergartners in familiar rhymes, poems, and chants as a means of building a different type of Word Wall: an ABC Wall.

Building a beginner's Word Wall: The ABC Wall

Our first familiar rhyme was "Jack and Jill." After reading, reciting, and dramatizing the nursery rhyme, we selected *Jack*, *water*, and *pail* as first key words for our ABC Wall. I emphasized the beginning sound of each word, helping students hear and say the sound and notice how they made the sound with their mouths and tongues. We then practiced writing the first letter in each word and evaluated other words for like beginnings. After "playing" with words and sounds for a short time, we reread the whole rhyme, putting the words back into a meaningful context. During the week, I heard Ezzie quietly reciting it to herself in a sing-song voice while working at her desk. This delighted me. "Jack and Jill" was revisited throughout the week in repeated shared readings.

We worked with the new letter-sound correspondences for one week through varied word play activities, then added them to the ABC Wall. The words were boldly written on different colored construction paper, carefully cut along letter boundaries (for an additional visual cue), and stapled on the Wall with an accompanying illustration (see Figure 1). Once on the Wall, the key words served as references for reading and writing new words all year long.

Note that 3 weeks would have been required to cover the three letter-sound correspondences from "Jack and Jill" in a Letter of the Week classroom. Using an ABC Wall as described here doubles or triples the pace of instruction. Two instructional emphases help students feel comfortable with this pace. First, their letter-sound knowledge is reinforced through appropriate word play. Second, daily reading and writing activities allow students to continuously use their growing knowledge in purposeful ways.

Word play

Word play activities are designed to build students' phonemic awareness and knowledge of letters and sounds. Each activity is fast-paced and short in duration, which maximizes the use of class time for reading and writing connected text. Given the ABC Wall word *Jack*, for example, I tell students the word begins with the letter *j* and this letter will be seen and heard in a lot of words like *jam*, *jacket*, and *jelly*. Students are asked to respond positively (i.e., with thumbs up) to words I say that begin with the same sound as the ABC Wall word, or negatively (thumbs down) to words beginning with a different sound. We then practice writing capital *J* and lower case *j* in the air, on dry erase boards, and on scratch paper. I ask students to volunteer words that begin with *j*. We listen to volunteers and decide if the word offered does indeed begin with *j*. We may make *j* words with magnetic letters or add *j* words to a chart through interactive writing (Button et al., 1996).

We proceed in the same fashion with other key words, letters, and sounds (i.e., *water* and *pail*). During reading workshop, students may be asked to hunt for words that begin with *j*, *w*, and *p* and add them to letter charts or write them on index cards. Later, these words can be sorted for beginning letters or other salient features.

As we read and reread the familiar rhyme, chant, or poem from a large chart during the week, we review and apply our knowledge. We read chorally, working on one-to-one correspondences, concepts of print, and fluency as commonly done with shared reading. Students volunteer to identify words on the ABC Wall and other known words by placing an index finger in front and behind the word on the shared reading poster. By Wednesday, the students are very familiar with the rhyme due to our repeated readings. I give each student a copy of the rhyme to illustrate and put in their "favorites folders." Students pair up and read from their folders, using pointers to work on one-to-one correspondences. Rereading familiar material like this is a critical part of building beginners' confidence and fluency.

The ability to hear and manipulate sounds in spoken words is an important phonemic awareness component. This capacity facilitates writing development since children must hear sounds in order to represent them with letters. During a repeated reading of our rhyme, we sometimes substitute sounds in words as one way to build this ability. For example, with "Jack and Jill" we may substitute /p/ for some of the words, reading, "Pack and Pill went up the pill to petch a pail of pater," etc. This type of oral language play reinforces the sounds represented on the ABC Wall.

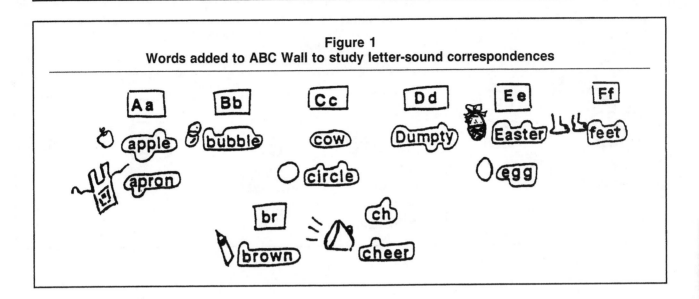

Figure 1
Words added to ABC Wall to study letter-sound correspondences

At the end of the week, I place the chart with the rhyme on an easel, chart stand, or affix it to a classroom wall. The chart remains visible so students may choose to revisit it during reading workshop time. As the next week begins, a new rhyme, poem, or chant is selected, and two or three new key words are highlighted for the ABC Wall.

Applying learning in varied contexts

I want my students to apply their growing knowledge of letter-sound correspondences in meaningful reading and writing contexts. One such opportunity occurs during the morning message (Routman, 1991). Before reading the message with students, I encourage them to read as much as they can. We talk about their attempts, how they are able to identify words, and what parts of the message are particularly troubling. One strategy we work on is making associations to key words on the ABC Wall to figure out unknown words. For example, Ezzie reported, I see *p* like in *pail*" at the beginning of the word *paint* in the morning message sentence, "In art, we will paint." This sparked a discussion:

> Teacher: How does knowing the word *pail* help you figure out this word?
> Students: It starts with the same letter.
> Teacher: So, if you know *pail*, (orally stretching and segmenting the word) /p/—-ail, you know the beginning sound is /p/. What else will help here?
> Students: Think of what makes sense.

> Teacher: Yes, (rereading from the message) "In art, we will /p/---." What makes sense and fits there?
> Students: Paint!
> Teacher: So, using what you know helps you figure out what you don't know. That's why we build and use our ABC Wall.

Discussion like this, initiated within a meaningful context, encourages students to use the ABC Wall in purposeful ways and to derive meaning using all three cueing systems (semantic, syntactic, and graphophonic). Records from student conferences indicate that children use the Wall during independent reading. Ezzie recently commented, "I know [read] some words because they start like words on the Wall."

The ABC Wall is referenced regularly during daily writing. As a minilesson, I often think aloud as I write a story in my journal or in the context of modeled writing. I might say something like, "Snydley, my cat, jumped in the garbage can again last night. I am writing the word *jumped* in my story. First, I hear /j/, just like the word *Jack*. I must need to start the word *jumped* with the letter *j*." As I write aloud and elicit help from students, I review stretching and segmenting words orally and making associations to key words on the ABC Wall. Letter-sound correspondences not yet represented on the Wall are also briefly introduced. This type of modeling naturally carries over to writing workshop. My anecdotal records have frequent accounts demonstrating students' use of the ABC Wall. For example, as

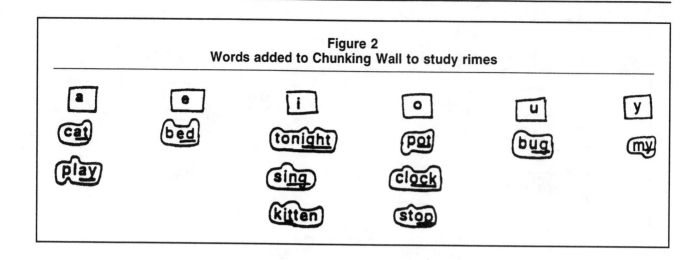

Figure 2
Words added to Chunking Wall to study rimes

a
cat
play

e
bed

i
tonight
sing
kitten

o
pot
clock
stop

u
bug

y
my

Philip wrote about his family trip to the beach, Ezzie helped by referencing the key word *bubble*. "*Beach* starts like *bubble*. You need a *b*." Students use this strategy independently as well, recording initial, final, and medial sounds with increasing accuracy and understanding throughout the year.

The same kind of activity takes place as the students and I work cooperatively to write the daily news (Routman, 1991). Once students share happenings in their lives and we choose one to record for the day, I elicit their help in deciding which letters are needed to spell the words in the news. Volunteers come forward and share the writing task. During activities like these, I make a point of asking students how they know which letter(s) is needed for a sound in the word we are writing. I want them to be able to describe their strategy use and share it with others. In one debriefing session, Lena shared her strategy, "If you don't know how to write a word, you can look up [on the ABC Wall] to find a word that sounds the same."

Other Word Wall possibilities

Once the ABC Wall is built, key words that begin with common digraphs like *sh*, *th*, and *ch* may be added. As students demonstrate facility with identifying and utilizing letters and sounds, similar methods may be used to build a Word Wall with common rimes (Wagstaff, 1994; Wagstaff & Sinatra, 1995). By the third and fourth school quarters many kindergartners are ready to use more than initial and final sounds to decode and spell. Thus, it becomes

appropriate to demonstrate and reinforce looking for the chunks in words to assist students in moving beyond a letter-by-letter strategy. I focus my students' attention on simple, frequent rimes like *an*, *at*, *ell*, *it*, *op*, and *ug*, again, taken from rhymes, poems, and chants. We create a separate Chunking Wall with key words containing these chunks (see Figure 2). The chunks, like the letter-sound correspondences, are learned, reinforced, and applied through short word play sessions and meaningful literacy activities.

During the first months of school, many first-grade teachers review the alphabet and basic letter-sound correspondences. Building an ABC Wall from the context of shared reading or writing is an appropriate way to revisit what first-grade students know and to create a classroom reference for use throughout the year. Depending on students' needs and abilities, an ABC Wall may be built more quickly than recommended here for kindergarten. From this starting point, classes may move into building a Chunking Wall.

Concluding remarks

I chose the course of action summarized here to advance my students' phonemic awareness, letter-sound knowledge, and facility with reading and writing. As I look around my classroom, I am surrounded by proof of lessons learned. This morning's daily news proudly boasts, in a variety of 5-year-olds' handwriting samples, "Last night Ralph's hamster had four babies. They look like pink jelly beans." On my desk is a pile of checkout papers, crowded with names of motivated readers and titles of favorite books. A stand holds today's poem, "Little Bo Peep has lost her sheep...." I study the ever-growing walls of words around us. They are reflections of learning proudly constructed with ownership shared between students and teacher.

Ezzie writes in her journal. She scans the Word Wall until she finds the letters she needs, then resumes writing. Her grasp on the pencil is secure. And the fears of the first day of kindergarten are a faded memory.

Currently a clinical instructor at the University of Utah, Wagstaff has also worked as a classroom teacher and reading specialist. She may be contacted at the University of Utah, 307 Milton Bennion Hall, Salt Lake City, UT 84112, USA.

References

Adams, M. (1990). *Beginning to read: Thinking and learning about print*. Cambridge, MA: MIT Press.

Allington, R.L. (1995). Literacy lessons in the elementary schools: Yesterday, today, and tomorrow. In R.L. Allington & S.A. Walmsley (Eds.), *No quick fix: Rethinking literacy programs in America's elementary schools* (pp. 1–15). New York: Teachers College Press.

Anderson, R.C., Hiebert, E.H., Scott, J.A., & Wilkinson, I.A.G. (1985). *Becoming a nation of readers: The report of the Commission on Reading*. Washington, DC: National Institute of Education.

Brown, K.J., Sinatra, G.M., & Wagstaff, J.M. (1996). Exploring the potential of analogy instruction to support students' spelling development. *The Elementary School Journal, 97*, 81–99.

Button, K., Johnson, M.J., & Furgerson, P. (1996). Interactive writing in a primary classroom. *The Reading Teacher, 49*, 446–454.

Clay, M.M. (1991). *Becoming literate: The construction of inner control*. Portsmouth, NH: Heinemann.

Cunningham, P. (1995). *Phonics they use: Words for reading and writing* (2nd ed.). New York: HarperCollins.

Downer, M.A., & Gaskins, I.W. (1991). *Benchmark word identification/vocabulary development program*. Media, PA: Benchmark Press.

Fountas, I.C., & Pinnell, G.S. (1996). *Guided reading: Good first teaching for all children*. Portsmouth, NH: Heinemann.

Gaskins, R.W., Gaskins, J.C., & Gaskins, I.W. (1991). A decoding program for poor readers—and the rest of the class, too! *Language Arts, 68*, 213–225.

Holdaway, D. (1979). *The foundations of literacy*. Sydney: Ashton Scholastic.

McGill-Franzen, A. (1992). Early literacy: What does "developmentally appropriate" mean? *The Reading Teacher, 46*, 56–58.

Richgels, D.J., Poremba, K.J., & McGee, L.M. (1996). Kindergartners talk about print: Phonemic awareness in meaningful contexts. *The Reading Teacher, 49*, 632–642.

Routman, R. (1991). *Invitations: Changing as teachers and learners K–12*. Portsmouth, NH: Heinemann.

Smith, J.W.A., & Elley, W.B. (1994). *Learning to read in New Zealand*. Katonah, NY: Richard C. Owen.

Stahl, S.A. (1992). Saying the "*p*" word: Nine guidelines for exemplary phonics instruction. *The Reading Teacher, 45*, 618–626.

Teale, W.H., & Sulzby, E. (1989). Emergent literacy: New perspectives. In D.S. Strickland & L.M. Morrow (Eds.), *Emerging literacy: Young children learn to read and write* (pp. 1–15). Newark, DE: International Reading Association.

Wagstaff, J.M. (1994). *Phonics that work! New strategies for the reading/writing classroom*. New York: Scholastic.

Wagstaff, J.M. (in preparation). *Working word walls: A book of integrated literacy lessons*.

Wagstaff, J.M., & Sinatra, G.M. (1995). Promoting efficient and independent word recognition: A new strategy for readers and writers. *Balanced Reading Instruction, 2*, 27–37.

Parents, You Teach Reading

by Susan Wargai Keskeny

1st Grade Teacher, Horace Mann Elementary, Detroit, MI

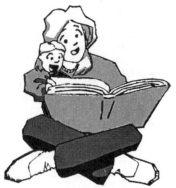
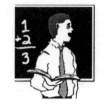

As parents you will often ask
"How can I help with the great task?"
"What task?" is my reply.
"With my child's reading!" is their cry.

Books, magazines and so much more
Should clutter your learning floor.
Some with pictures, some with print
Then sometimes stories he'll invent.

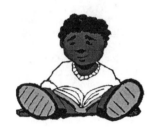
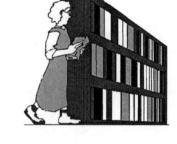

"I haven't the money!" is your call.
But books are free as I recall.
Corner librarians charge no fee.
They'll even select if need be.

"I haven't time!" another cry.
"Oh, but you do," I reply.
Read daily at the close of day
This way you'll show the way.

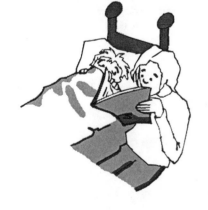

Questions, questions they will ask.
Replying is a vital task;
For in their heads wheels are turning,
Churning with desire for learning.

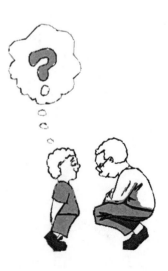

"You tell us, travel and explore!
We have no money for this chore."
But this is easy I implore,
For book adventures open doors.

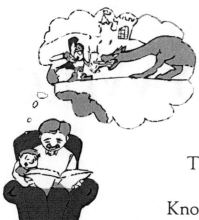

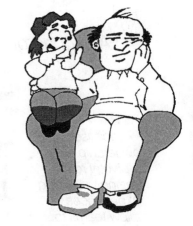

The trips to zoos, the mall and shore
Each add to their internal store.
Knowledge brought to the classroom door
Makes learning a much simpler chore.

"All they do is talk endlessly!
Frankly, listening tires me."
Listen you must is my reply,
For therein seeds of thinking lie.

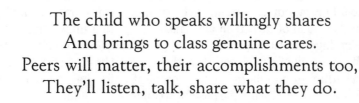

The child who speaks willingly shares
And brings to class genuine cares.
Peers will matter, their accomplishments too,
They'll listen, talk, share what they do.

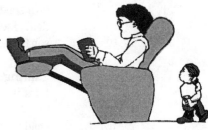

You're their teacher; if you read,
They'll read too; they'll see the need.
Enjoy, explore, plant the seed,
Talk, read, be in the lead.

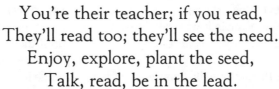

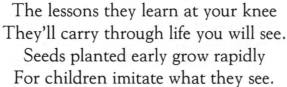

The lessons they learn at your knee
They'll carry through life you will see.
Seeds planted early grow rapidly
For children imitate what they see.

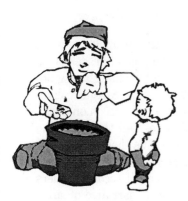

by Susan Wargai Keskeny
1st Grade Teacher, Horace Mann Elementary, Detroit, MI

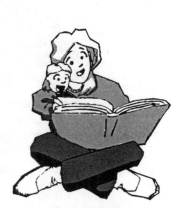

A Playful Way to Write

A second grade project that transforms kids into pint-sized playwrights

BY DIANE TREDENNICK

"Because ownership plays a pivotal role in setting up writing experiences, allow teams to select their favorite fairy tale to rewrite."

Each spring, my excited second graders write, produce and perform their own marionette plays. From the first sharing of a play to the publication of an anthology for our school library, our classroom reverberates with the sound of turned-on apprentices investigating the writing process.

We meet all of our objectives and special curriculum demands in an environment which fosters creativity, purposeful writing and a love of learning. Why not sow your own seeds in this experiential approach garden? Jack's beanstalk will pale in comparison to the bounty you'll harvest.

Sharing. Build students' knowledge of fairy tales in a team setting. Begin by searching for stories. Your school librarian can have children work in pairs, using on-line computers to locate literature. This is a time for children to share with one another. Encourage them to read aloud the stories they find and then to read them again and again.

In small groups, let students develop sequencing skills by brainstorming events from a fairy tale plot, writing them on chart paper and gluing them back together in the proper order.

Teach them to make character maps by placing a name in the center of a web and listing character traits on the spokes.

left handed — tall — **KIRSTY** — funny — cooperative

Looking for traits in a thesaurus is a happy challenge when partners share the task.

Prewriting. Structure prewriting activities to create enthusiasm, team spirit and ownership. Your author teams will work together for a long time, so establish rules that will shelter feelings and promote teamwork. Because ownership plays a pivotal role in setting up writing experiences, allow teams to select their favorite fairy tale to rewrite. Group members may create character maps for the major characters they choose.

By identifying many events, the groups make the eventual writing of their plays easier. So create a playful atmosphere for brainstorming story events. Cheer your teams on until their lists overflow. When the students sequence these events, they create a perfect guide for the script to their play.

Writing. Getting writing to make sense is hard, whether you're a second grader or an adult. Direction at the beginning and guidance along the way ensure carefully composed work. Present a mini-lesson on deciding upon an audience. Tell the class the elements you'll look for as they define their plot. Next, lay the groundwork for dialogue.

Dialogue in the hands of second graders easily becomes a lengthy narrative of story. Make a rule: no narrator role allowed. Students must use the characters' conversations to move their stories forward. If they get stuck, suggest they role-play and write down what they say.

Post reminders for your neophytes: an ogre saying something evil to show dialogue developing the character, a quote with wheels to show dialogue moving the story along. Begin searching for ways to inspire a creative mass of dramatists grappling with ideas, words, pencils, paper and one another.

Responding and revising. You must now set the stage for the authors to re-enter their work. I type each day's writing on a computer. Once I format the plays on a disk, parents or other volunteers help with the typing. Students relish making changes on their script, especially when they realize that they'll have a clean copy the next day. This means updating the plays after every writing session.

When typing the first draft of the plays, I correct misspellings and make side notes recording what instruction the class or a child needs. Leaving the rest of the writing intact protects the voice of a piece and gives students the opportunity to correct their own mistakes. As children gather to read their words in print, some changes take place spontaneously. Peer editing will catch others.

When you model the procedures you want the children to follow in responding and revising, you help the work advance smoothly. Establishing this cycle in the beginning provides a clear road map for independence in the days to follow. Your playwrights will adopt an important routine: share, respond, revise and continue writing.

Editing. Your guidance begins with the role of diagnostician. As you read the plays, determine your students' strengths and weaknesses. Write your prescription in the form of a mini-lesson and include how you want students to mark changes. Preventive or curative, a whole class presentation solves many problems quickly.

Diane Tredennick teaches second grade at Forest Creek Elementary School, Round Rock, TX.

From the beginning, peer-editing takes place daily. Model what you want student editors to say and how you want them to say it. In conferencing, highlight the good points you see and, when necessary, encourage writers to try again.

I conference with teams about any changes that might clarify meaning. The authors edit for every improvement they can find, and I take notes on future needs for teaching and reteaching. I complete the final editing, and we go to press.

Evaluating. Have the class set up self-evaluation criteria. As part of our assessment, we read every play aloud for the whole class. I evaluate my second graders on process, not product. To help keep track of the classroom contributions and interactions, I write comments on sticky notes, date them and write the students' name. I use them to help me write anecdotal records for portfolio assessment.

You must also appraise the value of this endeavor as it relates to the curriculum. Did the writing and reading meet your goals? Have your students internalized the writing process? Did your mini-lessons satisfy educational objectives as well as the personal needs of your children?

Publishing. There are many paths to choose from once a play is published. We donate our anthology of plays to the school library for our peers to read and perform.

We also perform plays for peers, parents and the community. Performing for an audience may be an elaborate event or a simple Readers Theater presentation. My students make their own marionettes and scenery, add music and songs, and pre-record their voices on a sound track.

Whatever path you choose, I hope you'll celebrate this happy and successful learning experience with gusto. ↓

"We meet all of our objectives and special curriculum demands in an environment which fosters creativity, purposeful writing and a love of learning."

Nurturing the Language of Art in Children

Judith Dighe, Zoy Calomiris, and Carmen Van Zutphen

The child has a hundred languages, a hundred hands, a hundred thoughts, a hundred ways of thinking, of playing, of speaking.

—Loris Malaguzzi

We three American educators visited the municipal early childhood system founded by Loris Malaguzzi in Reggio Emilia, Italy, or attended a symposium presented by Reggio leaders. These experiences challenged our beliefs concerning art for young children. We want to share our search and tell our sto-

Judith Dighe, the education specialist for a large Head Start program (99 classes), has been with Head Start many, many years. She holds a master's degree in early childhood education.

Zoy Calomiris, an art specialist, holds a bachelor's of fine arts from Maryland Institute College of Art and a bachelor's in education from the University of Maryland.

Carmen Van Zutphen holds a master's degree in early childhood education. She was a Head Start teacher with a degree in special education and early childhood education when she coauthored this article. She is currently a Head Start instructional specialist.

All three authors are with Montgomery County Public Schools in Maryland.

ries in the hope of starting dialogues with our colleagues across the country. We want to make clear that although the images and words that introduced us to the Reggio Emilia schools were our inspiration, we do not presume to call what we are doing the Reggio approach.

Judith: Within a few months of my visit to Reggio Emilia, I was asked to give a workshop on creative art. I had led this type of workshop many times previously. This time, in the midst of assembling materials for gadget printing, dip-and-dye, and medicine-dropper blots (never pattern art!), I was struck with a wave of uncertainty. Were these activities "creative" or even "art"? I started on a quest to reformulate my thinking about art for children and to delve into the theory and practice of art education here and in Reggio Emilia.

I found on this quest—and this has helped immensely—two colleagues, Zoy Calomiris, an art specialist, and Carmen Van Zutphen, a Head Start teacher, who were also struggling with questions about art for children. Carmen and Zoy were presenting art experiences in new ways and learning, Reggio-like, from observing children. The three of us started to talk together, question everything, read about art theory, and reflect jointly.

Our growing understanding of art for children

The beauty of the children's work in Reggio's Hundred Languages of Children exhibit notwithstanding, art is not the emphasis of the schools in Reggio Emilia; the child is. Reggio educators speak of projects that utilize children's symbolic languages, which include drawing, painting, constructing, clay modeling, and creative dramatics. These processes are imbedded in the total curriculum; they are children's way of making sense of the world through representation (Edwards, Gandini, & Forman 1993.)

Lasky and Mukerji (1980) summarized art theory and research to reach a similar conclusion: Art is an important way of knowing and communicating; in art children use "symbols that assist them in creating meaning for themselves about the world" (p. 3). This vision of art as symbolic representation for understanding, communication, and expression became the foundation for our attempts to provide experiences that we hoped would nurture some of our children's hundred languages.

Zoy: I never thought of children's art as something to decorate the hallways. My main task is to keep children thinking, experimenting, trying, changing, and moving things—going beyond what's obvious to seeing and expressing relationships.

We started with four basics: an atmosphere of respect with freedom for exploration and risk taking; a rich experiential curriculum; adequate space for children's projects and materials; and sufficient, or at least flexible, time. With these as a foundation, we set about finding ways to provide a supportive environment, encouragement, and guidance.

Dighe, Judith; Calomiris, Zoy; and Van Zutphen, Carmen. "Nurturing the Language of Art in Young Children." *Young Children,* January 1998.
Reprinted with permission from the National Association for the Education of Young Children.

The environment

Beauty

We were inspired by the beauty, light, and openness of the Reggio Emilia schools. Carmen made some inroads into making her Head Start classroom more attractive, adding tablecloths for lunchtime, artistically arranging displays of children's work, filling her library with beautifully illustrated children's books, and bringing in more of the natural world— flowers, shells, and plants.

In her art studio, Zoy was careful to include "breathing spaces" to avoid visual overload from too many displays. She used art reproductions to make the connection between reality and art—someone's interpretation of reality.

Zoy: I placed a vase of real irises as well as a reproduction of Van Gogh's *Irises* on a table. The real flowers caught the children's interest first. As soon as they entered the room, they started feeling and smelling them. We talked about the differences and similarities between the two objects and about the colors that Van Gogh used—the dark and light greens. I showed the children how to mix paint in order to get these variations of color. The children's paintings captured irises in their individual ways (see Figure 1).

Materials and tools

We had always stocked lots of open-ended types of materials, but the question of what, if anything, to put out for the children provoked a lot of discussion as well as "expert opinion" research. Broad brushes, thick crayons, watercolors, and fingerpaint are advocated by some art educators, denigrated by others (Seefeldt 1987). Most early childhood art activity books and workshops (the "creative" kind, not the cute craft/pattern art variety) feature painting with marbles, straws, spray bottles, bubbles, even brushes attached to a helmet!

Zoy, with her art education training, had not fallen for the allure of novel techniques, but the other two of us had. In most art education texts, however, we

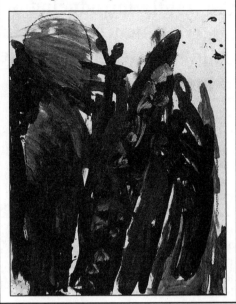

**Figure 1.
Irises painted by a four-year-old.**

found criticism of such techniques and constantly changing media. "Constantly introducing or changing art materials may actually stand in the way of a child's mastering the material enough to express his own feelings" (Lowenfeld & Brittain 1975).

We drew up our own list of basics: paint, clay, chalk, fingerpaint, pencils, crayons and markers of many sizes and colors, glue, paste, and all kinds of collage materials, especially natural objects such as shells and collected seeds. We wanted quality tools: brushes of many types and sizes, scissors that cut. And we found that keeping drawing/writing materials in the block area, science lab, and house and other dramatic-play centers as well as the art center elicited art from children who seldom chose the art center.

Encouragement/guidance

Observing children

We are trying to follow the Reggio ideal of using our observation of the child as the source of our curriculum. Closely watching and listening to children working and playing also demonstrates a

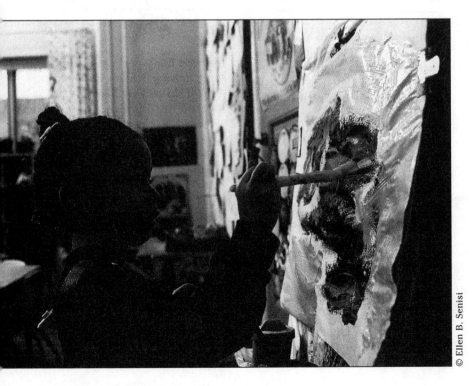

© Ellen B. Senisi

Constantly introducing or changing art materials may actually stand in the way of a child's mastering the material enough to express his own feelings.

valuing of the child's process; and it is the first step in knowing what kind of further encouragement—verbal or material—might be helpful.

Zoy puts out butcher paper the first day a new class is in her art room so as to record the children's interests and abilities. We have learned from Reggio to watch closely, preserve what we see with notes or camera, and listen, often with the aid of a tape recorder. We also encourage children to talk about what they are doing or making, and we are careful to listen.

Child-centered planning

We used children's words, actions, interests, and discoveries as the bases for short-term activities . . .

Carmen: Rodrigo screamed when he saw the spider on the rug near his foot. I picked it up, held it in a glass, and we talked about it.

"Maria, mira, mira, araña!" Rodrigo called to his friend to come and see. They watched and talked excitedly. I suggested they count the legs and so they did. As other children gathered around the spider, Rodrigo and Maria went to the chalkboard

and filled it with circles with radiating spokes.

"Spiders," Maria told me, though of course I knew.

"Would you like to make some on paper?" I suggested.

Lunch was delayed that day as Maria, Rodrigo, and twelve other children used paint, markers, chalk, and crayons to make spiders of all descriptions.

After lunch I read Eric Carle's *The Very Busy Spider* to the children; then we took the spider outside and watched it crawl away.

We have learned from Reggio to watch closely, preserve what we see with notes or camera, and listen, often with the aid of a tape recorder. We also encourage children to talk about what they are doing or making, and we are careful to listen.

The next day Rodrigo and Maria's spiders were still on the chalkboard. Numerous other spiders had been tacked or taped to the walls, and Rodrigo made a series of clay spiders.

. . . and long-range planning.

Zoy: On the Head Start children's first day in the art room, I rolled out the butcher paper; put out crayons, oil pastels, colored chalk, and markers; then stood back expecting to see an energetic composition of lines and color.

This didn't happen. Many of the children could not hold their drawing instruments properly. Others began wandering around the room after making a few marks on the paper. Few of

the children ventured to color beyond their immediate reach.

The children's teacher and I collaborated and drew up a three-phase plan to guide the children's art experience.

For the first few months, our emphasis was on exploration of a wide variety of materials. We worked to develop children's art vocabulary—color, shape, and texture words—and concentrated on mixing colors, filling the entire paper, gluing, and cutting. Children also learned to add textures by rubbing, printing, or splattering.

During the second phase, we guided the children in making representational images. [See the discussion of scaffolding that follows.] We chose the face and human body as our initial theme. In the classroom and the art studio, children observed body parts and tried them out, moving in many different ways.

By February we began what I saw as the third phase. The children needed less procedural direction. We focused on children's observational and analytical skills and encouraged individual expression. We worked with clay or drew every weekly art session and returned to familiar themes—self-portraits, families, trees. One week we would create a self-portrait in crayon and watercolors, the next week in clay. We were delighted with the spontaneity of the children's work and their verbal descriptions of their observations and creations.

We also incorporated visual representation into ongoing themes.

Carmen: One of our themes throughout October and November was the fall season. Children brought in lots of leaves and we commented on their colors and watched falling leaves.

In early December as we walked near the school, we shuffled through the fallen maple and oak leaves and halted before a small fir tree. With my encouragement the children felt, smelled, and talked about the tree. "It looks like a Christmas tree," said Dwayne.

We plucked a few twigs, brought them back to our room, and placed them on the art table along with magnifying glasses, pencils, and paper. I invited children to observe and draw the twigs.

Peter, a generally nonverbal three-year-old, was the first to sit and pick up the fir twigs. A few minutes later, when he seemed distracted, I joined him, asking, "How do the needles feel to you, Peter?" He touched the points and looked at me.

"You notice the thick line in the center that the needles come out of?" Again he nodded, picked up the pencil, and proceeded to draw the fir twig (see Figure 2).

In January, after our winter break, I noticed a pile of discarded Christmas trees near the school parking lot waiting to be collected by the county trucks. Wondering whether the children who had earlier shown an interest in the live tree would also want to observe some of the tinsel-looped branches in this pile, I took paper, pencils, and clipboards along when we went out.

Only Peter expressed an interest in recording his observations. We sat close to the aging Christmas trees. Peter felt the hardened sap on the tip of one of the branches and sketched a branch with a ball at the end.

We gathered a few branches to take inside, and I tacked one to the easel. Several children helped mix just the right shade of green, adding a little black to the green tempera. Peter beamed with joy at his remarkably realistic fir-branch painting.

Teacher-child interaction

We decided to teach or "guide" graphic representation in the same way that we teach language or social skills—by constructing occasions for it, nurturing its unique development in individual children, and teaching the component skills. We are feeling our way cautiously here, however, aware that there is disagreement in our field: some art educators advocate a hands-off, quiet observer approach; others propose more teacher facilitation (Efland 1990.) As learners we decided to experiment—trying an approach, observing, and rethinking.

Believing that sensory exploration and symbolic representation are intertwined, we encouraged children to notice the smell, taste, feel, and sound of things. We talked about the crunchy juiciness and sweet/tart taste of an apple, noticed how the plant in need of water was drooping, and compared the smooth and fuzzy sides of a magnolia leaf.

Carmen tried both a hands-off and hands-on approach in doing a self-portrait activity with her Head Start class. The first time she limited her role to putting out a choice of materials and making a request: "Would you make a picture of your-

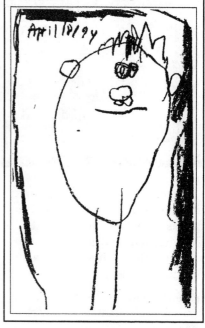

Figure 3.
Jamie's first self-portrait.

self?" Jamie, Amira, and Susan made self-portraits (Jamie's is pictured in Figure 3).

A few weeks later Carmen again asked these three children to make a picture of themselves. This time she placed hand-held mirrors on the tables with the art materials, and she sat with the children, observing and conversing with them as they worked.

As Jamie looked in the mirror, Carmen encouraged her to say what she saw and supplied the word "eyebrows." Both Jamie and Susan drew eyebrows and more facial parts than they had on their first drawings.

Amira drew dots on her ears: "Look at my earrings."

Jamie pointed to the two lines below her head and explained, "This is the neck."

"She looks happy," Susan commented about Jamie's self-portrait.

The next week Jamie and Amira chose the art center and without prompting sat together and made new self-portraits. Jamie took a circle stencil from the art shelf and used it to make an outline of her face; then she passed the

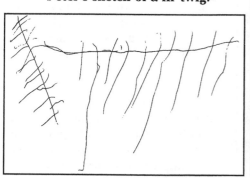

Figure 2.
Peter's sketch of a fir twig.

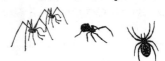

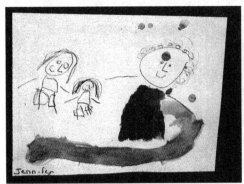

stencil to Amira. They kept most of the details of their previous pictures, this time adding teeth.

Carmen learned from her observations that guidance can also be unintentional.

Carmen: I had been working with three children intent on making clay faces. Dolores [almost four years old] didn't choose to join us but watched from the nearby puzzle table. After the three had left the art table and I also had moved to another part of the room, Dolores went to the art table. A short while later she approached me: "Teacher, teacher, I made this for you." She had in her hand a clay-sculpted gingerbread-person shape with three fingerprint holes adorning its middle.

Teaching skills

Some children need to be shown how to hold the scissors or crayon, or how to prevent unwanted paint drips. All children need techniques for dealing with clay, not making pieces so thin that they will break when dried or fired, not pounding it into the table so it will be impossible to pick up in one piece. We give this help matter-of-factly as needed. Our goal is to enable children to have enough control of the media to be able to use them to express their ideas and feelings.

We also taught printing, with sponges for example, as another technique for children to add to their

repertoire. After reading *Swimmy,* Zoy showed children how to tilt their paper so the wet watercolors would run together, resulting in approximations of the backgrounds Leo Llioni used in his illustrations for the book.

Scaffolding

With children who are just beginning to make representational figures, Zoy sometimes supplies a shape to be used as a focal point. When children wanted to make cats, she supplied a paper plate for the head. This stimulus was just enough (added to their experience with cats) to give children confidence and get them started (see Figure 4). It also provided them with a sense of scale, encouraging them to fill the page. When children in her first-grade art class drew cats (after reading *Have You Seen My Cat?* by Eric Carle), Zoy helped them analyze the cat's body in terms of shape and texture (see Figure 5).

We often use questions to lead children to doing their own problem solving. In helping children

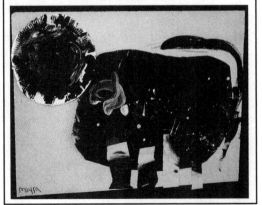

Figure 4.
Cat collage and painting by a four-year-old.

with their cat pictures, Zoy placed a paper plate in the lower corner of a paper held in her other hand. "If I put the cat's head here, will I have room for the cat's body?" she asked. The children giggled.

Modeling

No, we did not make pictures for children to copy; but we wanted children to see the care we took in artistically displaying their work and arranging materials. We also wanted children to see us drawing, so we drew to

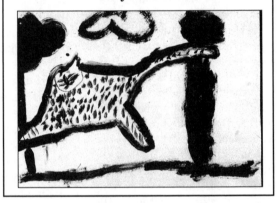

Figure 5.
Cat drawn and painted by a six-year-old.

recap a field trip, record children's words, or provide a recipe for cooking.

Zoy told of taking a sketch pad to the beach when her son was three: "Alex came and sat next to me with paper and pen, ready to draw the ocean. By the end of the week, I had a whole following of child-artists—children I hadn't known previously. They came with notebooks, pencils, and markers. Together we drew the landscape and mermaids."

* * *

This is where we are at present. Next year we will again listen to children, talk with each other (and with more of our colleagues), try new approaches, and question everything we do. We invite readers to join us in this process.

References

Edwards, C., L. Gandini, & G. Forman, eds. 1993. *The hundred languages of children: The Reggio Emilia approach to early childhood education.* Norwood, NJ: Ablex.

Efland, A.D. 1990. *A history of art education: Intellectual and social currents in teaching the visual arts.* NY: Teachers College Press.

Lasky, L., & R. Mukerji. 1980. *Art: Basic for young children.* Washington, DC: NAEYC.

Lowenfeld, V., & W.L. Brittain. 1975. *Creative and mental growth.* New York: Macmillan.

Seefeldt, C. 1987. The visual arts. In *The early childhood curriculum: A review of current research,* ed. C. Seefeldt. New York: Teachers College Press.

For further reading

Bettone, M. 1995. From our readers. Art education. *Young Children* 50 (4): 3.

Clemens, S.G. 1991. Art in the classroom: Making every day special. *Young Children* 46 (2): 4–11.

Dever, M.T., & E.J. Jared. 1996. Remember to include art and crafts in your

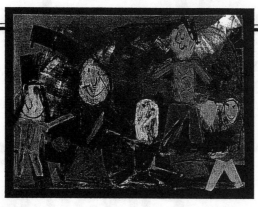

integrated curriculum. *Young Children* 51 (3): 69–73.

Edwards, L.C., & M.L. Nabors. 1993. The creative arts process: What it is and what it is not. *Young Children* 48 (3): 77–81.

Engel, B.S. 1995. *Considering children's art: Why and how to value their works.* Washington, DC: NAEYC.

Engel, B.S. 1996. Learning to look: Appreciating child art. *Young Children* 51 (3): 74–79.

Feeney, S., & E. Moravcik. 1987. A thing of beauty: Aesthetic development in young children. *Young Children* 42 (6): 7–15.

Lasky, L., & R. Mukerji. 1980. *Art: Basic for young children.* Washington, DC: NAEYC.

Marshall, S. 1963. *An experiment in education.* New York: Cambridge University Press.

Read, H. [1943] 1956. *Education through art.* 3d ed. New York: Pantheon.

Schiller, M. 1995. An emergent art curriculum that fosters understanding. *Young Children* 50 (3): 33–38.

Schirrmacher, R. 1986. Talking with young children about their art. *Young Children* 41 (5): 3–7.

Seefeldt, C. 1995. Art—A serious work. *Young Children* 45 (3): 39–45.

Swanson, L. 1994. Changes—How our nursery school replaced adult-directed art projects with child-directed experiences and changed to an accredited, child-sensitive, developmentally appropriate school. *Young Children* 49 (4): 69–73.

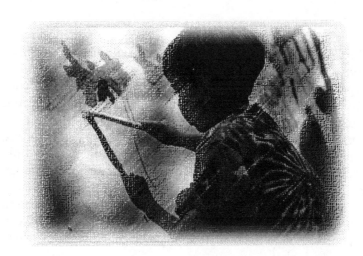

Creating and Managing Learning Centers

Creating Your Physical Environment

For the past two centuries or so, we have come to believe that what children need to know in order to become happy and productive adults can be learned by sitting in a crowded room and listening to an adult talk in an abstract language, while surrounded by other immature children. It takes a gigantic act of faith to believe that this is possible, but we seem increasingly willing to delude ourselves on this account, despite all evidence to the contrary.

— Mihaly Csikszentmihalyi, "Contexts of Optimal Growth in Childhood," from *Daedalus*, Winter 1993

The first stage in creating a child-centered classroom is to plan the physical environment. Choosing the centers you wish to incorporate into your plan, then designing a floor plan that meets all the needs of your situation, is both creative and exhausting.

It is helpful to try this step with another teacher. Often, we get stuck in old habits, leaving furniture and centers in their place simply because that's where they've always been. Another person helps in this stage of planning, offering a new perspective and fresh ideas.

Keep in mind that you do not need to remove all desks from your room, and you do not need to purchase all new furniture. In order to know what you need to remove, and what you may need to add, you first need to decide how you want your classroom to look.

Step One: Start With a Plan

First, decide what centers you wish to have in your classroom. I plan my year thematically, fitting the instruction of specific skills required by my school district into interdisciplinary units. This approach encourages the integration of curricular areas like math, science, and geography in order to teach a broad concept.

Excerpted from *Creating and Managing Learning Centers: A Thematic Approach*, by Phoebe Bell Ingraham. Peterborough, NH: Crystal Springs Books, 1997.

The curricular nature of my thematic planning directs my classroom environment: I teach a concept through experiences in these curricular divisions, so my classroom should be divided into these same areas. Reading and writing are utilized in every curricular area to encourage an understanding and a thoughtful application of these general concepts.

It may be easiest to begin with general areas, and become more specific as you gain experience in this approach. For example, divide your space into literacy development centers, cognitive development centers, creative development centers, physical development centers, and social and emotional centers (see Fig. 2-1).

It is important to note that every center in my classroom nurtures all of these developmental areas in some way, but I emphasize a particular domain when I place an activity into a center.

For example, while I include literacy interactions in every center of my classroom—children have opportunities to read and write while building with blocks, investigating a fossil, creating a work of art with paints, experiencing another culture, making an ABC pattern, and operating a grocery store—writing is such an important part of my students' total development that I have several centers designed specifically to encourage a variety of elements in writing:

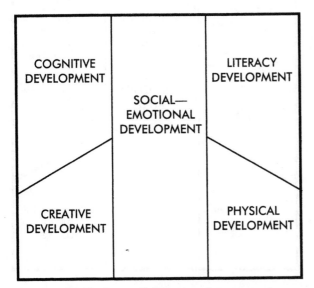

Fig. 2-1 Divide the available space into general areas for different types of centers.

• I want my children to take the time and effort to write creatively on a regular basis, so there is a specific center set aside for that task.

• I believe that legible handwriting is a skill that must be taught and practiced, but it must be connected to real-life activities in order for it to be utilized; so I incorporate handwriting activities into my creative writing center.

• My journal center involves the children in reflection and in recording their personal thoughts.

• I want my students to feel confident as readers and writers, and to do this, they must become fluent at these tasks. This takes practice in specific skills inherent in these activities. Therefore, I set up a language center for practicing specific reading, writing, and spelling strategies, as well as a library to encourage them to spend time reading.

Similarly, I design activities specifically to promote social and emotional development in the games, role play, and dramatic play areas, even though social and emotional development is nurtured in every center. And while math principles are used throughout our day and in many of our centers (blocks, cooking, science, geography, library, art, writing, and games), we set aside activities and spend time concentrating on the acquisition of specific skills within our curriculum in the math center.

Look at your classroom. Depending upon the size of the room and the number of students you have in your class, try dividing your room into the above five categories. Think about the needs each area will require. For example:

• Literacy centers will need plenty of light and electrical outlets so children can listen to tapes of books or make tapes of themselves reading. Areas for children to write need table or desk space.

I like my literacy centers close to the door, so the children and visitors notice that, first and foremost, we *read and write!*

• Cognitive centers also need electrical outlets, plus table space for students to work at writing tasks. There should be plenty of space for working with manipulatives in small groups, as well as for storing materials and a wide variety of resource books.

I like to incorporate a window near my science center, so the children will have opportunities to observe the world outside.

• Creative development centers should include space close to a sink and plenty of shelves to hold all the "junk" so necessary for creative projects. Plenty of table space is also important. If possible, it's nice to have two tables: one for teacher-directed activities and one for self-directed creations. In kindergarten and primary classrooms, an easel should be included.

• Physical development centers will need a lot of space, especially for kindergarten and primary classrooms. There should be room for a balance beam, bean bag toss, blocks, and large motor games. These activities will rotate through this area.

It is wise to place this center in a corner, away from traffic areas, and on a rug or carpeted area. It's best *not* to place your gross motor area against a thin wall, where another class might be disturbed by the noise of falling blocks.

For upper elementary children, fine motor development and eye-hand coordination need more attention than gross motor development. In these classrooms, it might be beneficial to incorporate the physical development centers into the social and emotional development centers. This will allow more space for the children to move within their groups. Manipulative games will encourage both areas of development simultaneously.

• Social and emotional development areas are more prevalent in kindergarten and primary classrooms than in upper elementary grades. As mentioned above, older elementary children participate in a variety of cooperative learning groups that nurture their social and emotional growth.

However, these areas are prime candidates for a temporary center in your class-room. Older children will benefit from occasional space to develop puppet shows, creative drama, and reader's theater. Allow ample opportunities for these experiences as your space allows.

Once you have established the general locations in your classroom for each grouping, you can divide them into specific centers that best meet the needs of your students and match your curriculum and the goals you have set for yourself and your students (Fig. 2-2):

• Math and science centers are the easiest centers for which to create experiential learning activities.

• Depending upon your writing program, you may wish to include an area for creative writing or journaling.

• Journals might be included within *each* center, particularly in late primary classrooms. For example, math journals might be included as an activity in the math center, while a round-robin journal could be kept on specific books of interest in your reading or library center.

A round-robin journal allows children to add their comments about a particular book or topic. Place a small journal in your read-

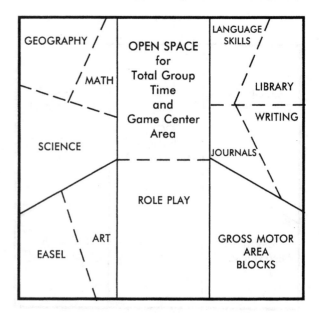

Fig. 2-2 Once you've divided your classroom into general areas, you can begin to place specific centers within each area.

ing or library center, and ask open-ended questions to start the conversation about the story. For example, in a journal for the book, *Stellaluna*, write the question:

"Have you ever done something that seemed normal for you, but attracted much attention from others? Why do you think that happened?"

Or you might simply ask, "Would you rather be a bird or a bat? Why?" Allow several children to react in writing before asking another question.

Journals designed for an author study might also be used in this manner. For example, during an author study of Mem Fox, place several of her books on a shelf, along with a "Mem Fox Books Journal." On the first page, list the books you've read together and have in your class library. Include blank pages for the children to write a response to their favorite Mem Fox book. When the author study is complete, this journal may be read aloud to compare and contrast the reading experiences and reflections that your students had when reading her books.

You do not need to begin with a great number of different areas. Start with the basics, and add new areas as you are ready to do so. It is much easier to establish procedures and rules when there are a few important areas well-stocked with exciting activities.

Including too many center areas before you have enough creative jobs to fill them will overwhelm you and invite off-task behavior during center time. Take it slow and plan carefully.

Step Two: Setting Up Your Classroom

Each center should include:

- shelves for holding needed materials and manipulatives
- floor area and table(s) and chairs for workspace
- wall space for displaying charts and student work
- materials to enable completion of the tasks and jobs assigned to the area, such as pencils, crayons, paper, scissors, stapler, tape, date stamp, letter stamps, envelopes, message board, hole punches, etc.

Think through each area you have chosen as a center, and note any materials you think are important to that area. Consider your style of teaching and your students' needs.

For example, in my library or reading center, I like to include a tape recorder with headphones. This is my listening area. However, many teachers highlight this skill, and so they choose to design a center specifically as a listening station. (More specific ideas are included in the chapters on each center area.)

In planning for each center, think first of what you already have in your room. Which centers could use desks pushed together to form a small table as the work space? (Try placing two table legs into a large coffee can when pushing desks or tables together to form a larger surface. This keeps them from constantly sliding apart.)

What centers should include a few isolated desks to form quieter work areas? There are some unique tables designed for special tasks, such as kidney-shaped tables that allow the teacher to sit across from each child.

You will want to utilize any special features your classroom has, and design your centers so that they function well in your particular setting. What shelves already built in to the room must be used to hold certain materials because of the location or size of the shelf? Consider the space you have, and the furniture you need and can obtain, in order to design the classroom that will work for you and your students.

For additional shelf space, check with your principal to see if there are shelves not currently in use either in your building, or in another building in your school district. You might be surprised at what you find. If you can purchase new furniture, shop wisely. Low shelving works well as center dividers, and still allows you to see throughout your classroom. Also, the tops of low-built shelves can be used to display tasks. Double-sided shelving units are perfect to use in centers, and they are less expensive to purchase than two separate shelves.

If you find that you need to provide much of the furniture, don't give up. Check out your basement, garage, or attic. You never know what is tucked away that might be useful if used another way. I have used old coffee tables as work areas for children to use while sitting on the rug.

Visit local thrift shops and garage sales. Check with neighbors and parents of children in your classroom who might be willing to donate old furniture. One year, a student's parent offered to build anything I needed if I would supply the materials. A teacher friend of mine had a parent who had refurnished her child's bedroom, and donated several beautiful bookshelves to her classroom.

Don't feel you have to have a large shelf for every area. Start with whatever you have, and add items gradually as you find a real need. It is probably a bigger mistake to fill your room with too much.

You can always use a bookcase to house a little of everything. Try painting each shelf a different color, and color-coding the items that belong on them to help the children replace materials in the correct spot. Or materials can be placed in different-colored tubs, depending on whether they deal with science, math, or language development. The shelf can have colored stickers to indicate what bins belong where.

This arrangement works well in a very small room. The children can take what they need from the appropriate learning center's shelves and work in a central location, and yet cleanup can be fast, with everyone able to help.

No matter how you set up your classroom, the most important thing is to be well organized. A workable structure within the classroom environment will provide a solid scaffolding to promote learning; and the children will be able to function independently and cooperatively, while learning what they need to know in the way they learn best. They will use the materials to complete your assigned tasks, and then create new learning activities and games for themselves that you never dreamed of! (See Fig. 2-3 for a sample room plan which incorporates learning centers.)

Adjusting Your Room Arrangement

As you proceed with your year, you may encounter difficulties with your center time that can be eliminated with minor changes to the room plan.

• **Too much noise:** Centers that produce much noise, even when children are working on-task, should be placed away from centers that contain quiet work stations. Try moving the quiet center to an out-of-the-way place in the room. Another option is to place a barrier between the noisy area and other centers of the room.

For example, I have my block center in a carpeted corner. It is near the science center, and that works well, for the children in the

(continued on page 32)

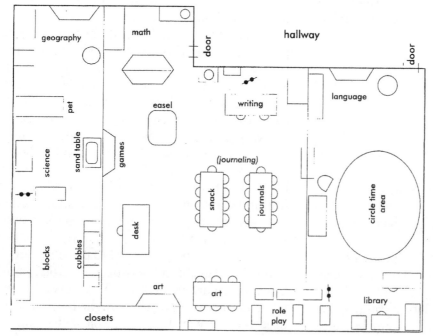

Fig. 2-3 A sample floor plan which incorporates learning centers into the classroom.

CHAPTER 2

Creating Learning Centers

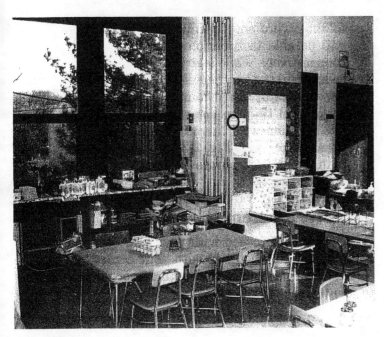

Art Table

The art table is located near shelves that hold art supplies for the children.

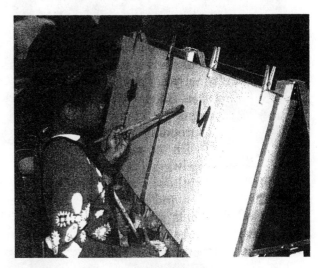

Easel

Our classroom has a two-sided easel with room on each side for two children. One side of the easel is devoted to assigned art tasks, while the other side is for art projects of the students' own choice.

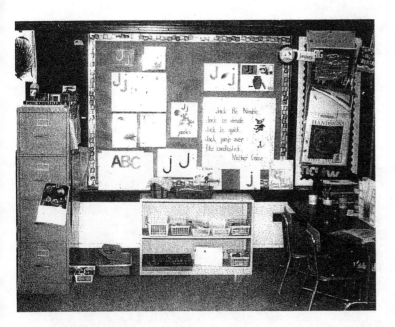

Language Center

Lots of activities that allow children to learn about the alphabet and the formation of words and sentences are included in the language center.

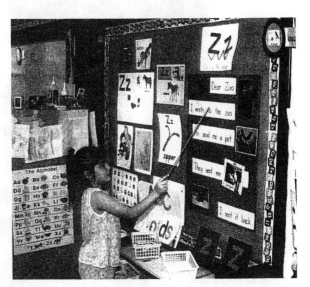

Here, a student works with an interactive chart in the language center.

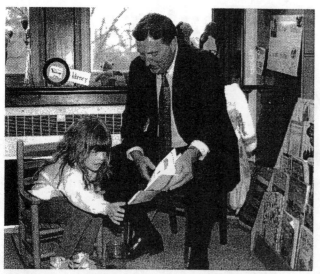

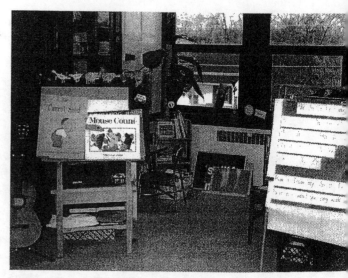

Library Center

The library center is a carpeted, out-of-the-way area with lots of books available for students to read. Here, a student demonstrates a task to Mr. Fox, our principal.

A stand in the library/circle center area can hold Big Books or interactive charts.

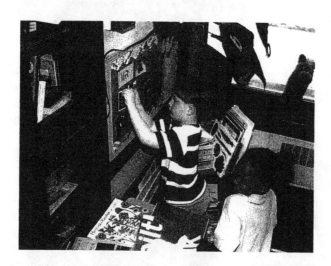

This boy is this week's Fabulous Friend; he tells a classmate about photos that he brought from home. The photos will stay in the library center all week.

Role Play Center

The role play center provides play activities related to current thematic units, as well as tasks that allow students to practice writing, math, and social skills in "real-life" settings. Here, the role play center has been turned into a pet store.

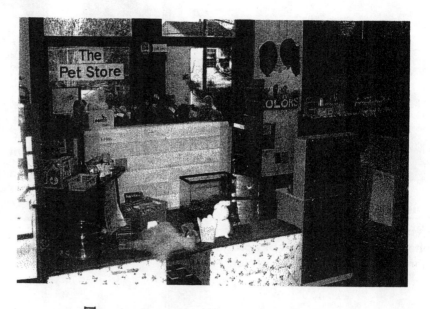

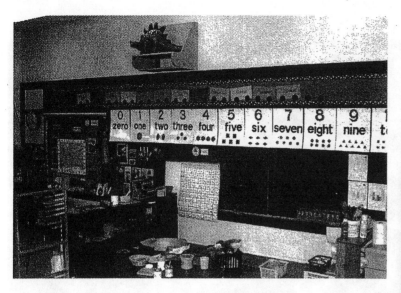

Math Center/Geography Center

The math center includes storage areas that contain manipulatives for counting and sorting activities, as well as activities that promote problem-solving and critical-thinking skills.

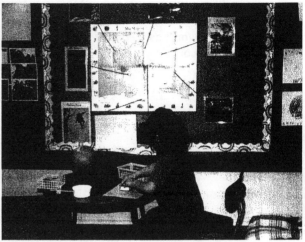

The geography center, located to the left of the math center, contains lots of mapping activities as well as activities that expose children to literature, music, art, and games from many cultures around the world.

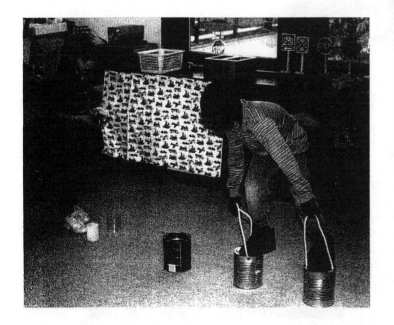

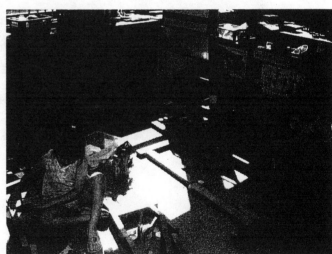

Gross Motor/Block Area

The block area should be out of the way, carpeted, and placed away from walls adjoining other classrooms or centers that require quiet concentration — block areas tend to be very noisy places!

Science Center

The science center has a shelf full of activities, a table with tasks to complete, and a chart stand for poetry or interactive charts. Locating the science center near the windows allows me to use the outside world as a subject for observation.

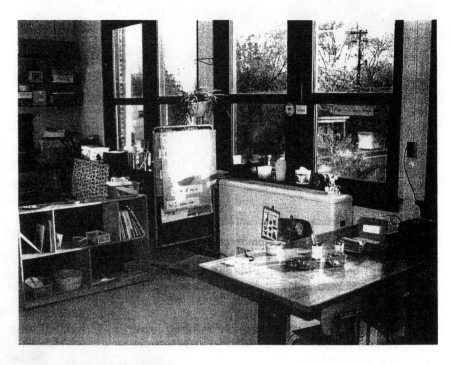

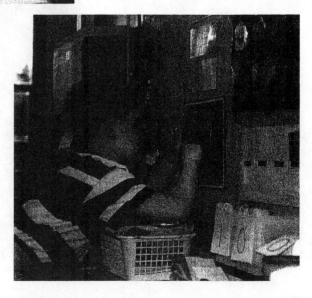

Calendar/Writing Centers

The writing center helps children develop specific writing skills, but also provides them with opportunities for creative expression. Two journal tables are included in the center.

Here, a student completes a calendar math activity in the calendar center (located to the left of the language center in the photo above, left).

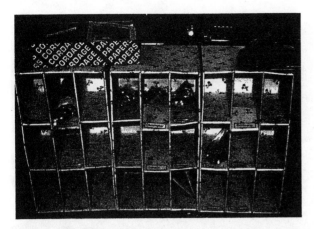

These cubbies are made from three nine-compartment shoe organizers, stood on end and lined up. They provide an accessible but out-of-the way place for children to keep their papers and other belongings.

science center are constantly moving around and discussing their work. Any activity that goes on in the block area can be tolerated by students working in science. I have also placed my cardboard cubbies next to the block center. They cushion the noise, and it provides additional space between the block center and another center that may be next to it.

• **Not enough space to children to work:** Children might need floor or table space, according to the specific tasks they choose in a center. If your room is small, do not fill each center up with furniture. Put a large table near the middle of the room, next to your open

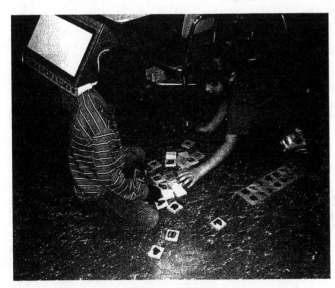

Two children play a memory game in the games center.

floor area. The children can bring work from any center to the table or floor and work alongside children from other areas.

I taught in a modular unit for several years which housed ten small centers. I set the room up in the manner shown in Fig. 2-4. To allow for a quick cleanup, I purchased plastic baskets to hold the activities for each center. The baskets were color-coded to a specific center, so that every child found it easy to help clean up and put things away where they belonged.

• **Constant disruption of children at work by others not in their center:** If children are constantly being disrupted in their work, check how you have positioned your centers. Placing quiet, cognitive centers next to more active social areas might be too much temptation for young children to stay focused on their work.

For example, children working in the art center are often mobile as well as social. Placing the art center in the middle of your room might require children to travel through another center to wash their hands. Their chatter as they create works of art would likely spread to all corners of the room. And carrying dripping glue or paint to a drying area, or to show an adult their work, can create a mess throughout the room. Such an active area should be placed near space needed for drying work, near the sink, and away from any quiet work station.

• **Difficulty with organization of materials within centers:** If your centers are constantly a mess, check to see if you have enough storage space for all materials necessary for the work at that center. Are the materials organized on a shelf, or do they sit out on the work area, so that messes occur and student work gets lost in the materials? Collect old baskets, cardboard shoe cubbies, file holders, and plastic stacking shelves used for mail. Use these to keep work areas neat and materials orderly.

• **Poor traffic patterns:** Do children have to travel through centers to get to their cubbies? Must they move through someone's work area to change centers, wash their hands, get a drink, or use the restroom? No center should be designed around busy traffic routes. Check to see that your shelves and tables are positioned to encourage children to walk around centers, rather than through them.

• **Completed work constantly being misplaced:** Is there a special basket that holds completed work? Is it located near the center of the room with the children's center charts, or where you might be working with children during center time? Placing it in the center of the room allows you as well as other children to note if children put completed work papers away before getting their center chart to change work stations. This also allows you the opportunity to quickly ask if they have remembered to put their name on their papers.

All of these problems can be alleviated by simply redesigning your floor plan. But before you begin to move the furniture around, take a careful look on paper.

Recently, a good friend who teaches a multiage primary class wanted to make some changes before the new school year began. Carla was concerned that the older children returning to her classroom would be bored by the same setup. Carla is an excellent teacher, and knows her students inside and out. However, it always helps to get another point of view.

First, I asked her if the room had worked the year before. Her answer was, mostly yes, but not completely. I suggested that the children would feel comfortable knowing some things had remained constant. Leaving the furniture and center areas in

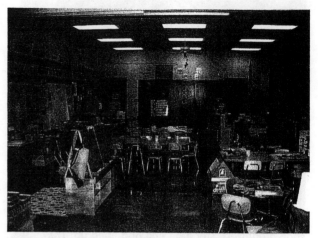

A view of my classroom. The easel, calendar math, writing, and language centers are on the left; games, art, and role play centers are on the right near the windows.

the same place, but changing several generic jobs, could help them recognize that their work would be expanded this year. I told Carla to think through her floor plan, listing things that worked very well and things that went wrong. If it worked well, she might be inviting trouble changing it just for the sake of change. But if there was a problem, maybe

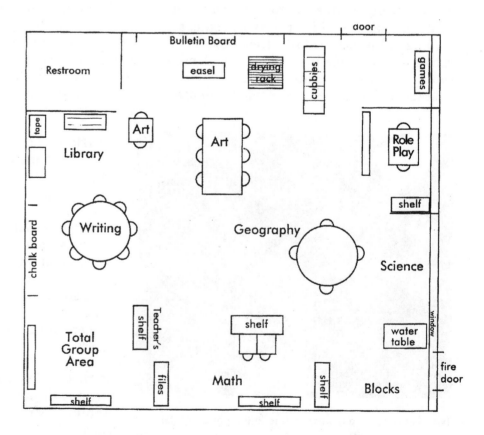

Fig. 2-4 Floor plan for a small, modular classroom.

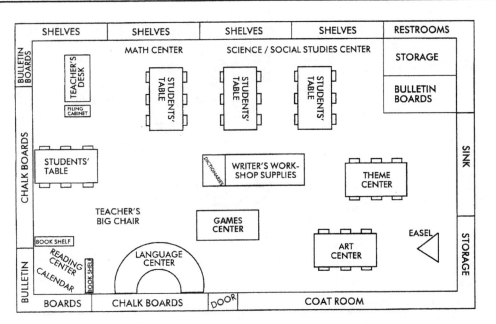

Fig. 2-5 Carla's room before she rearranged it. The games center located in the path to the doorway created problems; children brushing past it on the way home knocked puzzles onto the floor.

she could discover a better arrangement.

The next day, Carla came over set for the year. She had made a few simple changes, and now felt the room was perfect (see Fig. 2-5, 2-6, for Carla's before and after floor plans).

For example, she loved the art area near her sink, so that remained the same. However, she remembered that her daughter Chelsea had spent many an afternoon after school putting away puzzles. The games shelf was located near her doorway, and the puzzles often got knocked off the shelf as the class left in the afternoon. By thinking through what worked and what didn't, Carla was able to solve some problems without creating new ones.

Adding New Centers to Your Plan

Once you feel you're ready to add new centers, there are lots of ways to include them. The easiest is simply to observe the centers you already have in your classroom. Notice if any of them always takes your students an entire center time to complete the work. If so, you may have too many expectations for that one area. Think of ways you can break

that center into two different stations. What tasks would work well together, and be challenging and interesting enough to maintain the children's enthusiasm for that area?

I went through this several years ago. My art area consisted of a large table for specific art projects, a smaller table for "free" art experiences with materials such as play dough and paper scraps, and the easel. Too often, children would go to the art center and not have time for each task. So, my two art tables remained the art center, and the easel became a separate center.

In order to provide some choice in the easel center, I assigned one side of the easel to a specific task, while the other side contained different materials and could be used as the child wished. I later got a larger easel, with two places for painting on each side.

Another way to try out a new center is by setting up a temporary center based on the interests of your students. If it sustains their attention and can be easily assimilated into your room, it can become permanent.

For example, you could open an inventions center during a unit on simple machines or

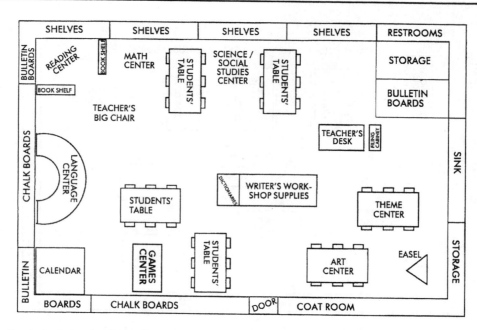

Fig. 2-6 Rearranging the room moved the games center out of the path of the children and provided a more secluded spot for the reading center. The students' tables are also placed more evenly throughout the room, creating several intimate environments for small group activities; previously, three of the tables had been bunched together at the back of the room.

transportation. The students could design and build simple inventions, constructing them with recycled materials, wood scraps, Legos™, or some other materials donated by students and local hardware stores. They could then write about their inventions' value, send away for a patent, and present their inventions to the class in order to promote their use.

If this area becomes popular, the class might ask to keep it going throughout the year. They could continue to invent products useful in other thematic units, such as weather gauges, solar vehicles, water-powered engines, or new uses of compost. The enthusiasm of the students determines whether or not the center becomes a permanent part of the classroom.

Another method for introducing a new center is to test it within an already existing center. My geography center is an example. It began as a portion of our science center. Each month, I created manipulative experiences to teach the children about people and places around the world. I started with only a few materials and books, and spent a year creating and locating enough activities to open a geography center the following year.

I was relieved to take this project slowly. It made it fun, rather than an overwhelming responsibility. Seven years later, my geography center continues to evolve as I change my focus from one particular country within a continent to another. But my young students still love to make maps and flags and study the habitats of their favorite animals. They love to play with the toys of children from other parts of the world. And together, we love the excellent books that teach us the folk tales and legends of other cultures.

Specific Activities in Centers

The activities in each area change throughout the year. It is most important to remember that each center should include numerous activities at a variety of developmental levels, in order to provide a developmentally appropriate environment for each student.

Books should be included in every center to demonstrate how they relate to our everyday lives. Joke books can be placed in the games center; number and shape books can be in the

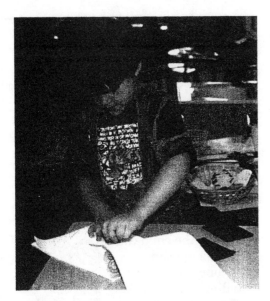

I have the children stamp the date on their journals after making an entry. Writing is a very important component of every center.

math center; coloring books and books with interesting illustrations can go in the art center; fiction and nonfiction books can be housed in science, geography, and language centers.

Writing should also be included in every center, for the experience of writing individualizes the instruction for each child. As children write, they reflect upon their own prior knowledge in order to assimilate or accommodate new information they have investigated. This reflective writing allows them to understand what they know, building the metacognitive skills they need in order to utilize their new knowledge.

I strongly believe that young children should have consistent opportunities to reread their own writing. Every time a young child writes, ensure that he can share his work with another person. In this way, he learns the power of literacy, and practices such skills as editing his own work and reading text with his own vocabulary, repeating activities specific to his stage of development.

Types of Activities

I have two main types of activities to complete in each center: specific tasks, which are jobs the children must do when working at the center; and work jobs, which are more generic in nature and are designed to offer opportunities to practice specific skills I have already taught to the class. The specific tasks come and go as students complete the work. The work jobs tend to stay for much longer periods of time in order to give children numerous chances to repeat the activities.

More specific examples of center tasks and jobs for each area of the room are given throughout the book, particularly in the chapters discussing each center area. Again, the "must do" tasks come and go, and are connected in some way to the thematic unit whenever possible. This allows students to make connections between concepts and across curricular areas, and encourages better use of the information when it comes time to solve problems.

This is an important element in an integrated curriculum. The jobs using the more generic materials allow for repetition of activities that reinforce key concepts within the curriculum. They are never designed to introduce a specific skill, but to reinforce a curricular objective that has already been taught. They should begin with the use of manipulatives, but opportunities to transfer the concept to abstract form should be available when students are ready.

For example, addition problems would be introduced by having the children count beads, then having them color those beads on paper, and finally by having them write the problems in number form.

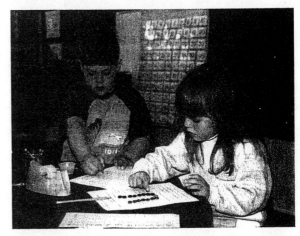

Children sort and count their m&m's for their graph. Each uses a different technique, one counting and marking the chart, the other placing candies on the graph.

Math Center Activity

This week, each child must complete one specific task: a bracelet made from a pipe cleaner and beads. The activity provides an opportunity to assess the children's patterning and counting skills. In a primary classroom, you might ask that they design their bracelet in an ABCD pattern, using a total of 20 beads. When they finish, they must write how many times they had to repeat their pattern in order to have the 20 beads.

For a more challenging task, design a more difficult problem. The children must use only 20 beads, but can choose from only three colors. What patterns can they create? Place a graph in the learning center showing the patterns the children created.

As a follow-up activity, divide the class into cooperative groups to discover how many different patterns it's possible to create with 20 beads and three colors. Many activities like this are open-ended, leaving the choice of pattern to the individual child.

Along with this pattern task are numerous other materials that each child can work with. He can:

- sort and classify postage stamps from a small plastic container
- make additional patterns with Unifix ™ cubes, beads, and tiles

- investigate sets of numerals using beads and cups (found in *Math Their Way*)
- seriate bottles of seeds from the least full to the most
- seriate mittens, shells, insects, or trucks (depending on the thematic unit) from the smallest to the largest
- count change according to the number of days the child has been in school (Example: on the 25th day of school, the child can use coins to count to 25 — one quarter, or two dimes and a nickel, or five nickels, etc.)

I assign the number of jobs that the children must complete. It is each child's responsibility to choose jobs which encourage her math development. I monitor her progress, assessing her completed work, reteaching when necessary, and directing her to try a specific job when she hasn't tackled a job she should have attempted.

Many of the materials stay in the center for the entire year (Unifix™ cubes, money, beads, junk boxes, tiles . . .), but the tasks the children complete with them increase in difficulty.

Part 3: Creating a Literate Environment *by Jean Feldman*

Children should be immersed in language so they can begin to appreciate its beauty and importance at an early age.

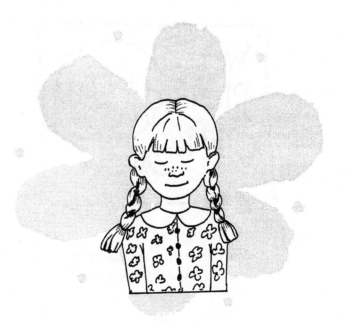

Part 3: Creating a Literate Environment. From *Wonderful Rooms Where Children Can Bloom! (K-2)*, by Jean R. Feldman. Peterborough, NH: Crystal Springs Books, 1997.

Signs

Signs can be used to encourage reading and writing skills, to demonstrate how functional language is, and to remind children of appropriate behavior.

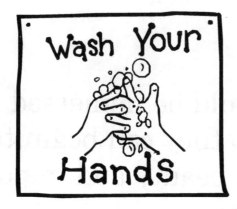

Put a reminder on the back of the bathroom door

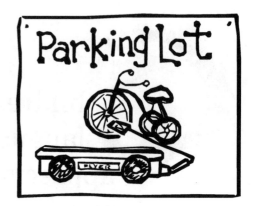

Use a sign to show where riding toys should be parked.

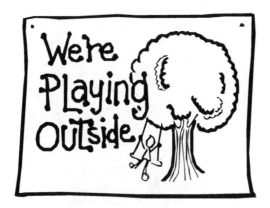

Use signs on the classroom door to show where you are.

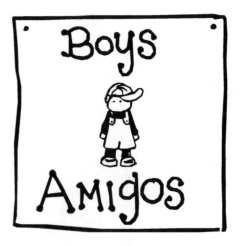

Create bilingual signs

Creating A Literate Environment ✵

Charts and Posters

Use charts and posters daily to reinforce the usefulness of reading and writing.

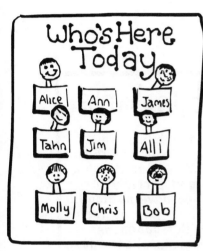

Sign In

Let each child draw her face on a circle and attach it to a popsicle stick. As the children come into the classroom each day, have each child select her stick from a basket, then place it in an envelope with her name on it. (Real photos of the children's faces can also be used.)

Job Chart

Write jobs on a poster, then write children's names on cutouts of hands. Attach Velcro to the backs of the hand cutouts and the poster so that each child can put his name by the job he would like to do.

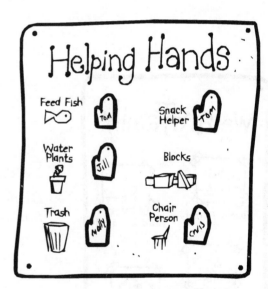

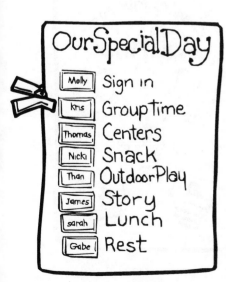

Daily Schedule

Write your daily schedule on a poster. Illustrate with real photographs of children participating in these activities or with pictures from school supply catalogs. (Use a clothespin to mark your progress through the schedule as you complete different activities.)

Top Tunes

- 🐟 Baby Fish
- ⭐ Twink a Link
- ⋔ McDonald's
- 🧱 Humpty Dumpty
- 🐊 Alligator

Song Chart

Let children tell you their favorite songs and write them on a poster. Add a picture clue for each song. When you need a song, ask a child to choose one from the chart.

Songs and Poems

Write words to songs, poems, or finger plays on charts. Point to the words as the children say or sing them.

Elephants

Elephants walk
like this and that.
They're terribly big
and terribly fat.
They have no hands.
They have no toes.
But goodness,
gracious what a nose!

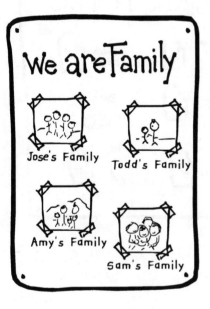

We are Family

Jose's Family | Todd's Family

Amy's Family

Sam's Family

Family Photos

Display photos of children's families.

Grandparents

Ask children to bring in pictures of their grandparents. Hang them on a poster and label.

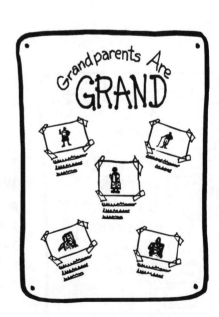

Grandparents Are GRAND

Creating A Literate Environment ✵

Language Experiences

Language experience charts reinforce the concept that, "What I say can be written down, and what is written down I can read."

Happiness Is...

Tasha - Spending the night with Granny.

Josh - Riding my bike.

Sami - Getting my new bird Tweetie.

Beth - My birthday party!

Complete a sentence
Ask children to complete an open-ended sentence.

The Pumpkin Patch

We went to Farmer Joe's Pumpkin Patch.

We rode a big yellow Bus.

We had a picnic.

Field Trip
Follow up a field trip with a story about it.

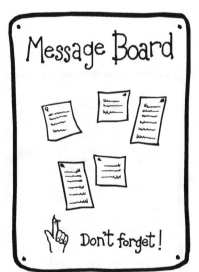

Message Board

Don't forget!

Messages
Use a message board with sticky notes as a reminder to you and the children.

When I Grow Up

Sadik - I might be a fire fighter.

Maria - I want to be a doctor.

Fritz - I'm going to be a baseball player.

Unit of study
Relate language experience charts to a unit of study.

❀ *Wonderful Rooms Where Children Can Bloom!*

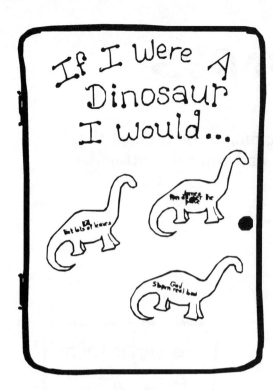

Cutouts

Write children's individual responses to questions on cutouts, then tape them onto a door.

Class Rules

Let children help formulate classroom rules. Refer to the rules when there is a conflict.

Class Rules

- Be kind to Friends.
- Take Care of yourself.
- Take care of our things at School.

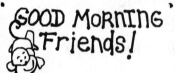

GOOD MORNING Friends!

What a great day we will have!

We're going to read a story about monkeys,

then make a monkey sandwich.

Today's Special

Write a message to the children each morning welcoming them. Include the special activities you will do that day.

Linesia Ray
Star Student

Linesia is five years old.

She likes to read and roller skate.

She has two little brothers.

Pink is her favorite color.

Star Student

Highlight unique qualities of a different child each week. Include her picture, likes, dislikes, favorite books, pets, etc.

 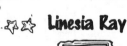

Daily News

September 29, 1999

We went to a puppet show in the library.

We sorted leaves,

then we made party pizzas for snack.

We played ponies outside.

Daily News

At the end of the school day, have the children recall the events of the day in sequence. Write down what they liked best or what they learned.

Homework

Write down a homework assignment or extension activity children can do each evening. Have the children read over it with you before they leave each day.

HOMEWORK

Bring in a sign of Fall.

Don't forget to bring in old newspapers for the paper drive.

Rebus Activity Charts

Rebus cards encourage children to "read pictures," follow directions, and work independently.

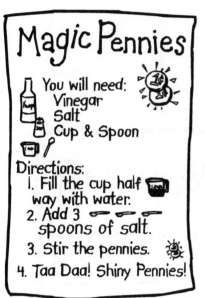

Magic Pennies

You will need:
Vinegar
Salt
Cup & Spoon

Directions:
1. Fill the cup half way with water.
2. Add 3 spoons of salt.
3. Stir the pennies.
4. Taa Daa! Shiny Pennies!

Science Experiments

Place directions for science experiments on charts.

Music

Have children construct their own musical instruments.

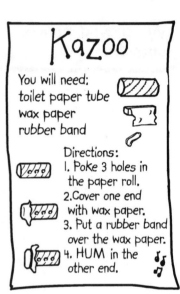

Kazoo

You will need:
toilet paper tube
wax paper
rubber band

Directions:
1. Poke 3 holes in the paper roll.
2. Cover one end with wax paper.
3. Put a rubber band over the wax paper.
4. HUM in the other end.

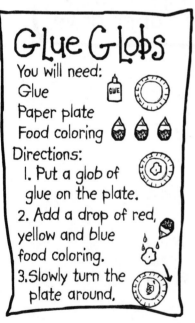

Glue Globs

You will need:
Glue
Paper plate
Food coloring

Directions:
1. Put a glob of glue on the plate.
2. Add a drop of red, yellow and blue food coloring.
3. Slowly turn the plate around.

Art Projects

Hang directions for art activities in the art center.

Manipulatives

Children will develop motor skills as they follow picture directions.

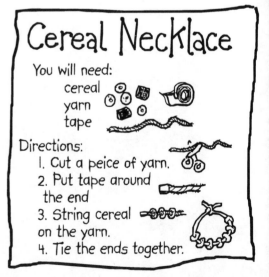

Cereal Necklace

You will need:
cereal
yarn
tape

Directions:
1. Cut a peice of yarn.
2. Put tape around the end
3. String cereal on the yarn.
4. Tie the ends together.

Walk-About Story

All children will be motivated to read the walk-about story.

Materials: . . . .

- ✹ butcher paper
- ✹ markers, crayons, or paints
- ✹ clear packaging tape

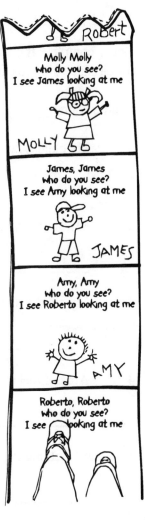

Directions: . . . .

Roll out a long sheet of paper.

Mark off 2' sections on the paper.

Let each child draw his picture and write his name in one of the sections.

Write the following chant in each section:

> (First name), (name) who do you see?
> I see (second child's name) looking at me.
>
> (Second name), (name) who do you see?
> I see (third child's name) looking at me.

And so forth....

Tape the paper to the floor with clear packaging tape. (You can also cover it with clear contact paper.)

Variations: . . . .

Let the children write and illustrate their own original stories using a similar format.

Have the children work together to write and illustrate a story. Hang the pages in the hallway. Tape a sheet of paper to the top of each page so other students walking down the hall will be curious and will want to lift the sheets and read the story.

✹ *Wonderful Rooms Where Children Can Bloom!*

PARENT CONFERENCE QUESTIONNAIRE

Please complete the statements below and bring this with you when you come for our conference. I'll look forward to the insight you will share with me on your child.

Child's Name_____   Date_____

1. My child's favorite activity at school is_____

    _____

2. My child expresses concern about _____

    _____

3. My child's strong qualities are _____

    _____

4. Areas I feel my child needs to work on are _____

    _____

5. Something my child would like to do at school is_____

    _____

6. Something I would like to see my child do at school is_____

    _____

7. Is there any special information about your child that you think we should know about?

    _____

    _____

*   Send home a list of multiple intelligences with a brief description of each. Ask parents to read over the list so they can discuss areas that they perceive to be their child's strengths.

Jean Feldman

PICTURE ME!

Name_____   Date_____

My favorite things to do are...

My special friends are...

Books I like to read are...

A song I like to sing is....

I like to eat...

My favorite center is...

This is a picture of me doing what I do best...

ASSESSMENT

Child's Name _____

Teacher _____

Birthday _____

LANGUAGE DEVELOPMENT	DATE	COMMENTS	DATE	COMMENTS
Recognizes colors				
Recognizes rhyming words				
Recognizes upper case letters ABCDEFGHIJKLMNOPQRSTUVWXYZ				
Recognizes lower case letters abcdefghijklmnopqrstuvwxyz				
Matches beginning consonant sounds				
Recognizes some sight words				
Says birthday, phone number, address				
Sequences several pictures				
Identifies opposites				
Speaks clearly				
Makes few grammatical errors				
Communicates well with friends and teachers				
"Acts out" and pretends				
Listens to story 10-15 minutes				
Follows 3 or more directions in order				
Retells story				

Jean Feldman

ASSESSMENT

Child's Name _____

Birthday _____

Teacher _____

MATH READINESS	DATE	COMMENTS
Counts to 50		
Recognizes numerals 0-20		
Makes sets 1-10		
Joins sets		
Separates sets		
Names shapes		
Separates coins		
Measures objects with standard unit		
Makes comparisons (more, less, equal)		
PHYSICAL DEVELOPMENT (LARGE MOTOR)	DATE	COMMENTS
Runs smoothly		
Throws ball with direction		
Gallops		
Skips		
Hangs by hands on bars		
Hops on alternating feet		

Jean Feldman

211

EMOTIONAL DEVELOPMENT	DATE	COMMENTS	DATE	COMMENTS
Maintains self control				
Verbalizes feelings				
Is aware of and responds to feelings of others				
Demonstrates self-confidence				
Works out own problems				
Shows pride in work				
Uses positive body language				

Additional Teacher Comments:

Date of Conference: _____   Parent Signature: _____

Additional Teacher Comments:

Date of Conference: _____   Parent Signature: _____

Jean Feldman

PHYSICAL DEVELOPMENT (SMALL MOTOR)	DATE	COMMENTS	DATE	COMMENTS
Writes first and last name				
Controls paint brush				
Draws person with detailed body parts				
Works 10-12 piece puzzle				
Stacks 10-12 blocks				
Cuts out simple objects				
"Handedness" established				
Writes some numerals, letters				
SOCIAL DEVELOPMENT				
Conforms to group				
Plays simple games				
Chooses friends				
Cooperates with adults				
Takes turns willingly				
SOCIAL DEVELOPMENT (SELF-HELP SKILLS)				
Ties shoes				
Dresses self completely				
Cares for personal hygiene (brushes hair, teeth, etc.)				
Helps prepare for activities				
Cleans up after self				

Jean Feldman

213

PORTFOLIO/YEARBOOK

Skills: assessment; children's progress

Materials: large paper grocery sacks (10 for each child), crayons, markers, pens, pencils, and other art supplies, hole punch, yarn or string

Directions: At the beginning of each month give children a grocery sack and ask them to decorate it with their picture and a sentence. (For younger children, the teacher will need to write the month and a sentence the child dictates.) As the children complete different projects during the month, file their work in their sacks. Examples might include self portraits, writing samples, drawings, art work, paintings, photos, anecdotal records, books read, interest survey, reading log, cutting and pasting samples, journal entries, etc.
At the end of the year give each child a blank sack to decorate for their cover. (A photograph can also be used on the cover.) Put the sacks in order, hole punch, and tie them together with string or yarn.

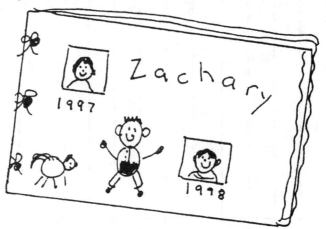

Adaptations: Use these books at your end of year conference with parents.

Clasp envelopes can also be used to make portfolios for the children. Simply have the children decorate an envelope each month and save samples of their work. At the end of the year, punch 2 holes in each envelope and put them together with book rings.

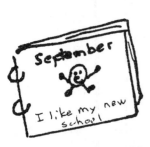

Hint!   Store paper sacks in a plastic milk crate with the open end up. Print each child's name near the opening so it can be seen.

Use a date stamp to date samples of work.

Jean Feldman

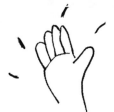 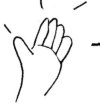

Creating a Children's "Discovery Museum" in Your Classroom

SCIENCE - <u>Muddy Bottle</u> - Put ½ cup of dirt in a plastic bottle, then add water. Glue on the lid and let the children shake the bottle and observe as the dirt settles. Experiment with sand, gravel, potting soil, etc. to see which one settles first. Have the children write relatives in other parts of the United States asking them to send a bag of dirt or sand from where they live. Compare.

BLOCKS - <u>"Me" Blocks</u> - Cut the top off two cardboard milk cartons (pint or quart size). Insert one carton inside the other. Glue the child's picture on one side, then glue paper on the other sides and let the child decorate. Cover with clear contact paper or clear packing tape. Use in the block center, then send home at the end of the year.

DRAMATIC PLAY - <u>Story Headbands</u> - Use felt or yarn to decorate plastic headbands for role-play or acting out stories. Glue on pink felt ears for a pig, yellow yarn for hair, brown ears for a dog, etc.

LANGUAGE - <u>Wipe Off Boards</u> - Purchase a sheet of "wipe off board" at a hardware or building supply store. Cut it into individual squares (12"). Write each child's name at the top in dotted lines with a permanent marker. Store in a plastic crate. Children can practice writing their names, draw pictures, or use as lap boards.

SENSORY - <u>Potato Dig</u> - Make potatoes by cutting off the foot from a pair of panty hose. Stuff the remainder of the panty hose in the toe of that foot and tie a knot around it to make a ball. Trim. Hide "potatoes" in the sandbox or put dirt in the water table and let the children "dig" them up with shovels and pails. (Use real potatoes, then let the children scrub, cook, and eat them!)

MANIPULATIVES - <u>Play Trays</u> - Place lunchroom trays on a table and put different textures and materials on them. You might use shaving cream, playdough and cookie cutters, scrap paper and a hole punch, colored water with eye droppers and cups, rice and plastic animals, pasta with holes and shoelaces, etc.

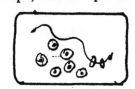 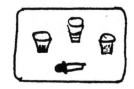

MATH - <u>Bean Ruler</u> - To make a bean ruler you will need clear packaging tape and large lima beans. Cut off a piece of tape (8" long) and lay it on the table sticky side up. Place 10-12 beans in the middle of the tape side by side, then fold over the tape. Let the children count "how many beans" long different objects are.

MUSIC - <u>Shaker</u> - Cut a slit in an old tennis ball with a utility knife. Insert beans, popcorn kernels, or pebbles and shake.

LIBRARY - <u>Big Book</u> - Use paper grocery sacks or poster board cut in half to make a big book. Take pictures of your school, community, or use local postcards. Incorporate the places on the pictures with this chant "<u>(place)</u>, <u>(place)</u> What do you see? I see <u>(another place)</u> looking at me."

ART - <u>Creative Brushes</u> - Let children paint with old make-up brushes, a shaving brush, pine needles, rubber bands tied together, a feather duster, car sponge, their elbows, Q-tips, a fly swatter, or anything else you can think of. To save paper, paint on old newspapers.

CONSTRUCTION - <u>Tin Punch</u> - Let children hammer nails in pie pans to create designs.

LARGE MOTOR - <u>Hand Ball</u> - Staple 2 paper plates together ¾ of the way around. Make a ball by wrapping masking tape around a wad of paper. Insert the hand in the paper plate and "bat" at the ball.

BOTTLES OF FUN

Children will have hours of fun shaking, observing, predicting, and playing with these bottles. Any type of plastic drinking bottle may be used. (Secure the lid with Super Glue.)

Muddy Water Bottle - Put ½ cup of dirt in the bottle. Fill it to the top with water. Shake, then observe as the dirt settles to the bottom. (Use peat moss, potting soil, clay, and other types of soil.)

Glitter Bottle - Add several tablespoons of glitter, 3 drops food coloring then fill to the top with water. Watch it sparkle!

Crayon Shavings - Shave old crayons, then add ¼-½ cup of the crayon shavings to the bottle. Fill with water, then turn the bottle upside down and watch the shavings slowly float around.

Bubble Bottle - Fill the bottle half full with water. Add several drops of detergent and food coloring. Shake. How long does it take for the bubbles to disappear?

Quiet Bottle - Pour ½ cup of clear corn syrup into the bottle. Add food coloring, then turn the bottle all around to coat the sides. Make bottles for different holidays by adding glitter or sequins to bottles. (This bottle can help a child who is upset to relax and settle down. That's why it's called the quite bottle!)

Beach Bottle - Put some sand in the bottom of the bottle. Add some small shells and fill half way with water. Squirt in some blue food coloring. To make a tiny fish, blow a little air into a small balloon and knot. Add eyes and a mouth to the fish with a permanent marker, then insert in the bottle.

Magnetic Bottle - Fill the bottle half way with sand. Add nails, pins, paper clips, tacks and other small objects that are attracted to a magnet. Tie a magnet to an 18" piece of string. Tie the other end of the string to the mouth of the bottle. Take the magnet and run it around the side of the bottle trying to attract the objects.

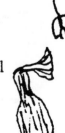

Mystery Sound Bottle - Add rice, beans, popcorn, and other materials to plastic bottles. Pull an old sock around each bottle. Have children shake the bottles and try to identify the objects by sound.

Tornado Bottle - Make several small aluminum foil balls by rolling up little pieces of foil. Put these in the bottle, then fill almost to the top with water. Add a small drop of detergent and some food coloring. Turn the bottle upside down and swirl it in a circular motion to create a "tornado" in the bottle.

HOMEMADE BOOKS

Children love to make books, which are a perfect way to reinforce reading and writing skills.

Baggie Book:

Cut construction paper to fit inside a plastic bag. Draw a picture, or glue on a photograph or magazine picture. Insert the picture in the baggie and zip it up. Put several of these together with a book ring, pipe cleaner, or ribbon to make a book.

Lunch Bag Book:

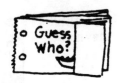

Take four or five lunch bags and fold the bottom over to one side. Glue an animal shape or other picture so part of it is hidden under the flap. Put the pages of the book together with a brad fastener or yarn. Children can try to guess what the animal is, then open the flap to see if they are correct. Older children can write riddles or other questions on the bag, then hide the answer under the flap.

Class Books:

Let everyone in the class draw a picture and write or dictate a sentence to go with it. Put the pages together and make a book the whole class can enjoy. Some topics might be:

> "The Magic Wish"
> "I Would Like to Tell the President"
> "If I Were in Charge of the World"
> "My Nightmare Looks Like"
> "Things to Be Happy About"
> "My Invention"
> "I Can Do Something Special"
> "When I Get Mad"
> "How to Save Our Planet Earth"
> "When I Grow Up"
> "If I Won a Million Dollars"

Let the children take turns checking these books out to take home and share with their families.

Teeny Tiny Book:

Sometimes children like big books, and sometimes they like little tiny books. Cut paper into 3" × 2" rectangles and staple together for creative book making.

Tag-Along Book:

Attach a pipe cleaner handle to a homemade book and it will "tag along" with you wherever you go.

Jean Feldman

Step Book:

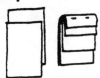

Take two sheets of paper and layer them about 2" apart as shown. Fold backwards, then staple at the top to make four pages. This is a good book for writing a story in sequence. (Add more pages according to the ability of your students.)

Big Book Joke Book:

Cut large sheets of posterboard in half. Divide children into pairs, and give each pair a piece of this posterboard. On the front they write a riddle, and on the back they draw the answer. Put all the pages together with book rings to make a class big book.

Grocery Bag Big Book:

Cut the front and back off grocery bags. Let the children draw pictures or write stories on these, then put them together with yarn to make a book. This is a fun book for illustrating songs or poems, such as "Frog Went a-Courtin'," "Old MacDonald's Farm," or "Five Little Monkeys."

Shape Books:

Cut construction paper and inside pages in various shapes to correlate with a unit of study, book, concept, and so forth.

Wallpaper Book:

Cover cardboard with wallpaper scraps to make the outside of a book. Staple blank sheets of paper inside.

Cereal Box Book:

Cut off the front and back of a cereal or other food box. Cut paper to fit inside. Punch holes and tie with yarn.

Fabric Book:

Glue fabric scraps to cardboard to make the outside cover for a book.

Self-Stick Vinyl:

Attach self-stick vinyl to the front and back cover of a homemade book.

Mylar Balloon:

Cut apart an old mylar balloon. Laminate it, then cut newsprint pages to fit inside. Use ribbon, a brad fastener, or book ring to put it together.

PLAY WITH ME
Home / School Activities

1. Take a walk together.

2. Say your phone number and address.

3. Help fold the laundry.

4. Count the doors in your house.

5. Look for something beautiful outside.

6. Can you find 10 things in your house that are red?

7. Read a book together.

8. Put on some music and make up a dance.

9. Find a picture in a magazine and make up a story about it.

10. Draw foods you like on a paper plate.

11. Can you hop, skip, gallop, and jump?

12. Say some nursery rhymes.

13. Practice what you would do if there were a fire at your house.

14. Find 8 objects that are smaller than your thumb.

15. Teach a song to your family.

16. Think of words that rhyme with "man" , "cat," "like," " big," "hot," and "bee."

17. Cook something for your family to eat.

18. Go on a shape hunt around your house; find squares, triangles, and circles.

19. Play a game like "Hide and Go Seek" or "I Spy."

20. Name the months in the year.

21. Draw a picture for someone you love.

WALLY GATOR

(Have a green piece of construction paper in your lap before you begin telling this story.)

Once upon a time there was a little girl
named Emalene who lived in Louisiana
in the bayou. She was very good friends
with all the animals who lived in the swamp-
especially Wally Gator. One day Emalene
left her house and went looking for Wally.

Fold the paper in half. Have the
fold at the bottom. Tear out half
a circle to be the door of Emalene's
house.

Emalene walked up and down the canals
in the bayou calling, "Wally. Wally Gator."
At last she came to the end of the swamp,
but still she did not see Wally.

Tear zig zags out of the fold as
shown.

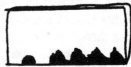

So slowly she walked back home.

Trace your finger over the zig zag
lines as she walks home.
Open the paper to reveal an alligator.

And guess who was waiting for her when
she got there? WALLY GATOR!

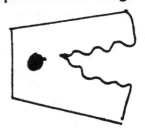

PICNIC BOOK

(Have a plain piece of paper in your lap as you begin to tell the story.)

Let's go on a picnic. Here's our picnic
basket.

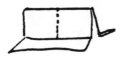

Fold the paper in half.

We'll need some hot dogs.

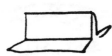

Fold the paper in fourths.

And let's take some hamburgers, too.

Fold in eighths.

Now we need a picnic bench.

Open the paper so it is folded
in half. Bend up the bottom sections
in opposite directions for a bench.

And we have so much food, it'd
be much more fun if we shared
this with a friend.

Tear down on the middle fold half
way to indicate dividing it in half.

And it be wonderful to have a book
to draw pictures of all our special
memories.

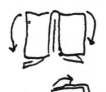

Hold the bench at the top, then bring
the bottom ends together. Fold the

BABY BIRD

(Have a piece of paper, scissors, and crayon in your lap before you begin the story.)

It was spring and time for the birds to build a nest. What do you think the birds used to build their nest? (Accept all answers from the children.) Did you know that birds are natural recyclers because they take bits of string, trash, sticks, and other things people throw away and use them to build their nests? The birds worked very hard carrying things in their little beaks to build their nest and this is what it looked like. (Fold paper in half and cut a semi-circle out on the fold as shown.) Mother bird sat on her nest a long time and she finally laid a beautiful egg. (Open the paper to reveal the egg.) She had to sit on the egg in the sun and in the rain and when the wind blew. Now she would have been very lonesome, but she made friends with two little bugs. This is what the bugs looked like. (Draw dots on either side of the shape.) Finally one day mother bird heard a little sound. She looked down and there was a crack in the egg. (Cut a slit toward the dots.) Then she heard a big crack. (Cut out the shape as shown.) And out of the egg came a baby bird! (Open the egg, bend out the beak, and fold up the bird.)

Cut two bodies out of felt. Cut out wings. Glue the beak in the head, then glue around the outside edges of the body leaving an opening in the bottom for your finger. Insert the wings in the slit on the top.

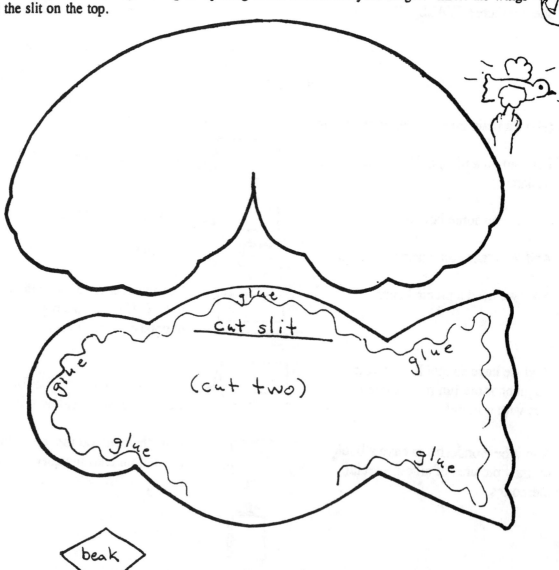

Jean Feldman

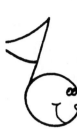

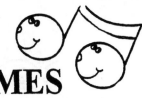

TUNES FOR TRANSITION TIMES

GUIDING CHILDREN WITH SONGS AND CHANTS

Hello Song
(Tune: Skip to My Lou)

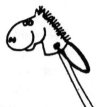

Hello, how are you?
Hello, how are you?
Hello, how are you?
How are you this morning?

I am fine, and I hope you are, too.
I am fine, and I hope you are, too.
I am fine, and I hope you are, too.
I hope you are, too, this morning.

Turn to your neighbor and shake their hand.
Turn to your neighbor and shake their hand.
Turn to your neighbor and shake their hand.
Shake their hand this morning.

VARIATIONS: Make up new verses, such
as "turn to your neighbor and give high five,"
or "turn to your neighbor and give them a hug."

Choo Choo Name Song
(Tune: A Tisket a Tasket)

Refrain:
Choo choo choo choo choo choo choo
Up the railroad track.
Choo choo choo choo choo choo choo
And then it comes right back.

First it goes to (child's name) house,
Then it goes to (second child's name),
Then it goes to (third child's name),
And then it goes to (fourth child's name).

Continue singing the refrain and verse
with the children's names as you go around
the circle.

I Wish I Had a Little Red Box
(Tune: Polly Wolly Doodle)

I wish I had a little red box
to put my mommy in.
I'd take her out and go
kiss, kiss, kiss,
And put her back again.

Daddy...hug, hug, hug.

Good friends... "How do you do?"

Activities: Have the children paint a big
box red. Let one child at a time get in
the box as you sing their name in the song.

Write children's names on index cards and
put them in a tissue box covered with red
paper. Pull out one name at a time and sing
the song using that child's name. (For
younger children glue their photograph
beside their name.)

Clippity Clop

Clippity clop, clippity clop,
On our way to (child's name) stop.
Hi (child's name).
Bye (child's name).

Clippity clop...
Continue singing different children's names

Special Me
(Tune: Twinkle Little Star)

Special, special, special me.
I'm as special as can be.
There is no one quite like me.
I'm as good as I can be.
Special, special, special me.
I'm as special as can be!

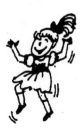

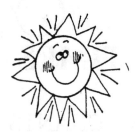

Weather Song
(Tune: My Darling Clementine)

Sunny, sunny, sunny, sunny,
It is sunny in the sky.
S - U - N - N - Y , sunny,
It is sunny in the sky.

(Substitute cloudy, rainy, or
other weather words in the song.)

Hi Ho Helper Song
(Tune: Seven Dwarfs' Song)

Hi ho, hi ho,
A cleaning up we'll go.
Put the toys away
For another day,
Hi ho, hi ho, hi ho,
Hi ho, hi ho,
A picking up we'll go.
So everyone
Join in the fun,
Hi ho, hi ho.

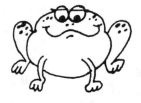

Jolly Good Helper
(Tune: Jolly Good Fellow)

(Child's name) is a jolly good helper.
(Child's name) is a jolly good helper.
(Child's name) is a jolly good helper,
He/she is picking up the blocks.
(Insert appropriate behavior.)

Handy Wash Song
(Tune: Row Your Boat)

Wash, wash, wash your hands
Play the handy game.
Rub and scrub and scrub and rub,
Germs go down the drain.

Everybody Do This
(Tune: Shortnin' Bread)

Everybody do this, do this, do this.
Everybody do this just like me.
Everybody stand up...
Everybody line up...
Everybody tip toe... etc.
(Sing the directions to the children
for whatever you want them to do.)

Ten Little Friends

Ten little friends came out to play
On a very bright and sunny day.
And they had a little talk.
Talk, talk, talk, talk, talk, talk.
And they took a little walk.
Walk, walk, walk, walk, walk, walk, stop!
Til they came to a great, big hill.
And they climbed to the top -
Do, do, do, do, do, do, do-
And they stood on the top
And were very still.
Til they all tumbled down.
Brrrrrrrrrm.
And they fell to the ground.
"We're so tired," they all said.
So they all went home and went to bed.
1-2-3-4-5-6-7-8-9-10.
Good night!

Miss Sue

Miss Sue, Miss Sue,
Miss Sue from Alabama.
Sitting in her rocker,
Eating Betty Crocker,
Watching the clock go...
Tick-tock-tick-tock banana rock.
Tick-tock-tick-tock banana rock.
Oosha mama - oosha mama - oosha mama
        Freeze!   (Children freeze in place.)

Jean Feldman

Cool Bear Hunt

(Children stand and act out motions.)

Chorus: We're going on a bear hunt.
We're gonna catch a big one.
With big green eyes
And a fuzzy little tail.

Look over there.
It's a candy factory.
Can't go over it.
Can't go under it.
Can't go around it.
Guess we'll go through it.
Yum, yum, yum, yummmm.
(Chorus)

Look over there.
It's a peanut butter river....
Guess we'll swim across it.
(Chorus)

Look over there.
It's a Jell-O swamp....
Guess we'll go through it.

Look over there.
It's a cave....
I guess we'll go through it.
It's cold in here.
I see two big green eyes
And a fuzzy little tail.
It's a bear!
HELP!
Go through the Jell-O swamp.
Go through the peanut butter river.
Go through the candy factory.
Run home.
Open the door. Shut the door.
We went on a bear hunt,
And we weren't afraid!

VARIATIONS: Change the words to going
on a dinosaur hunt, lion hunt, or to look
for other imaginary animals.

Tooty Ta

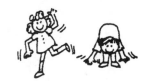

A tooty ta,
a tooty ta,
a tooty ta ta.
A tooty ta,
a tooty ta,
a tooty ta ta.

Thumbs up....
Elbows back....
Feet apart....
Knees in....
Bottoms up....
Tongue out....
Turn around....
Eyes closed.

(Add these different
motions to each
verse as you sing it.)

Concept Song
(Tune: Muffin Man)

Oh, do you see the color red?
The color red? The color red?
Oh, do you see the color red
Somewhere in the room?

(Choose a child to point to the color
and sing in reply.)

Oh, yes I see the color red,
The color red, the color red.
Oh, yes I see the color red,
Somewhere in the room.

Variations: Use this song to
reinforce shapes, letters, numerals,
words, etc.

Nursery Rhyme ABC
(Tune: 100 Bottles of Beer on the Wall)

ABCDEFG
HIJKL (clap!)
MNOPQRS
TUVWXYZ

Try singing different nursery rhymes
to "100 Bottles of Beer on the Wall."
Sing the letters of the alphabet
between each verse.

CLASS SONG
(Tune: Old MacDonald)

(Teacher's name) had a class
E I E I O.
And in his/her class,
He/she had a (child's name)
E I E I O.
With a "Hi, hi," here,
And a "Hi, hi," there.
Here a "Hi", there a "Hi,"
Everywhere a "Hi, hi."
(Teacher's name) had a class
E I E I O.

Continue singing the song with
other children's names and inserting
their suggestions for what they would
like to say.

Bubble Gum

Bubble gum, bubble gum,
chewy, chewy, chewy, chewy, chewy
bubble gum.

Bubble gum, bubble gum,
chewy, chewy, chewy, chewy, chewy
bubble gum.

I love it! I love it!
Chewy, chewy, chewy, chewy, chewy
bubble gum.

I love it! I love it!
Chewy, chewy, chewy, chewy, chewy
bubble gum.

Faster now...

Super fast...

Variations: Sing this song loud, soft,
slow, opera style, baby style, underwater
(put finger between lips and vibrate), and
other silly versions.

Creative Ways with Old Songs

Sing the names of the President's to
"Ten Little Indians."

Use the children's names in "The
Eency Weency Spider," "Five Little
Monkeys Jumping on the Bed," and
other songs.

Sing songs in loud "monster voices,"
soft "mouse voices," "fast speed,"
"slow speed," and so forth.

Learn phone numbers by singing them
to the tune of "Twinkle, Twinkle,
Little Star."

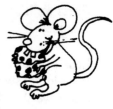

Love
(Sing in sign language.)

Love grows
One by one,
Two by two,
And four by four.

Love grows
Round like a circle
And comes back knocking
At your front door.

It Is Time to Say Good-bye
(Tune: She'll Be Coming Round the Mountain)

Clap your hands.
Stomp your feet.
It is time to say good-bye to all my friends.
It is time to say good-bye to all my friends.
It is time to say good-bye
Give a smile and wink your eye.
It is time to say good-bye to all my friends.
Good-bye friends.
Yee haw!

Jean Feldman

Individual Storyboards

Storyboards are a way of retelling where students re-create the setting and make paper puppets. There are a number of ways for students to make their own storyboards. Here are three of my students' favorites:

Paper Bag Storyboards

Each student will need his/her own paper bag. Holding the bag either horizontally or vertically, students illustrate the setting on the front of the bag. Students love this because the storyboard stands up while they are retelling. Puppets can be made out of paper and put on popsicle sticks.

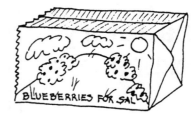

Another way to use paper bags is to cut them into the shape of a house, step 1. Staple on two paper doors, step 2. Students can then have two scene settings from the story, one on the doors and one inside the house. Puppets can be kept in back of the storyboard in the pocket that is formed when the doors are stapled on.

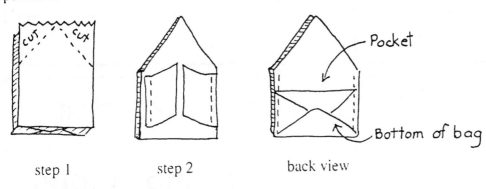

step 1   step 2   back view

Stand up Storyboards

Stand up storyboards can be made with a 9" x 12" piece of paper. If desired, cut the top of the paper into some kind of design, step 1. The paper can also be left alone so that it is rectangular in shape. I found that my students liked the idea of making the top different shapes. Fold the paper into thirds, step 2. Students can now draw the setting. Tape or glue a pocket onto the back of the 9" x 12" paper to hold the puppets.

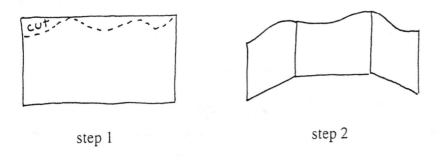

step 1   step 2

Use quality children's literature as the heart of your skills instruction

Skill(s)

Sight Vocabulary
multiple exposures
tally

Skill
modeled many times
limit 2-3

Books, Poems, Chants

Activities (skill)

Interactive Chart

Highlighting Tape with Books

Overheads from books

Literature Extensions (Book)

Book Innovations

Assessment
Depth of knowledge

Flip Books

Open-ended Sheets

Storyboards

Character Pictures

Literary Friends

Name _____ **Date** _____

Title of Book _____

Author _____

What was your favorite part? _____

Name: _____   **Date:** _____

Title:
_____

Author:
_____

Illustrator:
_____

This book was about

_____

_____

_____

_____

My favorite part was

_____

_____

_____

_____

    Patricia Pavelka

Literacy Centers

Writing Center
What can I do?

1. Shape Books
   story
   facts
2. Letters
3. Books
4. Poems
5. Pretend you were a __
6. Report
7. Literature Theme
8. Literary Friends
9. Quick Writes

Reading Center
What can I do?

1. Read
2. Use yellow tape
3. Use clear paper
   and marker
4. Make a flipbook
5. Retell a story
6. Watch a filmstrip
   Discuss it
   Write a script
7. Text Innovation

* Manipulating Text
* Teach Text Innovations

Performance Assessments for Literacy

* **Retelling** (Language, Comprehension)
Storyboards

  Puppets

  No manipulatives

  Flipbooks (Summarizing)

* **Running Records** (Three Cueing Systems)

* **Think Alouds** (Process and Strategies)

* **Show What You Know** (Skills)

* **Anecdotal Records** (Putting it all together)
Look for trends and patterns:
Individual and Whole Class

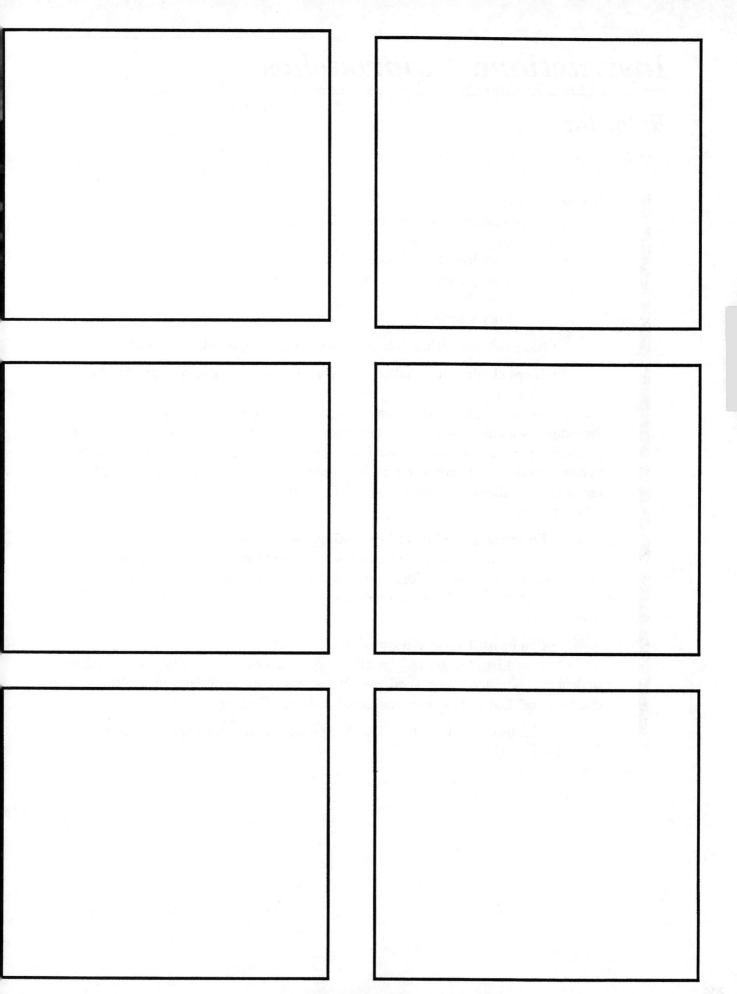

Instructional Approaches

Retelling

Retelling stories:
- **Helps children internalize story language.**

  Once upon a time . . . .
  They lived happily ever after . . . .
  They gnashed their terrible teeth and they roared their
     terrible roars . . . .
  They went out to seek their fortune . . . .

- **Increases comprehension of stories (beginning, middle, and end)**

- **Helps children internalize story elements (characters, setting, plot, theme, climax)**

  As children have many encounters with retelling, they learn to begin their stories with an introduction of the characters and the setting. They continue with the initial problem or events and retell the events/episodes in order. The idea of a story having a beginning (introduction), middle (series of events/episodes), and end (resolution) becomes internalized. Students begin to organize their thoughts and put the story into a coherent form.

- **Encourages confidence in speaking.**

  I notice the more often my students retell stories, the greater their confidence and self-esteem. For some children, speaking in front of a class is very scary. Have students start out by retelling aloud with no audience, then to a small group, and, finally, to the whole class.

- **Can be used as an assessment tool.**

  Listening to a child retell a story is a quick, easy way to assess whether a student has understood the general, overall meaning of the story. How many details did the child include? Did s/he use story language? Is the retelling organized?

- **Aids in vocabulary growth and expands and develops oral language.**

Excerpted from *Making the Connection: Learning Skills Through Literature* (K-2), by Patricia Pavelka. Peterborough, NH: Crystal Springs Books, 1995.

Barbara M. Taylor
Barbara E. Hanson
Karen Justice-Swanson
Susan M. Watts

Helping struggling readers: Linking small-group intervention with cross-age tutoring

The reading intervention program described in this study combined a modified enrichment program with cross-age tutoring and resulted in significant gains in reading for both students and tutors.

Providing the best reading instruction possible for children who are struggling academically remains a major responsibility for educators. Although the overall level of reading achievement in the United States has remained fairly stable since 1970 (Mullis & Jenkins, 1990) and is relatively high in international comparisons (Elley, 1992), we still have too many children and adolescents reading at low levels, which has a negative impact on their success in school (Williams, Reese, Campbell, Mazzeo, & Phillips, 1995). Recent data from the National Assessment of Educational Progress (NAEP) reveal that two fifths of the 1994 sample of fourth graders (age 9 to 10) failed to demonstrate even a basic level of reading ability. We also know that students who are struggling in reading come disproportionately from families of poverty (Mullis, Campbell, & Farstrup, 1993; Puma, Jones, Rock, & Fernandez, 1993) and that the gap in performance between middle- and lower-income children is not closing substantially.

Over the past 10 years we have learned a considerable amount about what works to improve the reading ability of young children at risk of reading failure. Early reading intervention programs, the most notable of which are Reading Recovery (Pinnell, 1989) and Success for All (Madden, Slavin, Karweit, Dolan, & Wasik, 1993), which focus on accelerating students' learning to prevent failure as opposed to remediating problems as they occur, have been found to be very effective (Hiebert & Taylor, 1994; Pikulski, 1994; Slavin & Madden, 1989). Programs that provide extensive one-on-one tutoring (Wasik & Slavin, 1993) and small-group models have also been successful (Hiebert, Colt, Catto, & Gury, 1992; Taylor, Short, Shearer, & Frye, 1995).

First-grade (age 6 to 7) early intervention programs have been widely incorporated into schools around the U.S. For example, Reading Recovery is now in more than 1,000 schools in more than 40 states (Shanahan & Barr, 1995). The rapid influx of programs as well as numerous recently published books and articles focusing on early reading intervention suggest that getting children off to a good start in reading is essential and that early intervention is a key factor in making this possible (Pikulski, 1994).

However, first-grade reading intervention alone is not sufficient. Educators have recently begun asking questions about what needs to be done to sustain the effects of early intervention and to help children, whether they did or did not receive first-grade intervention, who are struggling readers beyond the age of 6 to 7 (Hiebert, 1994; Hiebert & Taylor, 1994; Shanahan & Barr, 1995). Recent research on Reading Recovery, for example, indicates that the impressive learning levels achieved through the program are not sustained in subsequent grades to the level one would hope (Hiebert, 1994; Shanahan & Barr, 1995), that 10 to 30% of the children receiving the program in first grade (age 6 to 7) are not successfully discontinued (Shanahan & Barr, 1995), and that the high cost of the program may limit the number of children served out of the total who need help (Hiebert, 1994; Shanahan & Barr, 1995). Based on these findings, it is clear that even in elementary schools fortunate enough to have Reading Recovery, there are older children in Grade 2 and beyond who are in need of extra help in reading.

The purpose of this article is to describe Webster Magnet School's 2-year effort to go beyond early reading intervention. Webster Magnet, located in a large midwestern U.S. city, is a K–6 (ages 5 through 12) school with 1,100 children from diverse backgrounds. Of the student population, 56% are students of color and 49% receive subsidized lunch. Webster is a magnet school in a low-income neighborhood but attracts many middle-income students from nearby neighborhoods.

In October, 1994, 50% of the students age 7 to 8 at Webster scored in the lowest quartile on the Metropolitan Achievement Test (1993). Reading Recovery was in its first year of operation at Webster, but it was clear that there

Even in elementary schools fortunate enough to have Reading Recovery, there are older children in Grade 2 and beyond who are in need of extra help in reading.

would continue to be many 7-year-olds in need of special reading help. In response to this need to work with low-achieving readers, an effective, cost-efficient intervention program was developed. The program was supplemental to the non-ability-grouped regular reading program, which used a basal reader series and sets of trade books.

As a first step, the authors designed a small-group extension of the Early Intervention in Reading program (Taylor, Frye, Short, & Shearer, 1992) that could be implemented as a 7-week enrichment class for students age 7 to 8. This particular delivery model was used because it fit well with the enrichment model of the school in which children select specialty classes such as band, computer, and Spanish. For some of the children, the intervention program was supplemented with a cross-age tutoring program involving 9- to 10-year-olds as tutors in an attempt to maximize the effectiveness of the intervention.

As a follow-up to the 1994–95 project, willing teachers incorporated the reading intervention into their regular classroom routines the following year. This phase was developed to counteract the difficulty schools have in keeping innovative programs going; typically, they are introduced, are effective for a few years, and then die out (Allington & Walmsley, 1995; Slavin & Madden, 1989). Furthermore, effective instructional strategies within classrooms are needed to sustain the effects of intervention programs that are external to the classroom.

Research base for the reading intervention program

The reading intervention program developed at Webster was based on a number of instructional components found to be effective in fostering reading growth: repeated reading, coaching children in the use of strategies to foster independence in reading, writing, and one-on-one tutoring. Repeated reading was emphasized because this has been found to be an effective technique to build word recognition rate, accuracy, fluency, and reading comprehension (Adams, 1990; Dowhower, 1987; Samuels, 1979). The repeated reading in the second-grade intervention program resembled the Shared Book Experience technique (Holdaway, 1981)

Teachers identified [for the program] 31 children whose mean score on the fall Metropolitan Achievement Test 7 was at about the 10th percentile.

described by Reutzel, Hollingsworth, and Eldredge (1994) in which children read intact stories repeatedly, first in a group with teacher support and then individually or with a partner.

The emphasis on coaching children to read for meaning and to become independent in word recognition through the use of decoding and self-monitoring strategies has been discussed as an important aspect of Reading Recovery (Clay, 1993; Pinnell, 1989) as well as in the small-group Early Intervention in Reading program (Taylor et al., 1992). As Clay (1991) explains, to become an independent reader, a low-progress reader will need help in learning to detect and self-correct word

recognition errors, to become aware of and able to use a repertoire of effective strategies for working on text, and, perhaps most importantly, to do these things within the context of reading for meaning.

The importance of writing in learning to read has also been stressed by Clay (1991) and others (Adams, 1990; Clarke, 1988; Ehri, 1989). Through writing, children learn to hear the sounds in words and to spell these sounds with letters. They also learn to pay attention to letter order, learn about regular sound-letter sequences in words, and learn to write and read frequently occurring words. Thus, sentence writing has been identified as an important component in many successful early intervention programs (Clay, 1993; Hiebert et al., 1992; Pikulski, 1994; Pinnell, 1989; Taylor et al., 1992).

The effectiveness of one-on-one tutoring by trained teachers in preventing reading failure has been documented in a recent review by Wasik and Slavin (1993). Sixteen studies evaluating five programs, including Reading Recovery and Success for All, found substantial positive effects for tutoring by trained educators. However, one of the biggest drawbacks to such models is the expense (Hiebert, 1994; Shanahan & Barr, 1995; Wasik & Slavin, 1993). A community volunteer tutoring program in Virginia directed toward young students at risk of reading failure, in which the tutors are carefully trained, has had impressive results (Invernizzi, Juel, & Rosemary, 1997). Cross-age tutoring programs (Heath & Mangiola, 1991; Labbo & Teale, 1990; Limbrick, McNaughton, & Glynn, 1985) have also been effective in increasing elementary students' reading achievement. In addition to benefiting the younger children who are tutored, older students who are themselves struggling readers have benefited when they serve as tutors (Devin-Sheehan, Feldman, & Allen, 1976; Labbo & Teale, 1990).

The reading intervention program

Participants. In 1994–95 teachers of second-grade students (age 7 to 8) were asked to identify approximately one third of their students who they felt would benefit from the reading intervention program that would be offered twice during the year as an enrichment class by the building reading coordinator. Children scheduled for the fall enrichment session also participated in the cross-age tutoring program in which fourth-grade students (age 9 to 10) served as tutors.

The teachers identified 31 children whose mean score on the fall Metropolitan Achievement Test 7 (MAT7, 1993) was at about the 10th percentile. In October a project assistant listened to these children (who also received Chapter I help) read from *Tiger Is a Scaredy Cat* (Phillips, 1986), an easy reader at the primer level, and verified that none of the children could read this with 90% word recognition accuracy. Twelve children who did not have conflicts with other requested enrichment classes were scheduled for the fall reading intervention class (intervention plus tutoring group), and 7 were scheduled for the spring class (intervention-only group). The remaining 12 children made up a control group. They did not receive tutoring.

Materials. The reading material for the intervention program consisted of picture books and easy readers selected for their appeal to 7- and 8-year-old children and their appropriateness to the intervention model that was being used. The books were categorized into 6 levels (A–F, see Appendix A).

Books in Levels A–D were picture books that were fairly easy for the younger children to read. Level A books were only 40–60 words long and consequently could be read successfully by almost all of the children at the end of 3 days of choral, partner, and individual repetitive reading. Levels B, C, and D books progressively increased in length. However, picture clues or some repetition in the text allowed the children to read these books successfully also (with 90% word recognition accuracy or better) by the end of the 3-day cycle of choral, partner, and individual repeated reading. Levels E and F books were easy readers selected so the children could practice independent, as opposed to choral, reading. Level E books were easier than Level D books, but the children were asked to read the Level E books on their own the first time, whereas Level D books were read to them first and then read chorally before they were read independently.

Instruction. For 45 minutes each day for 7 weeks, the children met for the reading intervention class taught by the building reading coordinator. For 20–30 minutes of each class, the children engaged in a 3-day cycle of activities pertaining to the intervention program (see Figure 1 and Appendix B). The group spent 3

days reading a book from one of the six levels identified in Appendix A. During the first 5 weeks the children read picture books from Levels A–D in which choral and partner reading of the book was initially stressed, followed by independent reading. During the last 2 to 3 weeks of the session the children read easy readers from Levels E and F in which initial independent reading of the book was stressed, followed by partner reading. This allowed the children to demonstrate to themselves that they could independently read a book they had never read before. The teacher circulated among the children as they were reading independently or in pairs to coach them in reading for meaning and in the use of decoding and self-monitoring strategies (see Figure 2).

For partner reading, the children were taught and reminded as necessary to be good helpers who gave hints, but did not automatically tell a word when their partner was stuck. They were encouraged to give their partner the first sound of the word or to tell their partner to look at the pictures for a clue. For example, to help David with *eating*, Joseph pointed to a picture clue and said, "What is he doing? What am I doing?" as he pretended to eat. On another word Joseph helped David by saying, "You read that word already, / c / – / an /."

In addition to these reading activities, the 3-day cycle included discussion and writing. The purpose of the sentence writing was to engage the children in a comprehension activity related to the story, to refine their phonemic awareness, and to help them to continue to develop their word analysis skills and knowledge of symbol-sound correspondences, especially for vowel sounds. The writing was typically based on a teacher prompt, such as "What are things that keep you from going to sleep?" or "Tell about a place you can go to be alone" in response to *Marmalade's Nap* (Wheeler, 1983), a story about a cat who could not find a quiet place to take a nap. (See Figure 3 for additional examples of prompts.) As each child finished writing his or her sentence, s/he read it to the teacher who gave feedback on one or two words not spelled correctly by directing the child's attention to a word that had a sound missing or to a word in which the vowel sound wasn't represented with an appropriate spelling. For example, if the child wrote *friend* as *fred*, the teacher would ask the child to say the word and try to

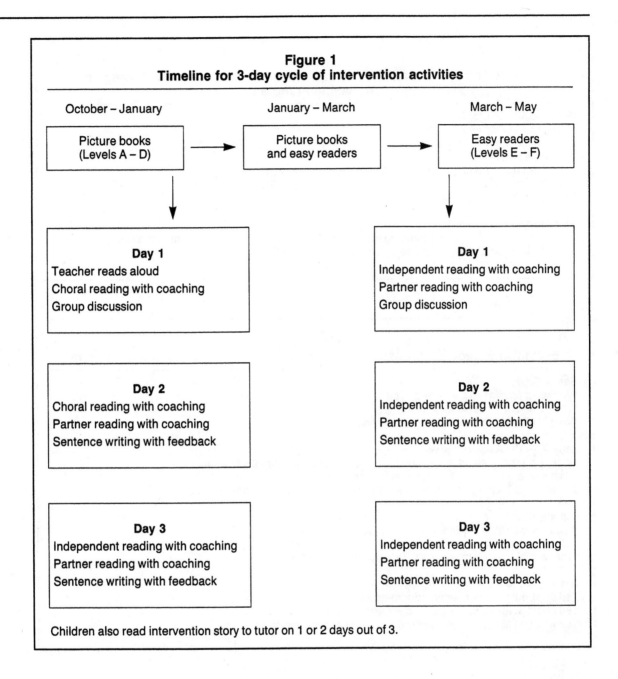

Figure 1
Timeline for 3-day cycle of intervention activities

October – January	January – March	March – May
Picture books (Levels A – D)	Picture books and easy readers	Easy readers (Levels E – F)

Day 1
Teacher reads aloud
Choral reading with coaching
Group discussion

Day 2
Choral reading with coaching
Partner reading with coaching
Sentence writing with feedback

Day 3
Independent reading with coaching
Partner reading with coaching
Sentence writing with feedback

Day 1
Independent reading with coaching
Partner reading with coaching
Group discussion

Day 2
Independent reading with coaching
Partner reading with coaching
Sentence writing with feedback

Day 3
Independent reading with coaching
Partner reading with coaching
Sentence writing with feedback

Children also read intervention story to tutor on 1 or 2 days out of 3.

figure out what sound was missing. Usually, the child could come up with the missing sound and the letter that represented that sound. If not, the teacher assisted the child. The purpose of this activity was to help the children refine their phonemic awareness. Or, if the child wrote *box* as *bax*, the teacher would ask the child to say the word slowly and try to figure out what other vowel spelled the sound heard in *box*. A child who finished the writing activity before the others either wrote another sentence or read from one of the earlier books in the program.

For the last 15–20 minutes of the enrichment class, the group engaged in other activities that involved language development and research skills. For example, the fall class created a calendar for the following year. They researched seasonal activities, holidays, and special events, and then students selected one month and developed a page of activities and pictures for the calendar. The spring class worked on shorter term projects that involved weekly art and writing activities centered around spring.

Figure 2
Decoding and self-monitoring strategies emphasized in the reading intervention program

---

Word attack strategies
Think about what would make sense.
Try to think of a word that starts with _____ that would make sense.
Look for a familiar rhyming part.
Sound out the word and think about what would make sense.
Use picture clues.
Read past the word and come back to it.

Self-monitoring strategies
Check to see if the word you come up with looks like what is on the page and makes sense.
Go back to a word you had trouble with if the sentence isn't making sense.

Figure 3
Examples of prompts for sentence writing in the reading intervention program

---

Sam's Cookie
Who/what is someone who made you angry and why?
What is a favorite snack or treat? When do you eat it?
What is something that makes you scared and why?

Lady With the Alligator Purse
Write a sentence about something in the story that couldn't really happen.
What was a part of the story that you thought was funny?
Tell about something that happened to you or someone in your family that was funny.

George Shrinks
If you were as little as George, what would you like to do?
Tell about a picture you like.
What would happen to George if he were as big as a giant?

Is Your Mama a Llama?
Tell us about your mother or grandmother.
Tell about something you lost and where you found it.
Tell why you liked a favorite picture. Describe a favorite picture.

The cross-age tutoring program

Participants. The younger children (age 7 to 8) in the fall enrichment session left their regular classroom twice a week for 25 minutes to participate in the cross-age tutoring program. Once the fall 7-week reading intervention class was over, these children continued to participate in cross-age tutoring through mid-April. The reading coordinator prepared the younger children for the book from the intervention program that they would be reading to their tutors (age 9 to 10) during a 10- to 15-minute period once a week.

The 12 older children selected as tutors met three criteria: (a) they had been identified by their teachers as being behind in reading and likely to benefit from the tutoring experience, (b) they did not have scheduling conflicts with other enrichment classes, and (c) they were able to read a 3^1 basal reader with at least 85% word recognition accuracy.

Materials. The reading materials for the cross-age tutoring program consisted of books from the intervention program (see Appendix

A). Also, the tutors read picture books to the younger children. A few of their favorites were *Miss Nelson Is Missing* (Allard & Marshall, 1977), *Another Mouse to Feed* (Kraus, 1980), and *The Cloud Book* (dePaola, 1975). The tutors also read aloud nonfiction material by authors such as Gail Gibbons and Joanna Cole.

Instruction. During the fall and winter enrichment sessions, the 12 older children in the tutoring class met for 45 minutes each day for 14 weeks with one of their teachers and the reading coordinator. This program was patterned after a similar cross-age tutoring program developed by Heath and Mangiola (1991). The children spent Mondays and Tuesdays getting ready to tutor. Their teachers modeled how to be a good coach who would hint but not immediately tell a child a word. There was considerable discussion about good word recognition strategies to teach the younger children to use (see Figure 2). Students kept an ongoing list of these strategies in a journal and referred to this as they were practicing or actually tutoring. The children also practiced reading the same books the younger children would be reading to them.

The younger children continued to participate in cross-age tutoring through mid April.

The tutors also chose a picture book to read to the young partners. They practiced reading this to themselves and to a classmate in the tutoring class. At the same time, they practiced being good coaches if someone got stuck on a word. They also planned with their teachers an extension activity focused on comprehension and based on the picture book they would be reading aloud. For example, one week the tutors prepared a character sketch activity. They helped their young partners identify a main character in the picture book and listed character traits. In another activity, tutors and their partners made a story map in which they decided on the main idea and listed supporting details. The tutors also regularly listed

generic and specific questions for discussion in their journals so they could refer to them when working with their partners.

On Wednesdays and Thursdays, the children and tutors met for 25 minutes during the tutors' enrichment class time. Each day the younger children read the book they were working on in their intervention program to their tutor. The tutors would coach with prompts such as, "Look at the picture" or "It starts with / p /." One example was Tom, helping Nate who was reading, "And most of all because it might be very…" (Barrett, 1970). Tom said, "Sound it out in chunks." Nate replied with, "Em… Embarrassing," and Tom said, "Yup," as he smiled and nodded his head. Tara helped Amber by covering up the end of the word and saying, "Sound this first part out." After Amber said, "Wal-," Tara covered it up and said, "Now say this last part." Amber said "-rus" and then "walrus."

Across the 2 tutoring days, the tutors read the picture book they had practiced to their young partners. They used the questions in their journals to have discussions about the story, talked about words with which the younger children might be unfamiliar, and then engaged the younger children in the comprehension extension activity related to the picture book.

Following the tutoring sessions on Wednesdays and Thursdays, the tutors had oral debriefing sessions on what went well and what were problems or concerns pertaining to the tutoring sessions. The children often reported that they liked working with their young partners and that their partners read well. They also frequently mentioned problems such as their partners talking too softly, not paying enough attention, or not sitting still. The teachers shared positive things they had noticed as the partners worked together and helped the tutors think of ways to solve problems that arose.

On Fridays the tutors wrote a letter to an adult mentor (one of the authors or the project assistant), using their debriefing discussions to help them decide what to write about. They typically would write about what had gone well that week when they met with their young partners, what problems they had had, and how their partners were doing in reading. The mentor wrote back by Monday of the next

Table 1
Number of 7- to 8-year-old students able to read at various levels with at least 90% accuracy (May, 1994–95 study)

		Highest level read		
Group	n	Primer or lower	1^2	2^{2*}
Intervention plus tutoring	12	2	1	9
Intervention only	7	4	1	2
Control	12	10	2	0

*All children could also read from *Frog and Toad All Year* with at least 90% accuracy.

week, praising the tutors for their efforts, giving advice, asking questions, and providing encouragement.

After the fall and winter enrichment sessions were over, the tutors continued to meet with their young partners once a week for 25 minutes through mid-April. The reading coordinator brought them a copy of the partners' intervention book in advance so the tutors could practice reading it. They also selected a picture book from the tutoring project collection and practiced reading this book in their regular classroom in preparation for reading it aloud to their young partners.

Results and discussion

In May a project assistant listened to the younger children read independently to determine whether or not they were able to decode second-grade material. First the children were asked to read a segment of a story from *Frog and Toad All Year* (Lobel, 1976), which was considered to be at a beginning level for most 7- to 8-year-olds. If they could read this with at least 90% word recognition accuracy, they were also asked to read a passage from *How My Parents Learned to Eat* (Friedman, 1984), which was from the 2^2 basal, but which had not yet been read in the regular reading program. Those who could not read the passage from *Frog and Toad All Year* with at least 90% word recognition accuracy were asked to read a passage from *The Three Wishes* (Aardema, 1989), which was in the 1^2 basal.

In May, 75% of the students in the intervention plus tutoring group, less than 30% in the intervention-only group, and none in the control group could read the passage from the 2^2 basal with at least 90% word recognition accuracy. The reading levels in May for children in all three groups are in Table 1. A Yates-corrected chi-square test revealed that significantly more children in the intervention plus tutoring group than in the control group were reading on grade level by the end of second grade ($X^2 = 11.38$, $p < .001$).

The means and standard deviations on fall Grade 2 and Grade 3 raw scores from the reading subtest of the MAT7 (1993) are shown in Table 2. An analysis of covariance on the Grade 3 scores, with the Grade 2 raw scores serving as the covariate, revealed a significant difference among groups, $F(2,24) = 3.66$, $p < .05$. Further comparisons revealed that the mean score of the intervention plus tutoring group was significantly higher than that of the control group, $F(1,24) = 6.45$, $p < .05$. The mean difference between the intervention plus tutoring and intervention-only groups approached significance, $F(1,24) = 3.85$, $p = .06$). In other words, after controlling for any differences in fall Grade 2 reading scores between groups, we found that the intervention plus tutoring group scored significantly higher on the MAT7 in fall of Grade 3 than the control group.

In May, the project assistant also listened to the tutors read independently. Each child read from *Rufus M.* (Estes, 1944), a story at the end of the fourth-grade basal reader, which they had not read before. Students in the tutoring class were reading below grade level at the beginning of fourth grade; their mean word

Helping struggling readers: Linking small-group intervention with cross-age tutoring

Table 2
Student scores on the MAT7 in the fall of Grade 2 and fall of Grade 3
(1994–95 study)

Group	n		Grade 2 (age 7 – 8)		Grade 3 (age 8 – 9)	
			Raw score	Percentile rank	Raw score	Percentile rank
Intervention plus tutoring	10	$\bar{x}$	34.50	(12)	41.40	(19)
		SD	7.79		7.41	
Intervention only	7	$\bar{x}$	35.00	(12)	32.57	(11)
		SD	8.54		12.30	
Control	11	$\bar{x}$	31.91	(9)	29.36	(8)
		SD	6.43		10.60	

Note. Two intervention plus tutoring children and one control child are missing because they moved between second and third grade. Their pretest standardized reading scores were 28, 41, and 28, respectively.

recognition score on a narrative passage from the 3[1] basal was 94.3%. In May of Grade 4 all 12 children could read the narrative passage from the end of the fourth-grade basal with at least 95% word recognition accuracy ($\bar{x}$ = 98.5%). In addition, in the fall the 12 children in the tutoring group had a mean raw score on the reading subtest of the MAT7 corresponding to the 12th percentile. In the fall of the following school year, the children in the tutoring group had a mean raw score on the MAT7 corresponding to the 19th percentile.

Together, the oral reading and standardized test results suggest that both younger and older students made progress in reading during the school year. Compared with a control group, younger children who received the 7-week intervention and 21-week cross-age tutoring programs made significant gains in reading ability. Furthermore, 75% of the children in the combined reading intervention/tutoring program who entered second grade unable to read at a primer level could decode a passage from a grade-level (2[2]) basal with 90% accuracy or better by May. None of the control group children could read this well, and only two of seven children in the intervention-only group could read at this level.

The 7-week intervention class that started in the spring without a one-on-one component was not sufficient to improve the reading ability of students arriving unable to read. Since the impact of this intervention is confounded with the fact that it took place relatively late in the year and did not include opportunities for one-on-one reading practice, further study is needed to determine whether an intervention plus tutoring program beginning in the second half of the school year can be effective.

On the other hand, the 7-week intervention program commencing in the fall and supplemented with a 21-week cross-age tutoring program was effective. The fact that we were able to help such a high proportion of nonreaders reach grade level in decoding ability by the end of the year with this particular intervention package is encouraging, particularly because the program did not take a great deal of student time and, relatively speaking, did not require much instructional time provided by teachers. This intervention was also relatively inexpensive. Approximately US$30 per child was spent on books for the intervention and tutoring projects. Averaged out across the year, the two intervention programs required approximately one sixth of the reading coordinator's time, resulting in a total instructional cost of about US$400 per child served. The reading coordinator was free to work with additional enrichment classes during the year and to spend the majority of her time on her primary responsibilities, which involved teacher training and support, working with parents, and providing administrative assistance to the principal.

Adaptations to classroom instruction

Although the results of the 1994–95 project were positive for many of the children who participated, we wanted to determine if it had any major impact on classroom instruction at Webster. As we describe below, the project did, in fact, lead to important changes at the school.

The reading intervention program within regular classrooms. During the 1995–96 school year, the reading intervention program was used in classrooms as supplemental instruction for all 7- to 8-year-olds. One of the teachers, who had piloted the program in her classroom the previous year, assumed the role of mentor to the other second-grade teachers. After meeting with the teachers to explain the program, she invited them to her room to observe several times in the fall before they began using the program. During the year, the teachers came to the mentor teacher or to the reading coordinator with questions as they arose. In addition to discussing the program at grade-level meetings and informally over lunch, the teachers met as a group with the reading coordinator and one of the other authors on a monthly basis to discuss their successes and concerns pertaining to the program.

In November each teacher selected a group of five to six struggling readers (reading below the primer level) to meet for 20 minutes a day. The group spent 3 days on a story, following the cycle of activities described previously (see Figure 1). A project assistant went to five of the classrooms once a week to coach the children individually as they read from their current intervention story. In two of these five classes the children also received help once a week through the cross-age tutoring program. In three others, a parent volunteer listened to the children read once a week.

One of the greatest challenges to teachers in providing the intervention program within the classroom was finding the time to do so. Four teachers taught the small-group lesson following the regular reading lesson while the other children in the room were engaged in independent reading, writing, or other projects related to the regular reading program. Another teacher taught her group while the other children were completing practice activities related to their math lesson. As they finished, they moved into independent reading and writing activities. This teacher actually met with all of her students in small groups each day on a literacy activity, so everyone had time to finish independent math work and to engage in independent reading and writing activities. One teacher reported that a trial-and-error process was needed to find a time that worked for him to provide the supplemental instruction. The after-reading class time didn't work, but he found that a 20-minute period directly after lunch worked well. During this time, the other children read independently.

Of 42 children in six classrooms with the yearlong intervention, 5 (or 12%) were reading on a 2^1 level and 19 (or 45%) were reading on a 2^2 level in May. All of the children had been reading below the primer level in September. Although the incidence of children reading on grade level by May was not as high as in the 1994–95 project, the results were encouraging as compared with the reading levels of control students from the previous year. Furthermore, teachers were very positive about the program. One teacher reported, "I really liked the program because it easily fit into the daily schedule. It worked; it got kids reading." Another said, "I liked it a lot. The poor readers really improved. The kids felt special to be in the group, and they felt very good about themselves." An added bonus of the program was that it made the teachers more aware of the importance of emphasizing reading strategies with all children.

The participating teachers plan to continue using the program, and as they become more experienced with it, we hope to see even more struggling young readers reading at grade level by May. Additionally, in the future, teachers plan to start the intervention in September instead of November to increase effectiveness.

The cross-age tutoring program within regular classrooms. Two fourth-grade teachers worked with two second-grade classrooms to provide the tutoring class within the classrooms. After meeting with the reading coordinator who explained the tutoring program, these two teachers identified six struggling readers for the program. These children met with the reading coordinator for two 30-minute sessions that focused on how to be a good tutor. The tutors practiced reading picture books aloud to a peer or to the reading coordinator in these initial sessions. Then, the classroom teachers helped their tutors prepare for each week's tutoring session.

On Mondays, the teachers gave the tutors the second-grade intervention book to practice and then gave the tutors time to select a picture book to read aloud to their second-grade partners. For 15–20 minutes on Tuesday through Thursday, the tutors practiced reading their picture books independently and with another tutor or with a parent volunteer. On Friday, the tutors met with their second-grade partners for 25–30 minutes for the tutoring session in the reading coordinator's room. On the following Monday, as they met to prepare for the next week's read-aloud book, the tutors discussed with their teacher what went well and what were problems to be solved pertaining to the previous week's tutoring session.

Teachers were positive about the tutoring program. One second-grade teacher reported, "Not all of my kids in the intervention program have a tutor, but I think they all should. Those who do are better readers. It really helps them with their learning." One of the fourth-grade teachers said, "The program helps the students improve in self-confidence in their reading. Their fluency and comprehension are improving. It puts them in the role of expert." Another said, "Many of the tutors show an increased responsibility with their own work because of the tutoring. They're building self-esteem and improving oral reading and vocabulary skills."

Conclusions

We are pleased that the combination of the reading intervention enrichment class and cross-age tutoring program carried out in this project made important differences in the reading ability of struggling readers at Webster, an urban school with high numbers of 7- to 8-year-olds in need of extra help in reading. Furthermore, the tutors, who were themselves behind in reading, made progress as measured by their ability to read from a fourth-grade basal and by their performance on the MAT7 (1993) at the beginning of fourth and fifth grades. We are equally pleased that the project was incorporated into other classrooms the following year. Thus, a number of teachers at Webster made significant changes in what they were doing for their struggling readers in the regular classroom.

It is important to point out that the reading coordinator was instrumental in developing and piloting the reading intervention and cross-age tutoring programs. Furthermore, she provided invaluable leadership in supporting and encouraging teachers who decided that they wanted to implement the intervention and tutoring programs in their classrooms. She provided materials for teachers, facilitated initial and ongoing staff development, and arranged for meeting times for children participating in the tutoring program. We do not believe the program would be operating without her support.

Beyond the need for a staff member in this essential leadership position, the two programs do not require much money to operate. What both programs do require are commitment and collaboration among classroom teachers. Second-grade teachers must find the time for 15–20 minutes of daily reading intervention if they are doing this themselves within the classroom. Fourth-grade teachers must find the time to help their students prepare for each week's tutoring session if they are playing major roles in the tutoring program. Also teachers must work together to find a time once or twice a week for their students to work together in the cross-age tutoring program. Most importantly, teachers must share the belief that these supplemental programs are worth the effort and that their struggling readers can make significant gains in their reading ability.

Changes at Webster have not occurred overnight and, in many ways, are just beginning. We believe that lasting change can be made only when classroom teachers, other staff, and administrators are willing to spend the time required to build support for struggling readers into the fabric of daily school life. As Allington and Walmsley (1995) so clearly state, there really is no "quick fix" for students who find learning to read difficult. Nonetheless, with little extra in the way of resources, but with the willingness to try, classroom teachers and a reading coordinator at Webster are working together to provide supplemental instruction for struggling readers that is having a positive impact on children's reading ability. We believe this type of school-wide effort is essential in preventing reading failure in elementary schools.

Taylor and Watts teach courses in reading education and children's literature at the University of Minnesota. Hanson is the reading coordinator and Justice-Swanson teaches second grade at Webster Magnet School in St. Paul, Minnesota, USA. Taylor can be reached at 338 Peik Hall, University of Minnesota, 159 Pillsbury Drive SE, Minneapolis, MN 55455, USA.

References

Adams, M.J. (1990). *Beginning to read: Thinking and learning about print.* Cambridge, MA: MIT Press.

Allington, R.L., & Walmsley, S.A. (1995). No quick fix: Where do we go from here? In *No quick fix: Rethinking literacy programs in America's elementary schools* (pp. 253 – 264). New York: Teachers College Press.

Clarke, L.K. (1988). Invented versus traditional spelling in first graders' writing: Effects on learning to spell and read. *Research on the Teaching of English, 22,* 281 – 309.

Clay, M. (1991). *Becoming literate: The construction of inner control.* Portsmouth, NH: Heinemann.

Clay, M. (1993). *Reading Recovery: A guidebook for teachers in training.* Portsmouth, NH: Heinemann.

Devin-Sheehan, L., Feldman, R.S., & Allen, V.L. (1976). Research on children tutoring children: A critical review. *Review of Educational Research, 46,* 355 – 385.

Dowhower, S.L. (1987). Effects of repeated reading on second-grade transitional readers' fluency and comprehension. *Reading Research Quarterly, 22,* 389 – 406.

Ehri, L.C. (1989). Movement into word reading and spelling: How spelling contributes to reading. In J. Mason (Ed.), *Reading and writing connections* (pp. 65 – 81). Boston: Allyn & Bacon.

Elley, W.B. (1992). *How in the world do students read?* The Hague, Netherlands: International Association for the Evaluation of Educational Achievement.

Heath, S.B., & Mangiola, L. (1991). *Children of promise: Literate activity in linguistically and culturally diverse classrooms.* Washington, DC: National Education Association.

Hiebert, E.H. (1994). Reading Recovery in the United States: What difference does it make to an age cohort? *Educational Researcher, 23(9),* 15 – 25.

Hiebert, E.H., Colt, J.M., Catto, S.L., & Gury, E.C. (1992). Reading and writing of first-grade students in a restructured Chapter 1 program. *American Educational Research Journal, 29,* 545 – 572.

Hiebert, E.H., & Taylor, B.M. (Eds.). (1994). *Getting reading right from the start: Effective early literacy intervention.* Boston: Allyn & Bacon.

Holdaway, D. (1981). Shared book experience: Teaching, reading, using favorable books. *Theory Into Practice, 21,* 293 – 300.

Invernizzi, M., Juel, C., & Rosemary, C.A. (1997). A community volunteer tutorial that works. *The Reading Teacher, 50,* 304 – 311.

Labbo, L.D., & Teale, W.H. (1990). Cross-age reading: A strategy for helping poor readers. *The Reading Teacher, 43,* 362 – 369.

Limbrick, E., McNaughton, S., & Glynn, T. (1985). Gains for underachieving tutors and tutees in a cross-age tutoring programme. *Journal of Child Psychology and Psychiatry, 26,* 939 – 953.

Madden, N.A., Slavin, R.E., Karweit, N.L., Dolan, L.J., & Wasik, B.A. (1993). Success for All: Longitudinal effects of a restructuring program for inner city elementary schools. *American Educational Research Journal, 30,* 123 – 148.

Mullis, I.V., Campbell, J.R., & Farstrup, A.E. (1993). *Reading report card for the nation and the state.* Washington, DC: U.S. Department of Education.

Mullis, I.V., & Jenkins, L.B. (1990). *The reading report card, 1971–80. Trends from the nation's report card.* Washington, DC: U.S. Department of Education.

Pikulski, J.J. (1994). Preventing reading failure: A review of five effective programs. *The Reading Teacher, 48,* 30 – 39.

Pinnell, G.S. (1989). Reading Recovery: Helping at-risk children learn to read. *Elementary School Journal, 90,* 160 – 183.

Puma, M.J., Jones, C.C., Rock, D., & Fernandez, R. (1993). *Prospectus: The Congressional Mandate Study of educational growth and opportunity. The interim report.* Washington, DC: U.S. Department of Education.

Reutzel, D.R., Hollingsworth, P.M., & Eldredge, J.L. (1994). Oral reading instruction: The impact on student reading development. *Reading Research Quarterly, 29,* 40 – 65.

Samuels, S.J. (1979). The method of repeated reading. *The Reading Teacher, 32,* 403 – 408.

Shanahan, T., & Barr, R. (1995). Reading Recovery: An independent evaluation of the effects of an early instructional intervention for at-risk learners. *Reading Research Quarterly, 30,* 598 – 996.

Slavin, R.E., & Madden, N.A. (1989). What works for students at risk: A research synthesis. *Educational Leadership, 64(5),* 4 – 13.

Taylor, B.M., Frye, B.J., Short, R.A., & Shearer, B. (1992). Classroom teachers prevent reading failure among low-achieving first-grade students. *The Reading Teacher, 45,* 592 – 597.

Taylor, B., Short, R., Shearer, B., & Frye, B. (1995). First grade teachers provide early reading intervention in the classroom. In R.L. Allington & S.A. Walmsley (Eds.), *No quick fix: Rethinking literacy in America's elementary schools* (pp. 159 – 176). New York: Teachers College Press.

Wasik, B.A., & Slavin, R.E. (1993). Preventing early reading failure with one-to-one tutoring: A review of five programs. *Reading Research Quarterly, 28,* 178 – 200.

Williams, P.L, Reese, C.M., Campbell, J.R., Mazzeo, J., & Phillips, G.W. (1995). *1994 NAEP reading: A first look.* Washington, DC: U.S. Department of Education.

Children's books cited

Aardema, V. (1989). *The three wishes.* Boston: Silver Burdett & Ginn.

Allard, H., & Marshall, J. (1977). *Miss Nelson is missing.* Boston: Houghton Mifflin.

Barrett, J. (1970). *Animals should definitely not wear clothing.* New York: Macmillan.

dePaola, T. (1975). *The cloud book.* New York: Holiday House.

Estes, E. (1944). *Rufus M.* New York: Harcourt, Brace, Jovanovich.

Friedman, J.R. (1984). *How my parents learned to eat.* Boston: Houghton Mifflin.

Kraus, R. (1980). *Another mouse to feed.* New York: Simon & Schuster.

Lobel, A. (1976). *Frog and toad all year.* New York: Harper & Row.

Phillips, J. (1986). *Tiger is a scaredy cat.* New York: Random House.

Wheeler, C. (1983). *Marmalade's nap.* New York: Knopf.

APPENDIX A
Children's books in the reading intervention program

Level A *(40–60 words)*
(Used in weeks 1 – 2 of enrichment class and in October with regular classroom model)

Title	Author
Who Is Coming?	Patricia C. McKissack
Sam's Cookie	Barbo Lindgren
Things I Like	Anthony Browne
Flying	Donald Crews

Level B *(60–90 words)*
(Used in weeks 2 – 4 of enrichment class and in November and December with regular classroom model)

Title	Author
Ten, Nine, Eight	Molly Bang
Marmalade's Nap	Cindy Wheeler
Sleepy Bear	Lydia Dabovich
The Cake That Mack Ate	Rose Robart
The Lady With the Alligator Purse	Nadine Bernard Wescott

Level C *(90–120 words)*
(Used in weeks 5 – 7 of enrichment class and beyond and in January with regular classroom model)

Title	Author
Sheep in a Jeep	Nancy Shaw
George Shrinks	William Joyce
Animals Should Definitely Not Wear Clothing	Judi Barrett
Hooray for Snail!	John Stadler
Who Is the Beast?	Keith Baker

Level D *(120–200 words)*
(Used in weeks 6 – 7 of enrichment class and beyond and in February and March with regular classroom model)

Title	Author
The Happy Day	Ruth Krauss
Which Witch Is Which?	Deborah Guarino
Is Your Mama a Llama?	Pat Hutchins
Mr. Gumpy's Outing	John Burningham
The Little Mouse, the Red Ripe Strawberry and the Big Hungry Bear	Don Wood and Audrey Wood

Level E *(easy readers)*
(Used in weeks 5 – 7 of enrichment class and beyond and in January and February with regular classroom model)

Title	Author
My New Boy	Joan Phillips
So Sick!	Harriet Ziefert & Carol Nicklaus
Tiger Is a Scaredy Cat	Joan Phillips
Wake up Sun	David Harrison

Level F *(easy readers)*
(Used in weeks 6 – 7 of enrichment class and beyond and in March, April, and May with regular classroom model)

Title	Author
Fox All Week	Edward Marshall
Four on the Shore	Edward Marshall
There Is a Carrot in My Ear and Other Noodle Tales	Alvin Schwartz
Mouse Tales	Arnold Lobel
Frog and Toad Together	Arnold Lobel
Frog and Toad Are Friends	Arnold Lobel

APPENDIX B
Intervention procedures

Levels A–D (October – March)

Day 1   Teacher reads story, perhaps to the whole class.
Group reads story twice with the teacher.
Group discusses the story.

Day 2   Group reads story as a group once with the teacher.
Partners take turns reading the story once while the teacher circulates to provide coaching.
Children write individual responses in complete sentences to a question on the story posed by the teacher and then share these with the teacher.
The teacher provides individual feedback focusing on children's ability to represent all sounds and to represent short vowel sounds correctly in one or two selected words in their sentences.

Day 3   Children read the story individually, and partners take turns reading the story as teacher circulates to provide coaching.
Children write individual responses to the new question posed by the teacher.
The teacher provides individual feedback to the sentences as in Day 2.

Levels E & F (January – May)

Day 1   Teacher reads story first, only if necessary. This is phased out when possible so that the emphasis is on reading independently.
Children read to themselves first and then read in pairs. The teacher coaches individuals. Group discusses the story.

Day 2   Children read to themselves and then in pairs. The teacher coaches individuals. Children write individual responses to the story and share these with teacher.

Day 3   Children read to themselves and then in pairs. The teacher coaches individuals. Children write individual responses to the story and share these with teacher.

The labeled child

Karen Morrow Durica

Durica teaches at Carl Sandburg Elementary School, Littleton, Colorado, USA.

I pray for the labeled child;
That child who is gifted and talented.
No longer can she be lazy and idle
Or a daydreamer.
So much more is expected
Of those as gifted and talented as she.

I pray for the labeled child;
That child who is learning disabled.
No longer will the world expect brilliance
No longer will someone tell him to reach for the
   stars
Because that is where greatness will be found.

I pray for the labeled child;
That child who is dyslexic.
Reading — oh, the joy of reading!
Will always be hard for her to find.
No matter that she can recite — no *sing* —
Mary Had a Little Lamb,
She won't be able to read it,
At least not without difficulty.
She will learn that all her friends
Who laugh and cry and wonder about books
Can do so because they are not dyslexic.

I pray for the labeled child;
That child who is A.D.D.
An unorganized bubble of hyperactivity.
No longer will someone teach him to cope in a
   world
That values compliance.
No longer will someone say "You can do this;
Oh, it may be hard, but it is within you to do this."
A dose of medicine now replaces the need for
   that inner effort
And eliminates the possible victory.

I pray for the labeled child;
That child who is emotionally handicapped.
That child who rebels
Because she *should* rebel.

The child who acts out
Because there is nowhere else
For the hurt and anxiety and fear to go.
The child who is diagnosed "sick,"
When perhaps her actions are the one true sign
   of sanity
In the demented world in which she is forced to
   live.

I pray for the child of no label.
In a system which marks so many special,
This child neither shines nor demands.
For this child life has been neither harsh nor
   generous.
This is the one who "makes" the teacher's day
Because there are so many children who need
   real attention.

I pray most of all for some magic day
When the tests, the labels, and the names
Will disappear — will be forgotten.
When each child who enters a classroom
Will be an apprentice of learning.
When each classroom will be a safe place
To discover — on your own —
What will be the struggles of your life,
And the victories.
When the feeble and the bright,
The gregarious and the shy
Will all find their place
In the great adventure of education.
When the only label that will be attached to
   anyone is
                    LEARNER.

Durica, Karen. (March 1994). The labeled child. *The Reading Teacher*, 47 (6), 503. The International Reading Association. Copyright © 1994.

Chapter 4

Better Note Taking

Getting It All Down

Background

Although there is no one best way to take notes, research suggests that the very act of note taking, in any form, promotes retention of information. Note taking increases concentration. It helps the individual to organize, process and encode information and it provides material for the student to study later on.

High school teachers expect their students to be able to take

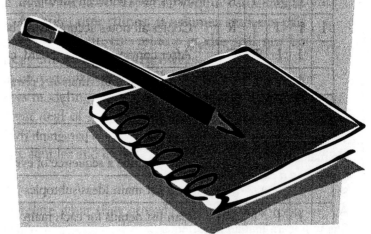

notes during class, but that assumes a great deal. Where and when have students been given the instruction and repeated opportunities for practicing note taking? Instruction in organizing notebooks and recording topics that have been studied can begin early in elementary school. Even students in second and third grade can be shown how to label and date any work recorded in their notebooks. Teaching this habit early will make keeping notes organized later much easier.

Most of what goes on in classrooms is auditory. The teacher introduces a topic or leads the class through an activity. Students discuss their experiments, describe steps in solving a math problem or respond verbally to something they have read. Since most of our students are visual learners, this method of instruction does not match their learning style. It is imperative, therefore, that we help students take the great amount of auditory input received during class and transcribe it into some visual form.

Be sure to model several note-taking strategies during the course of the year. Additional opportunities for practice should be provided, both during class and for homework, in order for students to use and improve this skill.

I have included on the next page a suggested scope and sequence of subskills for the middle grades which will lead to improved note taking later on. While I will illustrate several methods of note taking, I will provide many suggestions for using a favorite note taking strategy of mine, the Cornell Method, or Column Note Taking.

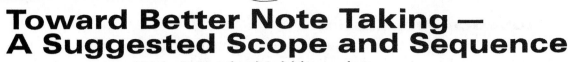

Toward Better Note Taking — A Suggested Scope and Sequence

Key: I - Introduce/Model frequently
T - Teach (provide many opportunities for student practice)
R - Review (extend, students apply independently when developmentally ready)

4	5	6	7	8	**Getting Started:**
I	I	T	T	R	Writes title/heading on page correctly
I	I	T	T	R	Labels all notes in notebook-date, topic, page
I	I	T	T	R	Leaves a wide 3" margin (recall column)
I	I	T	T	R	Skips lines between subtopics
I	I	T	T	R	Copies all notes accurately off board, leaving a wide margin on the left
	I	I	T	T	After copying notes off board, can generate questions in the recall column
	I	I	T	T	Circles and underlines key phrases in notebook when studying
					From Text:
I	I	I	T	T	Can paraphrase a paragraph that has been read
I	I	I	T	T	Can describe a sequence of events, steps, or ideas
	I	I	T	T	Can list main ideas/subtopics
	I	I	T	T	Can list details for each main idea/subtopic
	I	I	T	T	Can make a "semantic map" which shows main ideas/subtopics
	I	I	T	T	Can categorize details under subtopics
		I	I	I	Can write a summary of a section
					From Classroom Discussion:
		I	I		Can paraphrase what has been said
		I	I		Can describe a sequence of events, steps, or ideas
		I	I		Can list main ideas/subtopics
		I	I		Can list details for each main idea /subtopics
		I	I		Can make a "semantic map" which shows main ideas/subtopics
		I	I		Can write a summary
		I	I		Can use a "semantic map" to outline an essay with three main ideas/subtopics and two details for each
			I		Can identify the speaker's or writer's organizational plan, such as: simple listing, chronological pattern, cause and effect, generalization with examples, comparison and contrast

Grades

Advance Preparation

As you prepare for each unit of study (your content curriculum), develop several examples of note-taking strategies based on upcoming class assignments to model on the overhead or blackboard.

Have on hand copies of the following reproducibles:

✔ **K-W-L Chart** *(page 46)*
✔ **Topic-Subtopics Map** *(page67)*
✔ **Noting What I've Learned** *(page 47)*
✔ **Column Note Taking Outlines** *(pages 48 and 49)*

Strategies

The Traditional Outline

Traditional outlining is really quite an advanced concept that requires students to use many higher-level thinking skills. Among other things, it assumes students can use complex organizational skills. Most students in the middle grades will not be developmentally ready to use this strategy effectively on their own.

If you choose to introduce this form of note taking, you will need to walk students through the process step-by-step, always modeling your own notes on the overhead or blackboard. Students will need a great deal of guidance as they begin to identify the various parts of an outline.

In my opinion, the strategies below are simpler and more effective for most students.

K-W-L Chart

A K-W-L Chart can help students relate what they already know about a topic to the new information they are about to learn. It is through connections that we make meaning from what we learn and improve the likelihood that we can retrieve the information later from our memory. The chart may be used to record new information gathered through research, class discussion, viewing films or reading the textbook.

Mapping

Most students prefer creating semantic maps to using traditional notes and outlines. A map, or graphic organizer, is a visual representation of ideas that the student organizes and designs. (See Chapter 9, *Learning Through Visualization*, for more information on graphic organizers.) Main ideas are attached to the topic and details are attached to the main ideas. This "word map" show relationships of concepts to one another. The **Topic-Subtopics Map** trains students to think critically as they judge how ideas are related to one another and which ideas are more important than others (main ideas vs. details.) Creating maps helps students integrate the thinking-reading-writing processes.

For students to commit themselves to creating and designing maps during study time, they need to be convinced of the maps' usefulness. To accomplish this, provide students with a map you have created of an upcoming unit. They should not be familiar with the material. Have students in pairs discuss what they can learn from the map. Then, as a class, ask them to share what the pairs have learned. Discuss whether a map would be useful for taking notes from future textbook assignments. Most students will admit that they learned a great deal from your map. They will, therefore, be more eager to try it out as a study tool for themselves.

Noting What I've Learned

The easiest form of note taking for a student is to write a simple list of new ideas that he or she has learned. Usually, the list has no particular form, but it provides a record of important facts. Using the **Noting What I've Learned** outline, you can provide a structure for a simple list. Discuss the general topic of an assigned reading with your students and have them record the topic on the top of the page. Since this is probably a first experience with note taking, present students with three or four subtopics included in their assignment. Have them write the subtopics in the boxes provided. As they read the assignment, students should record two or three details (definitions, explanations, examples and so on) about each subtopic. A completed outline is shown below. Students also will enjoy drawing pictures in the boxes to aid visual memory.

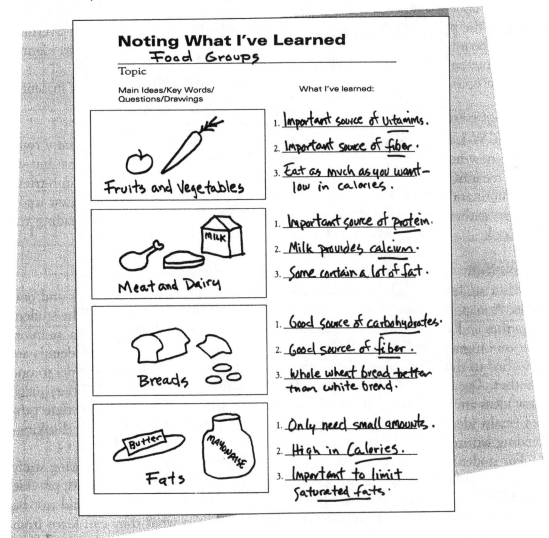

Column Note Taking

General Subject _U.S. Regions_ Date _6/9/94_

Recall Column Subtopics/Main Ideas	Note Column Supporting Details
[drawing of city buildings] Northeast	New England; Mid-Atlantic; Many large cities; cold during the winter; an important manufacturing region.
[drawing of sun and road] Southeast	A growing region; sometimes called the sunbelt; Lots of agriculture; tourism is important.
[drawing of barn and tractor] Middlewest	Great Lakes States; Plains; lots of farms; manufacturing near Detroit and Chicago; cold during winter.
[drawing of cactus, sun, buildings] Southwest	Land of open spaces; deserts; cactus and plateaus; mining is important; large cities such as Phoenix continue to grow.
[drawing of mountains] West	High and dry; 2 sections— mountain states and Pacific states; ranching and mining are important; lots of air industry in the Pacific states.

Column Note Taking

My favorite note-taking strategy is adapted from Walter Pauk's Cornell Method, Column Note Taking. Developed for college students, this method calls for students to take notes on the right-hand side of the page in the Note Column. Afterwards, they create marginal comments, questions or key phrases which they record in the left-hand column, called the Recall Column. This is one of the most effective note-taking strategies because it provides an excellent independent study tool for students. By covering the Note Column, students can quiz themselves by reciting information triggered by notes in the Recall Column. By uncovering the Note Column they can get immediate feedback about the accuracy and completeness of their memory.

I have adapted the **Column Note Taking** outline for a variety of purposes. The form on page 48 has boxes in the Recall Column which can be used in many ways. Main ideas, questions, drawings, key words and problems can be written in the boxes. Pictures can be drawn to illustrate key ideas. A description of the picture can be written in the Note Column. In Science classes, students can draw what they observe at different stages in an experiment, and then write a description in the Note Column. Language Arts and English teachers like to use the boxes to list literary terms. Math teachers have used the boxes to write word problems which their students solve on the line to the right. Above is a completed sample from a Social

Studies class. A summarizing paragraph can then be written on the back of the page.

Using the form on page 49, students can copy or take their own notes in the Note Column. After doing so, they can generate and record questions based on their notes in the Recall Column. Younger or less able students can decide what the notes are describing and they can label the main idea or subtopic in the Recall Column.

Cooperative Note Taking

Cooperative note-taking activities help students learn new ideas from one another. Provide frequent opportunities for students to take notes. One way to do this is to prepare a five-minute lecture (be sure your presentation is organized, including: three to four subtopics with details for each). Have students listen and take notes in the right column (using **Column Note Taking**). After the lecture, ask each student to individually spend five minutes clarifying his or her notes and writing questions or key words and concepts in the Recall Column. Then have pairs of students discuss what they have noted and how each partner has organized the information. Encourage students to borrow at least one idea from their partner's notes. As a class, discuss the process of note taking while the teacher shows his/her notes for the lecture on the overhead or blackboard.

Teaching Suggestions and Extension Ideas

1. Remember when you review the Suggested Scope and Sequence that developmentally there will be a great range of abilities within one grade level. You and your colleagues need not be locked into the exact time frame suggested. Instead, review your unique school population and its needs, and just be sure to build upon the subskills in a unified approach for the best long-term outcomes.

2. The **K-W-L Chart** is especially helpful at the 4–6 grade level. Using it at the beginning of each new unit of study will activate prior knowledge and provide motivation to investigate a topic further. Some students will resist and say, "I don't *want* to know anything more." In that case, smile, change the **W** to an **N** and ask, "What do you *need* to know? in order to fully understand the topic?"

3. The **Noting What I've Learned** outline can be used in any classroom. For example, in Science and Art classes, students can record information about equipment, safety, steps to follow, ingredients, types of materials and so on. They can draw pictures in the boxes to help them remember the way things should look. A summary can be written as a follow-up.

In Social Studies, Science, and Health classes students can prepare brief oral reports to present to the class. Insist that the reports be organized and include three to four subtopics/main ideas with two or three details for each. Student listeners at their desks can take notes using this outline. A summary of one of the reports can be written for homework with students using only what is recorded in the notes.

In English classes, students can employ this outline to keep track of information when they prepare for a book report. Tell them to staple two outlines together and label each box with the parts of a story, such as, Main Characters, Setting, Theme,

Conflict, Resolution and so on. As students read, they can record details that are related to each part. Younger students can draw pictures in the boxes which illustrate important events or ideas from the book. Details about the picture can be noted to the right.

4. In addition to the many suggestions given for using **Column Note Taking**, one additional strategy comes to mind which has broad applications among the varied disciplines. After your class has completed reading a piece of literature from a particular time period or culture or a chapter from a text, have students generate a random list of important ideas and concepts gleaned from the reading. Record these ideas and concepts on the blackboard. Then pair off the students and have them group the ideas by category (family customs, food, education, daily life, geography and so on.) Instruct them to use Column Note Taking and record the categories, or subtopics, in the Recall Column, and the specific ideas and concepts in the Note Column.

5. The best way to benefit from note taking is to interact with the notes *soon after taking them*. Visual learners should be encouraged to write marginal notes or questions as they review their notes nightly. They can use highlighters to emphasize important information, draw boxes around key concepts and enumerate details listed. Occasionally, you should ask them to transcribe their notes into some other form (a chart, Venn diagram, matrix, summary and so on) for homework. Auditory learners should be encouraged to recite the information from their notes. They can use a tape recorder if that makes it more fun, or they can simply close their door and pretend they are teaching someone else. Long-term memory is increased by engaging in *review soon after the first exposure* to information.

6. Another way to engage students in cooperative note-taking activities is to prepare another five-minute lecture. (Again, be sure your presentation is organized and includes three to four subtopics with details for each). Students listen and take notes in any form (simple listing, Column Note Taking, Mapping, Traditional Outlining and so on). After the lecture, each individual spends five minutes editing, clarifying, reorganizing the notes. Then students switch papers. Each student writes a summary—using only what is provided in the notes. Do not grade these papers. Use them only as a means of identifying the best note-taking strategies. Discuss which type of note taking led to the most complete summary. Provide frequent opportunities to try again.

(Topic) _____

K

(List what you already **know** about the topic.)

W

(List questions about what you **want to know** about the topic.)

L

(Using your questions as a guide, write all the information you have **learned** in this column. Use the back of this page if necessary.)

Noting What I've Learned

Topic _____

Main Ideas/Key Words/
Questions/Drawings

What I've learned:

1. _____

2. _____

3. _____

1. _____

2. _____

3. _____

1. _____

2. _____

3. _____

1. _____

2. _____

3. _____

Column Note Taking

General Subject _____ Date _____

Recall Column Subtopics/Main Ideas	Note Column Supporting Details

Column Note Taking

General Subject _____ Date _____

Recall Column Subtopics/Main Ideas	Note Column Supporting Details

Comprehension

As I began leaving the basal and workbook and moved toward literature-based reading, comprehension was an area that concerned me, especially with my older students. I wanted to make sure they understood everything the chapters were saying, so I made up comprehension questions. I wrote about 6–12 questions per reading assignment, and gave them to my students every day. When I look back and analyze those questions, two things stick out in my mind:

1. Most of the questions were literal, and
2. This was the reason my students defined reading as "answering questions."

My students had been given little or no instruction in knowing how to answer questions.

One strategy I discovered to be extremely effective in helping students successfully deal with comprehension questions is called Question-Answer Relationships (QARs), developed by Pearson and Johnson (1978). QARs help students learn about the process they use to formulate answers. It helps students become aware of the different methods or information sources needed for answering different types of questions. I have seen this heightened awareness increase some of my students' abilities as they answer comprehension questions about both narrative and expository texts.

There are three basic question-answer relationships:

Literal

These are just that, literal questions. The answers are *Right There*. The answer is directly written and stated in the text (right there). The words used to make up the question are the same words that are in the answer.

*Students are actually **reading the lines.***

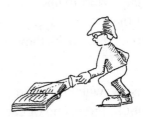

Interpretive

When faced with these questions, students will constantly come up to me and say, "The answer is not there." And they are right! The answer is not there in black and white. They need to make inferences in order to come up with the answer. Students need to *Think and Search* to find the answers.

*Students are actually **reading between the lines.***

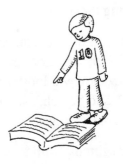

Applied

These are questions that need to be answered using your own experiences. These answers are not in the book. You must find the answers *On Your Own*.

*Students are actually **reading beyond the lines.***

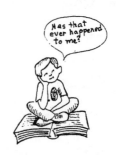

Excerpted from *Making the Connection: Learning Skills Through Literature* (3-6). Peterborough, NH: Crystal Springs Books, 1997.

When I begin teaching students how to use QARs, I start with very easy materials. I ask students to tell me some of their favorite books when they were young. Usually *Goldilocks and the Three Bears* is mentioned. I take that book and make a copy of some pages and put them on the overhead. We read the page on the overhead and then I ask some *literal* (Right There) questions. I write the questions on the board so students can see that the words used to make up the question are the same ones that contain the answer. For example, this question is written on the board:

What did Mama Bear pour into the bowls?

We find the answer on the page and underline the same words in the question and answer:

Mama Bear poured porridge into the bowls.

I use the last page of the book to illustrate an *interpretive* (Think and Search) question. It states that when Goldilocks opened her eyes and saw the bears, she screamed and ran out the door. I ask the question:

How did Goldilocks feel when she saw the bears?

My students usually laugh and say scared, afraid, petrified, etc. I then ask them how they knew, because it didn't tell them on the page. This is a great way to begin to help them see what it means to read between the lines. When teaching this strategy, I tell my students that I'm more concerned about them knowing *what kind of* QAR they are looking at rather than knowing the answer.

When my students come up to me with a question and say, "I don't get it," or "I can't find the answer," my first response is to tell them what kind of question it is. They then need to tell me how they will look for the answer. Students start coming up to me saying, "I know it is a "Think and Search," so the answer is not right there on the lines, but I need help knowing what paragraphs or pages I need to put together." That is very different from, "I don't get it!"

Beginning with a very easy and familiar book ensures that all students are successful and can really start to understand the concepts. I use easy, familiar materials for at least a week or two. I then start to apply this strategy to more detailed books, and finally to grade-appropriate materials: the books they are reading for enjoyment, as well as their science and social studies texts.

Now, when I write questions to go along with reading assignments, I usually limit the amount to three, one of each kind. On the facing page is an example of the questions students were asked to answer while reading *James and the Giant Peach*. Notice that there is one kind of each QAR.

James and the Giant Peach

Pages 28-47

1. What happened to Aunt Sponge and Aunt Spiker?

2. How did all the creatures feel when the peach started to roll? Prove it!

3. Where do you think they will end up? Why?

Another way to use QARs is to have students write their own questions after reading. My students have traveling strategy folders that they can take and use anywhere they are working: at their desk, in the hall, at a table, in the resource room, at home, etc. (Manila file folders work well.) On the inside of the folder is the reproducible found on the following page. I find that if students have this information right at their fingertips, they use it!

Once a month we look at the folders, and those students who need clean copies get new ones. Usually by the end of each month the QAR sheets are full of "chicken scratches," which shows me they are really using these.

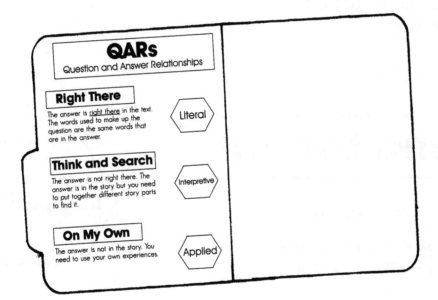

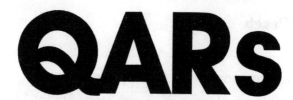

QARs

Question and Answer Relationships

Right There

The answer is <u>right there</u> in the text. The words used to make up the question are the same words that are in the answer.

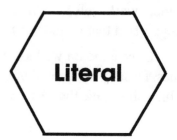

Literal

Think and Search

The answer is not right there. The answer is in the story but you need to put together different story parts to find it.

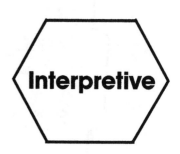

Interpretive

On My Own

The answer is not in the story. You need to use your own experiences.

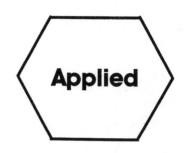

Applied

Home and School Reading Contract

	Independent	Read Aloud
Monday	☐	☐
Tuesday	☐	☐
Wednesday	☐	☐
Thursday	☐	☐
Friday	☐	☐
Saturday	☐	☐
Sunday	☐	☐

Successful Readers

Before Reading

* think about what they already know about the subject
* know their purpose/are motivated
* have a general sense of how the BIG ideas will fit together

During Reading

* attend to both words and meanings
* concentrate well while reading
* willing to "risk" -- guess, fill in meanings using context clues
* stop and use "fix it" strategies when confused
* construct efficient strategies to monitor comprehension

After Reading

* understand how the pieces of information fit together
* able to identify the BIG ideas and why they are critical
* interested in reading and finding out more, asking questions, raising issues

Struggling Readers

Before Reading

* begin to read without thinking about the topic
* do not know why they are reading/ lack of motivation
* have little sense of how the BIG ideas will fit together

During Reading

* overattend to individual words -- miss meanings
* trouble concentrating
* read slower, stop frequently
* easily defeated by difficult words and text
* seldom use "fix it" strategies, just plod along--just finish
* unable to monitor their comprehension

After Reading

* do not understand how the parts form the whole
* often focus on details--don't see what is essential
* view reading as "no fun", just what to be done

Beverly Eisele

Teaching Implications

Before Reading

* help students form a reading "roadmap" before beginning
* Introduce the book through the cover illustration, pose questions

During Reading

* use student reading level books to promote fluency
* encourage students to read like talking
* teach "fix it" strategies
* pose questions to encourage frequent student comprehension checks

After Reading

* lead student discussion of :

  * literary elements
  * main idea
  * cause and effect
  * sequencing
  * prediction

Top Ten "Must Do" Elements for Reading Instruction

 Use **Flexible Grouping** for reading instruction
* Whole group
* Small group
* Buddies
* Independent

 Teach **Guided Reading** everyday to every child

 Insure 20 minutes of **independent reading** for each student with a book on his/her reading level.

 Shared Reading -- Teaching read-aloud everyday, books <u>above</u> the student's reading level.

 Actively teach **<u>reading strategies</u>** that include:
* word decoding
* using context for assistance
* use what you already know

Beverly Eisele

Use a **variety of materials** that insure success through scaffolding, step-by-step progress.

 Teach **Working With Words** everyday through hands-on materials.

 Construct semantic maps, graphic organizers.

 Emphasize and teach the top 10 **reading skills**:

* Vocabulary   * Compare and Contrast
* Decoding   * Inferencing
* Sequencing   * Literary elements
* Main Idea   * Draw Conclusions
* Important Details

 Assess student progress
1. Determine student reading level at beginning of the year
2. Re-evaluate at mid-year
3. Reassessment at end-of-year
4. Assess progress day-by-day using check lists and teacher observation

Beverly Eisele

Before Reading

* prepare students for reading or listening
* assess students prior knowledge
* provide a visual aid for brainstorming, clarifying, categorizing, and prioritizing (organizing thinking)

Graphic Organizers

During Reading

* make logical predictions
* develop a visual "roadmap" for following story development
* understand story patterns, connections

After Reading

* students compare and contrast one novel to another
* examine figurative language
* understand the author's craft

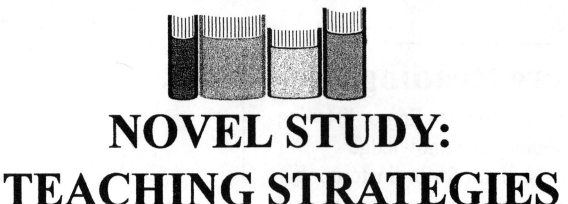

NOVEL STUDY:
TEACHING STRATEGIES

Novel: <u>Night of the Twister</u> by Ivy Ruckman

<u>**Pre-Reading Strategies:**</u>

* Teacher introduces book by showing front cover illustration

* Ask students to make predictions based on this visual information

* Teacher reads p. 2, the real story form Associated Press, June 1980

* Student Connection - any student related stories of their experiences with tornadoes should be shared at this time

* Read the dedication--What could this infer?

* On a U.S. map locate Nebraska and the Platte River

* Who was the President at the time the story takes place?

Beverly Eisele

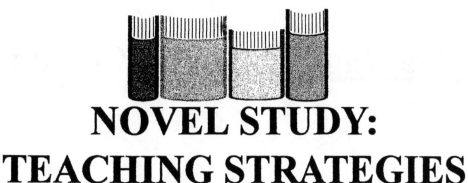

NOVEL STUDY:
TEACHING STRATEGIES

NIGHT OF THE TWISTER - CHAPS. 1 & 2 VOCABULARY

During Reading Strategies:

These are some vocabulary you may want to discuss or use for word games as you read the chapters. **Do not** review and explain these words before you read.

red-letter	dawned
merchandise	doomsday
via	indication
cirrus	cogitates
pining	authentic
backgammon	muttered
chortled	ambles
inhale	

Students learn vocabulary **best** through:
  * acting out the word
  * using the word in their speech, frequently
  * drawing the word in word games
  * knowing a synonym for the word
  * reading the word in context

Least effective methods for learning vocabulary:

  * look up the word in the dictionary, write the definition
  *copy the word several times
  * match the word with definition on paper

During Reading Strategies: Continued

Newspaper: Read the weather page in USA Today.
Find Nebraska on the weather map.
What's the forecast for today?
Find a location that has a similar weather forecast.

GAME: BE A DETECTIVE (skill: foreshadowing)
As the story progresses, what are some clues the author gives as to
what is about to happen?

> * clouds change appearance, sun disappears behind them p. 10
> * green sky p. 13
> * windy cold replaces hot, muggy day p. 11
> * trees and newspapers whipped by wind p. 13
> * strong blasts of air p. 15

Beverly Eisele

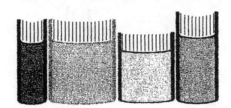

TEACHING STRATEGIES

"After" Reading Activities

Written Response--to a book, or story.

Student writes: title, author, and any of the following: a favorite part, a prediction, favorite character, scene or reason why he like the book. Illustrate as you wish.

Materials: A spiral notebook for each student. Write *Response Book* on front cover of each. Use same color for each notebook so these are easily recognized in a desk or basket.

Letter Writing--after reading any of the books on the letter writing bibiliography. Teacher uses one for the model. Students write their own.

Materials: Envelopes, writing paper, crayons, colored pencils, etc. Use the Tool Box for Writing that was shown this summer.

Postcards -- What are you studying in social studies? Write postcard back home from these locations and illustrate the front.

Materials: Show sample travel postcards and provide 4x6 index cards for writing. Use the Writing Tool Box.

Research Center -- Open the encyclopedia to anything you wish to study. Use books the same way. Write 5 facts about your subject that other people find interesting.

Materials: Encyclopedias and many books on a variety of subjects (include science and social studies), paper, writing tools.

Beverly Eisele

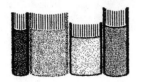 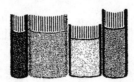 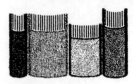

Write a story following a model shown from a famous book.

Example: The Important Book by Margaret W. Brown.
Teacher reads the book, shows and explains the model on chart paper.
Teacher models the writing and uses this chart for students to examine
and follow. Student responses could be from the areas of *science*: The
Important Thing About . . . electricity, magnets, symbiosis, mammals,
seeds, water, etc., or *math*: division, fractions, addition, grouping,
money, time--or *social studies*: explorers, colonists, Civil War, WWII,
government.

Compare words through writing. Pose questions on a chart like:
Would you eat a rhea? Explain. Where will you find a Periodic Table in
high school? Would you be happy if someone said you were feeble?
Does your mother live closer to Tampa or Munich? Would you wear a
fedora to school?
Materials: Chart paper and markers, a copy of today's story.

Categorize Vocabulary: Find 5 words from today's story. Put them in
the chart under appropriate headings. Long Word, Short Word, Dancy
Word, or Awesome Adjectives: Vexing Verbs.

Write an anagram with a word we have studied.
Died millions of years ago
Ice Age wiped them out
No human has ever seen a living dinosaur
Only continued study can discover cause of extinction
S
A
U
R

Beverly Eisele

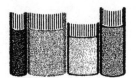 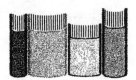 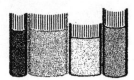

Bring an unusual object to class. Students touch, examine, feel and then write what it is. *I think the object is a ____ that is made of ____. It is used for ____ by ____.* Objects could be in conjunction with books being read.

Write growing sentences and use one word from your story today.

Cats walk.
Cats walk fast.
White cats walk fast.
Five white cats walk fast.
My five white cats walk fast.
My sister's five white cats walk fast.
My sister's five ferocious white cats walk fast.
My sister's five ferocious white cats walk fast homeward.

Write a rule book. Illustrate with pictures that show the rule. **Example:** Fraction--any number over itself equals one. Any number over one equals itself. A fraction with a higher numerator than a denominator is an improper fraction.

That's Good. **That's Bad**. Use science examples (ants, rain, ice, lions, electricity, disease, or social studies; Georgia, the Revolutionary War, Congress, or language arts topics; homophones, summaries, book reports, reading). **Follow the pattern:** *The good thing about_____. The bad thing about_____.*

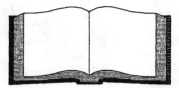

Highly Motivating--Low Readability Chapter Books

Books in a series--reading level indicated on back of boo

Magic Tree House Books

Stepping Stone Series

Bailey School Kids

Junie B. Jones--Barbara Park

Mary Marony--Suzy Kline

Tony Abbott Series

Cam Jansen

Encyclopedia Brown

Gary Paulsen--Action Adventure Series

ALPHABET BOOKS

A IS FOR ASIA	by Cynthia Lee
ANTICS	by Cathi Hepworth
HIEROGLYPHS FROM A TO Z	by Peter Der Manuelian
BUTTERFLY ALPHABET	by Kjell Sandved
A WALK IN THE RAINFOREST	by Kristin Joy Pratt
A IS FOR ANGRY	by Sandra Boynton
THE ALPHABET FROM Z TO A	by Judith Viorst
ALPHABLOCKS	by Kat Anderson
GEOGRAPHY FROM A TO Z	by Jack Knowlton
ASHANTI TO ZULU	by Margaret Musgrove
ABC OF ECOLOGY	by Harry Milgram
WE READ: A TO Z	by Donald Crews
THE Z WAS ZAPPED	by Chris Van Allsburg
Q IS FOR DUCK	by Mary Elting & Michael Folson
ABCEDAR	by George Ella Lyon
WILD ANIMALS OF AMERICA ABC	by Hope Ryden
ALLIGATOR ARRIVED WITH APPLES	by Crescent Dragonwagon
ANAMALIA	by Graeme Base
ILLUMINATIONS	by Jonathan Hunt
THE AMAZING ANIMAL ALPHABET BOOK	by Roger & Mariko Chouinard
AARDVARKS, DISEMBARK!	By Ann Jonas
GRETCHEN'S ABC	by Gretchen Simpson
THE HANDMADE ALPHABET	by Laura Rankin

THE ALPHABET SERIES BY JERRY PALLOTTA
(high interest / science facts / strong vocabulary)

THE BIRD ALPHABET BOOK
THE ICKY BUG ALPHABET BOOK
THE OCEAN ALPHABET BOOK
THE FLOWER ALPHABET BOOK
THE YUCKY REPTILE ALPHABET BOOK
THE FROG ALPHABET BOOK
THE FURRY ALPHABET BOOK
THE DINOSAUR ALPHABET BOOK
THE EXTINCT ALPHABET BOOK
THE DESERT ALPHABET BOOK
THE FRESH WATER ALPHABET BOOK
THE UNDERWATER ALPHABET BOOK
THE VICTORY GARDEN VEGETABLE ALPHABET BOOK

Third-Eighth Grade Reading Level

Reading
Level

2	Adler, David	*Cam Jansen* books
6	Armstrong, Sperry	*Call It Courage*
5/6	Armstrong, William	*Sounder*
7	Avi	*The True Confessions of Charlotte Doyle*
7		*Poppy*
7		*Something Upstairs*
7/8		*Nothing But the Truth*
4		*The Barn*
6		*The Blue Heron*
5	Banks, Lynne Reid	*The Indian in the Cupboard*
5		*The Secret of the Indian*
5	Bauer, Marion	*On My Honor*
3/4	Blume, Judy	*Tales of a Fourth Grade Nothing*
3/4		*Superfudge*
3		*The One in the Middle is the Green Kangaroo*
3		*Blubber*
3		*The Plain and the Great One*
4		*Otherwise Known as Sheila the Great*
6/7	Burch, Robert	*Queenie Peavy*
4/5	(Depression Era South)	*Doddie and the Go Cart*
4		*Ida Early Comes Over the Mountain*
5	Byars, Betsy	*The Burning Questions of Bingo Brown*
5		*Bingo Brown and the Language of Love*
4		*Trouble River*
4		*The Pinballs*
4		*The Cybil War*
3		*Tornado*
7		*Cracker Jackson*
3	Cleary, Beverly	*Beezus and Ramona*
3		*Henry and Beezus*
3/4		*Ralph S. Mouse*
5		*Dear Mr. Henshaw*
5		*Strider*
5		*A Girl From Yarnhill (autobiography)*
6/7	Cooney, Carolyn	*The Face on the Milk Carton*
5/6	Dahl, Roald	*The Witches*
5/6		*Matilda*
3/4		*The BFG*
3/4		*Fantastic Mr. Fox*
3		*James and the Giant Peach*
7/8		*Nothing But the Truth*
2/3		*George's Marvelous Medicine*
2		*The Twits*
6	Defelico, Cynthia	*The Apprenticeship of Lucas Whitaker*
6		*Weasel*
6/7		*Lostman's River*

Great Chapter Books: Third-Eighth Grade Reading Level

Reading
Level

5	Dixon, Franklin	*Hardy Boys* Series
4	Fitzhugh, Louise	*Harriet the Spy*
5/6	Fleischman, Sid	*The Whipping Boy*
4	Gardiner, John Reynolds	*Stone Fox*
6/7	George, Jean Craighead	*My Side of the Mountain*
7		*Julie of the Wolves*
3/4	George, Jean Craighead	*A Day in the Desert*
3/4		*A Day in the Rain Forest*
5/6		*Who Really Killed Cock Robin?*
4		*There's An Owl in the Shower*
2	Giff, Patricia Reilly	*The Beast in Ms. Rooney's Room*
2		*Henry Mudge*
2		*Happy Birthday, Ronald Morgan*
2		*Next Year I'll Be Special*
2		*The War Began at Supper*
2		*Ronald Morgan Goes to Bat*
2		*Today Was a Terrible Day*
2		*Watch Out, Ronald Morgan*
5	Hahn, Mary Downing	*M.C. Higgins the Great*
5		*Brother Brown*
5		*The Planet of Junior Brown*
7/8	Hinton, S.E.	*The Outsiders*
7/8		*That Was Then, This Is Now*
3	Hope, Laura Lee	*Bobbsey Twins* Series
3	Howe, James	*Bunnicula: A Rabbit Tale of Mystery*
3		*The Celery Stalks at Midnight*
3		*Howliday Inn*
3		*Dew Drop Dead*
2/3		*The Fright Before Chrstmas*
6	James, Mary	*Shoebag*
5	Keene, Carolyn	*Nancy Drew* Series
5/6	Konigsburg, E.L.	*From the Mixed Up Files of Mrs. Basil E. Frankweiler*
6		*The View from Saturday*
5/6	L'Engle, Madeleine	*A Wrinkle in Time*
4	Lowry, Lois	*Anastasia Krupnik*
6		*The Giver*
5/6		*Number the Stars*
5	Macaulay, David	*Motel of the Mysteries*
6/7		*Unbuilding*
6/7		*Cathedral*
4	MacLachlan, Patricia	*Arthur for the Very First Time*
4		*Sarah, Plain and Tall*
4	Mikaelsen, Ben	*Rescue Josh McGuire*
5	Naylor, Phyllis Reynolds	*Shiloh*
6	O'Dell, Scott	*Sing Down the Moon*
5		*Island of the Blue Dolphins*
4	Park, Barbara	*Mick Harte Was Here*

Reading Level		
5	Patterson, Katherine	*Jip: His Own Story*
8		*Park's Quest*
5/6		*Bridge to Terabithia*
5/6	Paulsen, Gary	*Hatchet*
5/6		*The River*
5/6		*Brian's Winter*
4/5		*Mr. Tuckett*
5		*Voyage of the Frog*
5		*Tracker*
6		*Dogsong*
6		*Dancing Carl*
4/5	Peck, Robert Newton	*Soup and Trig Books*
5	Rawls, Wilson	*Summer of the Monkeys*
5/6		*Where the Red Fern Grows*
4	Ruckman, Ivy	*Night of the Twisters*
3	Sachar, Louis	*Sideways Stories from the Wayside School*
3		*Sideways Arithmetic from the Wayside School*
2	Sharmat, Marjorie	*Nate the Great* series
2		*Rich Mitch*
4	Smith, Doris Buchanan	*A Taste of Blueberries*
4	Smith, Robert Kimmel	*The War with Grandpa*
3		*Chocolate Fever*
3		*Jelly Belly*
2/3		*Bobby Baseball*
2/3		*Mostly Michael*
3	Sobol, Donald	*Encyclopedia Brown* series
8	Speare, Elizabeth George	*The Witch of Blackbird Pond*
5		*The Sign of the Beaver*
6	Spinelli, Jerry	*Maniac Maghee*
6		*Crash*
5	Taylor, Mildred	*The Gold Cadillac*
5		*Roll of Thunder, Hear My Cry*
5		*Song of the Trees*
7/8	Taylor, Theodore	*The Cay*
3	Warner, Gertrude	*Boxcar Children* series
4	White, E.B.	*The Trumpet of the Swans*
3/4		*Stuart Little*
5		*Charlotte's Web*
6	Yolen, Jane	*The Devil's Arithmetic*
6	Zindel, Paul	*The Doom Stone*
5/6		*Loch*
8		*My Darling, My Hamburger*

HOW DO WE COLLECT *Baseline Data?*

What Constitutes Baseline Data?

Because the work included in a portfolio represents a student's learning over time and provides evidence of its breadth, it is important to carry out an initial reading and writing assessment during the first and second months of the school year. This baseline information is the first component of the portfolio preparation process. *Baseline data* consists of any sample work that demonstrates what students can do in a certain area when they arrive in the classroom. This information serves as a starting point from which we can measure a child's progress, just as we put a mark on the doorpost in order to measure a child's physical growth.

How do we collect baseline data in reading?

During September and October we give individual students a diagnostic reading performance test, which consists of a reading miscue analysis or running record (Clay 1993) and/or a listening assessment. For the reading assessment, we select passages from graded texts or from publisher-produced sources such as *The New Sucher-Allred Reading Placement Inventory* or the *Burns/Roe Informal Reading Inventory*. The student reads aloud a short, untitled passage and retells the story in his or her own words. Another useful resource is the district reading specialist, who may be able to suggest other materials on this order. We also ask the student questions to elicit evidence of various types of comprehension — making inferences, thinking critically, identifying the main events, and synthesizing the story by giving it a title. We sometimes ask questions about vocabulary or background knowledge to verify whether the student has indeed understood the text.

We record the entire process on audiotape, analyze the tape, and then discuss it with the student. With students who are not yet reading — young children in the primary grades, English-as-a-Second-Language students, or students with learning problems — we check comprehension by reading to them. This listening sample then serves as the baseline data.

In analyzing this information, we look for signs of the student's strengths as well as for strategies the student uses to understand the text, and record this information on the form. We also note problem areas and any strategies a student needs to learn. Although grade level is not the issue in this analysis, we do want to know whether students can handle the texts we will be using. Figure 3-1 shows a sample of a filled out Reading and Listening Baseline information sheet (a blank version appears as form A-1 in Appendix A). We generally use the key included in Figure 3.1 to fill in these forms, but we advise you to design your own marking system if that would be better suited to your needs. If you are not accustomed to analyzing reading data, a resource like *The Whole Language Evaluation Book,* edited by Ken Goodman, Yetta Goodman, and Wendy Hood, is an excellent guide.

The following day, the students have a chance to listen to their tapes for a performance evaluation.

This is the students first opportunity to try self-evaluation.

We ask students to fill in a form (see A.2 in Appendix A) containing open-ended questions intended to help them assess their reading before the conference with the teacher. When students listen to themselves read on the tape while following along in the text, they become aware of their own reading behaviors and are more prepared to discuss their evaluation with the teacher. Student and teacher share their findings with one another and launch their assessment partnership.

What does this conference sound like?

During this first conference of the year, the teacher's attitude is key to the students' first success at self-assessment. We are careful not to focus on deficits or the students will clam up. Instead, we focus on the strengths and strategies already in place. We also

look at the strategies needed if the student is to become an even more effective reader. The dialogue might sound like this:

Teacher: Billy, I wanted you to read and retell the story on the tape recorder so we can have a record of your reading at the beginning of the year. Since I don't know much about you, I need to find out what strengths you already have and what strategies you still need to improve your reading. In January and June you will read on the tape again and then we can compare your progress in reading since the beginning of the year. It will be very exciting because you will be able to hear how much you have improved this year. Your parents will also be able to listen to the tape and hear how much you've improved. Won't this be nifty?

Billy: Yeah.
(The discussion turns to Billy's performance on the tape.)

Teacher: What did you learn about your reading when you listened to yourself?

Billy: I read lots of words wrong and I should read better.

Teacher: I noticed that you had trouble with some words, but I saw you beginning to do some things that good readers do. Did you hear yourself stop when you read a word that didn't make sense?

Billy: Yeah.

Teacher: When you stopped to think about that word you indicated that your brain was listening to the story, and when you read a word that didn't make sense, you stopped to fix it. Did you know that good readers use that strategy? Poor readers would just keep going and not pay any attention to whether they are making sense or not. So let's mark that strategy on this form. What do you think, Billy? Did you correct yourself every time you got stuck?

Excerpted from *Portfolios in the Classroom* by Beth Schipper and Joanne Rossi. York, ME: Stenhouse Publishers, 1997.

Billy: Not every time, 'cause sometimes I couldn't figure out the word.

Teacher: So what were you doing to figure out the word? Could you hear yourself on the tape? You were whispering.

Billy: Yeah! I was sounding it out.

Teacher: Yes, you were! Good readers use this strategy too. In fact, you did a beautiful job. You kept sounding and blending the sounds together until you recognized a word that made sense in the sentence. When you did that I said to myself, "Yay, for Billy! He uses sounds and context clues together!" Let's mark that on the form under strategies you use. How do you think you did when you retold your story in your own words?

Billy: Good. I only missed the part about the baton because I didn't get it.

Teacher: I agree with you. You retold the story and covered all the main points in sequence. The baton part was difficult because if you've never seen that word in print, you may not know what to say when you retell that part of the story. Do you know what a baton is now?

Billy: Yeah, it's that stick thing that runners give to each other when they race.

Teacher: How did you figure that out?

Billy: Well, it says that she won the race even after she dropped the baton. So I figured that that must be the stick. I saw a relay race on TV once.

Teacher: I'm really impressed, Billy. You just explained to me another strategy that good readers use. You used your background knowledge, things you already knew, to give meaning to the story. Let's mark that on the form also. Did you know you were using strategies that good readers use?

Billy: No, I just do 'em, I guess.

Teacher: Yes, you do. How do you do with the questions?
(They go on to discuss the different questions.)

Teacher: Do you have some goals for reading? Let's put them down here on the form.

Billy: *(Thinks and finally responds)* I want to read bigger words and chapter books, and um, remember more about the story after I read.

Teacher: Those are excellent goals. I have some goals for you also. I wrote them here. Number 1, become more consistent in monitoring your sense-making. Number 2, develop your vocabulary. Number 3, by January, learn to enjoy reading more. Is there anything else you want to add?

Billy: No, it looks good to me.

Teacher: Thank you for helping me learn about you and your reading. I think you've got a good start. *(Billy smiles with pride and walks to his desk.)*

Conferences like this one help to establish a classroom environment that invites students to participate in their own learning. During the conference the teacher asks questions to focus on the student's use of strategies while reading. This language may or may not be new to the student, but it will develop awareness and encourage students to monitor their own reading behaviors.

How do we collect baseline data in writing?

Most teachers are more familiar with collecting baseline data because students usually do a writing sample during the first few days of school. In the past, we collected and graded it, but we suggest instead that you treat it like the reading baseline data. We ask the student to write a story or a paragraph on something he or she knows a lot about. To determine which developmental writing skills the student has already mastered, we take the writing sample home and analyze it, then schedule a conference with the student, just as we do for the reading sample. Here again, we look for strengths over weaknesses. For example, Chris, a third grader, wrote the following sample. His former teacher allowed him to type it on the computer because he had such difficulty expressing himself using a pencil.

TREES ARE GID BEACUSE THEY GIV ASAJANT [OXYGEN] TO PEOPLE. SOM PEOPLE DOT BLEV IN TREES GIV ASJNET TO PEOPLE. SOM PEOPLE COT TREES DOWN. ANNAMLS LIV IN TREES AND WIHN THE TREES GIT COT DOWN THE ANNAMLS HAF TO LIF AND GOT A NOW HOME BECAUSE THEY OLD HOME IS DESROED.

Figure 3.2 shows the Writing Baseline Information Form we filled in for Chris. A blank version appears in Appendix A (See A.3).

The conference about this piece of writing might sound like this:

Teacher: Chris, what do you think about your writing?

Chris: I don't like to write.

Teacher: Why don't you like to write?

Chris: 'Cause it's hard to hold the pencil and I can't think of anything to say.

Teacher: But you had some good ideas here and you've done some things that good writers do. Can you tell what they are?

Chris: *(Shrugs his shoulders)*

Teacher: One thing good writers do is to write about the subjects they know. You seem to know a lot about what happens when people cut down trees. Where did you learn about it?

Chris: I like to learn about things in science. I talked about this with my dad.

Teacher: Oh, terrific! Let me show you something else you did that good writers do. I marked it on the sheet. *(Shows form)* You gave the reader some interesting information. It's like a small report. You had a main idea and you support it with details. Look, I was able to mark many of these ideas under organization. You didn't just put the ideas in any order. You told what happens first, next, and last. This is a cause and effect paragraph. Did you know that?

Chris: No.

Teacher: Well, now you know. Let's look at some other things you did. You had sentences with periods at the end and you used some sounds to spell some words you had never spelled before, like *oxygen* and *destroyed*. I'm curious. Why did you use all capital letters?

Chris: 'Cause it's easier.

Teacher: Hmmm. Oh, you mean you're not always sure when to use capital letters?

Chris: I suppose so.

Teacher: Should we put down capitals as something we need to work on?

Chris: I guess.

Teacher: You wrote a report instead of a story. Most kids wrote stories. Why do you think you did that?

Chris: 'Cause I hate to write stories. I only like to write about real things.

Teacher: Oh, I see. What kinds of things would you like to be able to do in writing this year?

Chris: Maybe spell more words and get faster on the computer.

Teacher: OK, we'll put that down. I'm going to add another couple of goals for you. I noticed you didn't do any brainstorming even though you practiced it last year in Mrs. Simmons's class.

Chris: I hate brainstorming. It takes too long. I just like to write sentences.

Teacher: This year I'll show you some ways to make it easier for you. OK?

Chris: I guess.

Teacher: The other thing I'd like to add is that you become more comfortable writing stories. Maybe you can use some information you know to write some interesting stories?

Chris: Maybe.

Teacher: Even though you don't like writing, weren't you surprised you did so many things that good writers do?

Chris: Uh huh.

Because of his spelling difficulties, Chris's writing has received a lot of criticism. Few people can see past his spelling mistakes.

Once again, the baseline conference has two major aims. One is to create a student-teacher partnership that encourages the student to take an active part in the conference and to assume some control over the evaluation process. The teacher points out students' strengths as a basis for building the writing skills but without ignoring weak areas. These she addresses through lists of areas needing work or goals. The second aim is to help the student become aware of their own strengths and weaknesses in writing. Unless they have some awareness of these underlying elements, they regard their writing as simple as a series of isolated assignments. The baseline conference is the first step in giving students the language to consider and select portfolio pieces.

We found these conferences a little awkward at first, but using a checklist makes the process easier and helps keep the focus on naming the strengths first. We still reminisce about the reactions of some kids during these conferences, most of whom had never before heard or talked about their strengths. Not surprisingly, they couldn't wait to have another conference.

Assessments are drawn primarily from the Reading and Listening Baseline Information checklist and the Writing Baseline Information checklist completed in September. Although children will be familiar with their baseline strengths and needs because of their conference, they should keep their first reading and writing samples in their portfolio all year. Without these first reading and writing samples for comparison, students will not be able to see the extent of their growth or reflect on the significance of this new learning.

Some teachers keep the first samples in their own folders and hand them out before students write self-assessments. Others staple the first writing sample to the portfolio cover, where it is available for comparison each time students write a self-assessment. In addition, we staple a photocopy of the baseline checklists on the inside cover of the portfolio to remind students of their starting point.

What about baseline data in the content areas?

We've focused on the language arts, but that does not mean that the same process can't be used in the content areas. We aren't content area specialists, but we've worked successfully with many content area teachers who have adapted this process for their own subject. If the purpose of baseline data is to establish a starting point, what students know before instruction begins, the one thing these teachers had to decide was what baseline data would be most meaningful for their purposes.

Two math teachers looked at their curriculum for the year and decided what background knowledge and skills students needed in order to be successful in their classes. One gave students several word problems to solve and asked them not only to give the answers but also to tell, in writing, the process they used to solve the problems. He also checked their straight computational skills by giving them some problems in several different categories, such as fractions, decimals, percentages, and so on. The other teacher found a math placement test that matched the district's curriculum and the text she would be using. Both teachers gave a simple survey to check students'

- interest
- study habits
- attitude toward the subject
- sense of competence in the subject areas

Although the baseline measurements were different, both teachers gained information about students they could share with them. This information is the foundation for conferences and for the portfolio process.

Science and social studies teachers have told us that they need information about their students in the following areas:

- background knowledge of the subject area
- reading skills
- writing skills
- study skills
- attitude

During the first few weeks of school, one of the ways teachers have measured students' background knowledge is to ask them to write down what they know about certain topics in their journals or learning logs. Sometimes the responses are in narrative form and sometimes in the form of a semantic map or a brainstorming list. Teachers can get a sense of a student's ability to write coherent paragraphs from this activity. The following samples of journal entries from a fifth-grade class concern children's background knowledge in photosynthesis.

- "I think photosynthesis is a photo or picture and a thesis statement. I really have no clue what photosynthesis means."
- "I think photosifies is something to do with a computer. Something like holloghans. I saw a T.V. show that had this computer that can make hollergram. Or it could be like something to do with photos."
- "I think it is when you guess how a picture would look like."
- "I thing photosynthesis are pictures because the word photosynthesis has the word photo and synthesis is like someby studies about picture drawings of art or something like that."
- "I think a photosynthisi is a graph you did and experament like a copy of something a graph is a brainstorming your thoughts."

Teachers can get a sense of students' reading ability and background knowledge by using an assessment strategy called *cloze* procedure. A cloze passage might look like this:

Photosynthisis is a process by which green _____ make their own _____. They get water from the _____ using their _____. They use the _____ in their leaves and the _____ from the sun to make _____. As a result _____ is released into the air. If green _____ do not get _____ they die.

(*Answers: plants, food, soil, roots, clorophyll, light, food, oxygen, plants, light*)

To generate a cloze passage,
1. Select short passages that reflect some of the main concepts you will be covering during the semester.

2. Delete key words or every word a

certain regular intervals (every 6th or 8th word, for example). Teachers often use nonstick tape (3M makes Post-it tape) to mask the words before they run off copies.

3. Ask students to fill in the blanks with words that make sense to them, based on what they know. Do not give them a list of words from which to select.

4. Scan the passages to see whether student have a grasp of the concepts. Even if students have not inserted the exact word, they may supply one that reflects some knowledge.

For information on study skills and attitude, teachers have used short student surveys or inventories similar to the one used by math teachers.

Is it realistic to try to have conferences in content areas with 120 students? Ms. Murdock didn't think so, but she was determined to develop portfolios in her seventh-grade science class. We told her about the "have chair, will travel" version of conferences. Once she had collected her baseline data and analyzed it, she made notes about each student on a checklist. Then she assigned students a project that involved reading and writing at their desks. She moved from desk to desk with her chair and had a five-minute conference with each student. Some conferences were longer or shorter depending on the student. She discussed the strengths and the needs of each student, and together they set some goals.

We should put in a word about Ms. Murdock's classroom management during these conferences. She set up the expectation that this was a sacred time between her and the student that was not to be interrupted unless someone was dying. She made sure the assignment she gave was engaging and that students were clear about what they needed to do. Once the conferences were under way, her students understood the power of discussing their individual strengths and needs. Students reported that they really liked setting goals together with the teacher. In fact, she overheard Ray tell his friend not to bother Ms. Murdock because this was really "bad" (translation — "cool").

Figure 3.3 shows a filled out example of the content area checklist. A

blank form can be found in Appendix A (See A.4).

What will be the focus of the portfolio?

We have spent September and October getting to know our students: we have acquired baseline information about them, and we have observed them for almost two months. We have used the language of assessment in our classroom instruction, made charts for new instruction together, and used language from the charts in our conferences. The students meanwhile have been completing assignments. We want to begin to keep some of this work at school so that student have a cross-section to choose from for their portfolios. Since teachers tend to focus on the subject with which they feel most comfortable, we felt less overwhelmed in the beginning when we focused on just reading and writing and added new subjects gradually.

Before we go any further, we have to make a decision about the focus of the portfolio:

- Will it be only a writing portfolio?
- Will it have reading and writing assignments in it?
- Will it have examples from content areas such as science, math, social studies?
- Will it also contain work from art PE, music?
- Will it encompass a mini-portfolio in each subject area that is combined at the end of the year?

What goes into a work folder?

The last component of the portfolio preparation process is gathering assignments and projects into the *work folder*. The work folder is a file that holds students' work temporarily, until they select items for their portfolio. Students choose work for the work folder at the end of each week by quickly culling items from the week's accumulated papers. We recommend that students keep no more than five to ten items in the work folder at a time. Students are much more discriminating about what has potential than we acknowledge. If a student has left out a piece of work we think represents a developmental milestone, we ask the student if we might keep it in our file for the time being. These papers remain in the work folder until the former portfolio selection. All other work is sent home.

Parents are accustomed to seeing their child's work come home, and we need to send it home or we will be submerged under accumulating paper. But we should also alert parents to the portfolio process so they understand that we really are assessing children's work. We communicate this to parents in two ways: we send a letter home explaining the process, and we explain it again at Back-to-School Night. The following letter is an example of one we've used.

Dear Parents:

We are all very excited to tell you about what's new in our classroom. We will be keeping portfolios that contain pieces that best show your child's learning over a period of time. We will still be sending work papers home, but we will keep selected pieces for the portfolio.

After a period of about six weeks, we will look through all the pieces together, and the student will decide which best represent his or her efforts as a learner over this period. Then we will send this "portfolio" home so that your child can discuss it with you and get your reactions. At the end of the year, your child will have a wonderful record of growth and achievement that we can pass to the next teacher. There will be all kinds of information — journal entries, reading tapes, reactions to readings, creative writing, informational writings from science, social studies, math, art, music, PE, etc. You will see portfolio pieces in all stages of production: some will be just ideas, some will be rough drafts (mistakes and all), and some will be finished products. Not all will be polished. There will be no marks on the papers; if another student and I make a comment or ask a question, we will attach a separate piece of paper to the writing.

I am using portfolios because I believe that students must take responsibility for their own learning and must therefore have a great measure of control along the way. Our job — yours and mine — is that of facilitator. For my part, I will do my best to create an environment in the classroom where students are free to take risks in learning, to work cooperatively, to be actively involved in their own learning and the assessment of their learning, to take pride in what they produce, and to learn strategies that will serve them long after they have left my class. For your part, we ask that you show an interest in what your child is doing, write a letter to your child and have a conference about his or her portfolio, and be supportive when he or she makes mistakes along the way. We'll give you more specifics when we send the portfolio home for the first time. In this process, we will be building on your child's strengths and helping him or her over the rough spots.

If you have any questions about the portfolio process or if you would like to see the work before it arrives in the portfolio, please come to the classroom and your child will be very happy to share it with you.

I thank you in advance for your support.

This is only one example of a letter that might go home. Teachers should send letters that reflect their own classroom and personal teaching style.

Summary
We have talked about the final steps before portfolio selection: gathering baseline data, showing students how to make charts of reading and writing strategies, modeling the "Criteria Talk" and sharing the criteria during instruction, deciding on the focus of the student portfolio, and the process of choosing pieces for work folders.

Now we move on to portfolio selection.

Exerpted from *Portfolios in the Classroom: Tools for Learning and Instruction* by Beth Schipper and Joanne Rossi. © 1997. Stenhouse Publishers, York, Maine.

Figure 3.1

Reading and Listening Baseline Information

Name ___Thomas_____ **Date** _9/28/95_____

Grade _3rd_____ **Teacher** _Mrs._____
                                                              Brown

Reading Section Level ___2.5_____ Independent

                       ___3.0_____ Instructional

Listening Level ___4.0_____

Key:	+	=	excellent
	✔+	=	very good
	✔	=	good
	✔ −	=	fair
	−	=	poor

Oral Reading Observations (Omit for Listening Selection)

___✔ −___ fluent
___+___ knows some sight words
___✔ −___ uses phonics
___no___ uses phonics exclusively
___✔ −___ uses context clues
___✔___ uses repetition

Retelling

___+___ main points
___−___ details
___−___ in sequence

Comprehension

___+___ main idea
___−___ details
___ESL___ vocabulary
___✔ −___ inference
___+___ critical thinking

Strategies Observed

___+___ uses background knowledge
___✔ −___ self-monitors and corrects
___+___ synthesizes information
___✔ −___ makes meaningful substitutions

Strengths:
- loves to read
- seems to get main events

Areas in needs of work:
- using context to self-monitor and correct
- vocabulary; continue work in English vocabulary development

Student's Goals
- "understand more words in English; read chapter books"

Teacher's Goals:
- develop strategies for monitoring comprehension & self-correcting
- strengthen vocabulary and sequencing

- ESL — English as a Second Language
- Non-English Proficiency
- Limited English Proficiency

Figure 3.2

Writing Baseline Information

Name ___Chris_____ Date _10/12/92_____ Grade _3rd_____

ESL _____ NEP _____ LEP _____ Teacher_____

Developmental Level _____ Drawing pictures

_____✔_____ Emergent writing

_____ Standard writing

Key:	+	=	excellent
	✔+	=	very good
	✔	=	good
	✔ –	=	fair
	–	=	poor

Writing Observations

____✔____ dictates text

_____ writes in first language

____✔____ writes with inventive spelling

____✔____ writes complete thoughts

_____ uses detail and descriptive language

____✔____ writes complex sentences

_____ writes for different audiences

Organization

_____ uses prewriting strategies

____✔____ states a main idea

____✔____ story has beginning, middle and end

____✔____ writes three related thoughts

____✔____ details support the main idea

____✔____ details in sequence

Process/Passion

_____ takes initiative for writing

_____ responds to teacher's questions

____✔____ has unique style, voice

_____ views self as writer

Mechanics

___✔ –___ uses punctuation correctly

____–____ uses capitalization correctly

___✔ –___ uses standard grammar

____–____ uses standard spelling

Strengths:
- background knowledge, sense of sentence, sequence, concept of cause and effect

Areas in needs of work:
- prewriting strategies, mechanics (caps, spelling), editing/proofreading strategies

Student's Goals
- spell more words, get faster on the computer

Teacher's Goals:
- become more comfortable with writing, acquire strategies for correcting spelling

• ESL — English as a Second Language

Figure 3.3

Content Area Baseline Information

Name Ricardo **Date** _____ **Grade** 6th **Teacher** _____

ESL _____ **NEP** _____ **LEP** _____ **Content Area** Math

Observations

✔	study habits
✔	interest in subject
✔ −	assignments completed
✔	participates in cooperative groups
✔ −	works independently
−	participates in class discussions
−	can read text
✔ −	has appropriate writing skills

Key:	+	=	excellent
	✔+	=	very good
	✔	=	good
	✔ −	=	fair
	−	=	poor

Skill Areas Needed for Competency (Here teachers list specific skills required for their subject area)

✔	whole numbers
✔	decimals
✔	fractions
✔ −	percentages

Problem-Solving/Thinking Skills/Concepts in Subject Area (Here teachers list specific concepts required for their subject area)

✔	operations
−	measurement
✔	time
✔ −	money
−	word problems

Strengths:
- strong computation skills; good grasp of concept of math and operations; works well in groups; hard worker; always attempts assignments

Areas in needs of work:
- lack of English proficiency slows progress in certain areas such as word problems; needs help reading the book

Student's Goals
- get better at reading and writing

Teacher's Goals:
- have Ricardo become familiar with key math terms and signal words in English

- ESL — English as a Second Language
- Non-English Proficiency
- Limited English Proficiency

By Brenda Power & Kelly Chandler

6 Steps to Better Report Card Comments

For years, the report card's little comment box has caused big headaches for teachers. It's too small for a detailed response, but too conspicuous to ignore. What's a teacher to do? Traditionally, we've resorted to bland, general statements about student performance, such as "Lisa is reading at grade level and actively participates in class." And our tone has sounded an awful lot like the parent's drone in a Peanuts cartoon—distant, distinct, and artificial.

Comments don't have to be that way, though, despite limited space. Try our six-step plan for improving your report-card writing. Soon your students, their parents, and even your colleagues will be noticing—and benefiting from—the precision and thoughtfulness of your written responses.

1 **Begin with an "adjective brainstorm."** Create a list of your students' names. Beside each name, jot down one or two adjectives that describe the student as a learner, challenging yourself to avoid repetition (see chart, page 80). Begin this process two weeks before you start filling in report cards so you have ample time to find just the right descriptors for each student.

2 **Take supporting notes.** Once you've completed your list of adjectives, make brief notes during class time that confirm your observations. Virtually any situation—an exchange during a workshop, a direct quote from a conference, an indication of growth through a piece of writing—could inspire notes. It's more effective to provide parents with concrete, relevant examples of their child's performance than with broad, generic statements.

3 **Use sentence stems.** This is an excellent way to get the juices flowing, especially for students who are difficult to describe. The following stems have worked well for us.
- Jessica's best work of the quarter was. . .
- Jonathan has shown improvement in. . .
- This term I was glad to see Connor. . .
- Ask Sarah to talk about. . .
- This term Melissa challenged herself by. . .

Varying stems will help you expand your range of comments, even for such a small space.

4 **Focus on the positive.** It's important to emphasize what students do well so that you, parents, and the students themselves can build from those strengths. Areas of improvement can be revealed through other report-card notations, such as letter grades or conduct codes. Most negative adjectives can be reworked to suggest strengths. For example, *restless* and *easily distracted* students can be characterized as *very energetic*. Regardless of how frustrating a student is, a comment space is not the appropriate place for a disciplinary referral. A phone call to or meeting with parents may be a better course of action.

STUDENT	DESCRIPTORS	EXAMPLE	REPORT-CARD NARRATIVE
Krista	caretaking, kind	Jeff's coming to class	Krista is such an important part of the class community. She is very sensitive to others' feelings. Recently, she helped a new student to feel more comfortable with our routine.
Martin	knowledgeable, curious	nonfiction read-alouds	Martin brings lots of prior knowledge about the natural world to our discussions. Recently, he shared the definition of "photosynthesis" with us during a read-aloud.
Marcy	mischievous, playful	writing workshop	Marcy's mischievous sense of humor comes through in her writing. She likes to write puns and jokes in her journal, and her playful "Once upon a bird" beginning to a story has been borrowed by several other classmates.
Sarah	diligent, hardworking	independent reading	Sarah works hard at improving her independent reading skills. After reading a book numerous times, she often seeks out an adult to listen to her read it aloud.
Angela	thoughtful, helpful	classroom transitions	Angela is always willing to help keep our classroom neat and orderly. She's also quick and thoughtful about assisting others with chores during pick-up time.
Johnny	creative, innovative	bird story in journal	Johnny recently wrote a wonderful piece in his journal called the "Never-Ending Bird Story." Twenty pages long(!), it was creative in its style and innovative in its illustrations.

Lois Pangburn, a first-grade teacher from Mapleton, Maine, generates descriptors and supporting examples for each of her students, then writes comments based on her observations.

5 Write the easy comments first. You will develop comment-writing skills more quickly if you start with students who are easy to describe. As your confidence grows, you'll probably find that you have more to say about those enigmatic students than you realized.

6 Ask colleagues for help. Once you've brainstormed some adjectives and incidents, you may want to elicit the support of colleagues in describing challenging students. Music, physical education, and art teachers might have been observing your students for years, and could have just the insights you need for that student you're struggling to describe. Instructional aides and student interns may also provide valuable observations about the students with whom they have worked.

Your Resources

Well-Chosen Words: Narrative Assessments and Report Card Comments by Brenda Power and Kelly Chandler (Stenhouse. 1998; [800] 988-9812)

Quick Tips for Writing Effective Report Card Comments by Susan Shafer (Scholastic, 1997; [800] 724-6527)

Report Card on Report Cards: Alternatives to Consider by Tara Azwell and Elizabeth Schmar (Heinemann, 1995; [800] 541-2086)

Brenda Power and Kelly Chandler teach at the University of Maine. Together, they wrote *Well-Chosen Words* (Stenhouse, 1998) and serve on the editorial board for *Teacher Research: The Journal of Classroom Inquiry.*

BRING SANITY TO YOUR LIFE —
Ten Ways TO USE YOUR TIME MORE EFFICIENTLY

BY IRV RICHARDSON

Do you wake up each morning and mentally make lists of all the things you need to do to prepare for your teaching day? Are you looking to put some sanity back in your life while you balance teaching in a classroom with the rest of your life? Well, it's about time — *your* time and how you spend it.

A wise time management expert once said of time, "We have all there is and there isn't enough." If there were an extra day in the week or an extra month in the year, somebody would have undoubtedly discovered it by now. Since there won't be any extra hours to get it all done, you need to look at the time you do have and make some different decisions about how to spend that time.

The following ten guidelines will help you reevaluate how you are spending your time and offer suggestions about ways to use what time you do have more efficiently.

1. Remind yourself that being an effective teacher doesn't mean being a perfect teacher. There is always more you can do to make your classroom a better place for children . . . create a new center, put up a new bulletin board, rearrange the classroom, invite in a new guest speaker. As someone who cares deeply about children it is easy for you to become "over-intended." All of these intentions are great, but if you consider yourself less of a teacher because you don't complete all of your intended classroom improvements, or if you complete them and then resent your job for taking up so much of your life, then these intentions are self-defeating.

Give yourself permission to be less than perfect. Set reasonable goals for your classroom improvements, either by setting a finite amount of time on which to work on them, or by limiting the number of classroom improvements you implement in a given period of time.

2. Focus on the things that will make a difference in your students' education. As a teacher your primary function is to teach students. This role involves planning for effective student instruction, teaching your students, and assessing student progress. While a visually attractive classroom is wonderful, spending time cutting out letters and cartoon characters won't have the impact that planning an effective lesson will. When making up your lists of things to do, be conscious of spending your valuable time on supporting quality instruction.

3. Get help for non-teaching tasks that take up your valuable time. Your community is full of people who want to support you and your students. Make a list of all of the things that need to be done for your students and your classroom *and* that can be done by someone else. Is there someone talented in graphic arts in your community who might help create a bulletin board? Could you send paper and staplers home to parents so they can create blank student journals? Can a parent go to the library or use the Internet to gather resources for the next unit? Could the students enrolled in the graphic arts program at the high school publish your student's work? While getting these volunteers organized can take time, establishing these support systems save a lot of your time in the long run.

4. Utilize technology to help save you time. There is a reason businesses have invested so much money in computers and software — it saves people time. Think about your lesson preparation and your assessment procedures. Do you find yourself writing the same information over several times? Do you copy your assessment notes from one page to another? Talk with the technology person at your school, or another teacher who uses technology, to see if there are ways that technology can free up your time.

Every day the Internet has more and more information available for teachers — everything from lesson plans to resources for your special units. Ask your technology coordinator or another colleague to show you websites created especially for teachers.

5. Explore ways to connect with your colleagues. You are not the only one who feels pressed for time. The other teachers at your school are also working hard to create lesson plans and classroom materials. Explore how you can work together to save time and effort. Would another teacher be interested in using the unit you worked so hard to develop? Can you share your great lesson plans? Can you make it known that you have a community volunteer coming in to laminate so everyone can take advantage of the outside assistance? How about posting a list of the materials you need near the staff mailboxes and including the information in the school newsletter?

6. Involve the students in classroom routines and in the management of classroom materials. Think about ways to appropriately involve your students in the day-to-day management of the classroom. After all, it isn't just your classroom, it's theirs too. Involving students in running the classroom will make your life easier, will give students the vital message that they are important, and will give them valuable skills.

Utilize attendance boards on which students mark themselves present and sign up for lunch. Assign students to add up the lunch count and check it for accuracy. Mark the outline of classroom materials like scissors, staplers, tape, etc., on posterboard and then laminate the posterboard. At the end of the day, assign students the responsibility of making sure all of the materials are back where they belong.

List all of the classroom functions that need to be accomplished and can be done well by students. Be sure to carefully explain what needs to be done and why it is important, and then monitor the work. You might even consider delegating the job of "supervisor" to students.

7. Overlap tasks so you accomplish more than one thing at a time. Are there times during the day that you can accomplish more than one thing at a time? For example, can you assess student reading during reading group? Can you write a positive note home using a clipboard while you circulate around the room? Can you combine tasks so that a trip to a different part of the school can accomplish more than one purpose?

8. Analyze how you spend your non-instructional time at school. Monitor what you do doing the times you aren't with students. Although there is no such thing as a "free period" for a teacher, most teachers' schedules allow for times without students. Do you make the most of this time to accomplish the important things that need doing or is this time spent socializing or getting a cup of coffee? I am not suggesting that you become a recluse, rather I am suggesting that you spend your time with colleagues thinking about the ways you can make each other's teaching lives easier.

9. Carefully consider school commitments that fall outside of your classroom responsibilities. As anyone who has ever taught knows, teaching is enough of a full-time load. Schools often require teachers to work outside of the classroom on curriculum, accreditation, and other important school projects. If these assignments are not required, carefully consider your time before you volunteer for additional work outside of the classroom. Make sure this project will be worth your time and effort. As a professional, you should be involved in the school beyond your classroom, but limit your involvement to your areas of passion or the areas that will provide the most benefit for students. When volunteering for such activities, see what times might be provided for this work. Sometimes working after school hours can be more efficient than being re-

leased from classroom teaching, because you don't have to write plans for a substitute teacher.

10. Remind yourself why you teach and that what you are doing is vitally important. Sometimes we get so involved in the many different daily demands that we forget to reconnect with our purpose for being in the classroom. Teaching today is a demanding profession. Take heart in the fact that you are building a future, one life at a time. Take the time to remind yourself why you are teaching young children:

- Put up an inspirational quotation at the back of the room that you can read regularly.
- Read a professional book or journal.
- Take a seminar to learn new information and connect with colleagues.
- Enjoy a visit from a former student and ask him what he remembers about your classroom.

Irv Richardson is a former multiage elementary teacher and principal; he is now the program director for The Society For Developmental Education.

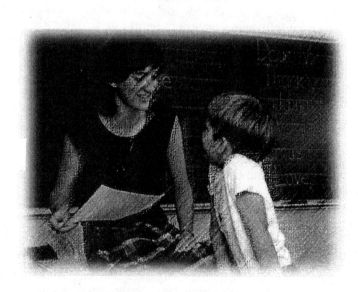

Harvey Silver, Richard Strong, and Matthew Perini

Integrating Learning Styles and Multiple Intelligences

What does it mean to express kinesthetic intelligence in an interpersonal way? Integrating styles and intelligences can help children learn in many ways—not just in the areas of their strengths.

In the 20th century, two great theories have been put forward in an attempt to interpret human differences and to design educational models around these differences. Learning-style theory has its roots in the psychoanalytic community; multiple intelligences theory is the fruit of cognitive science and reflects an effort to rethink the theory of measurable intelligence embodied in intelligence testing.

Both, in fact, combine insights from biology, anthropology, psychology, medical case studies, and an examination of art and culture. But learning styles emphasize

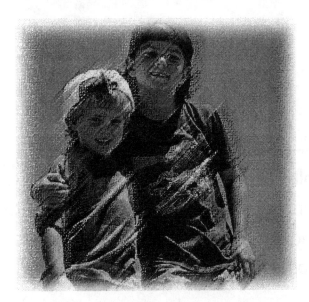

the different ways people think and feel as they solve problems, create products, and interact. The theory of multiple intelligences is an effort to understand how cultures and disciplines shape human potential. Though both theories claim that dominant ideologies of intelligence inhibit our understanding of human differences, learning styles are concerned with differences in the *process* of learning, whereas multiple intelligences

center on the *content* and *products* of learning. Until now, neither theory has had much to do with the other.

Howard Gardner (1993) spells out the difference between the theories this way:

> In MI theory, I begin with a human organism that responds (or fails to respond) to different kinds of *contents* in the world. . . . Those who speak of learning styles are searching for approaches that ought to characterize *all* contents (p. 45).

We believe that the integration of learning styles and multiple intelligence theory may minimize their respective limitations and enhance their strengths, and we provide some practical suggestions for teachers to successfully integrate and apply learning styles and multiple intelligence theory in the classroom.

Learning Styles

Learning-style theory begins with Carl Jung (1927), who noted major differences in the way people perceived (sensation versus intuition), the way they made decisions (logical thinking versus imaginative feelings), and how active or reflective they were while interacting (extroversion versus introversion). Isabel Myers and Katherine Briggs (1977), who created the Myers-Briggs Type Indicator and founded the Association of Psychological Type, applied Jung's work and influenced a generation of researchers trying to understand specific differences in human learning. Key researchers in this area include Anthony Gregorc (1985), Kathleen Butler (1984), Bernice McCarthy (1982), and Harvey Silver and J. Robert Hanson (1995). Although learning-style theorists interpret the personality in various ways, nearly all models have two things in common:

■ *A focus on process.* Learning-style models tend to concern themselves with the process of learning: how individuals absorb information, think about information, and evaluate the results.

■ *An emphasis on personality.* Learning-style theorists generally believe that learning is the result of a personal, individualized act of thought and feeling.

Most learning-style theorists have settled on four basic styles. Our own model, for instance, describes the following four styles:

■ *The Mastery style learner* absorbs information concretely; processes information sequentially, in a step-by-step manner; and judges the value of learning in terms of its clarity and practicality.

■ *The Understanding style learner* focuses more on ideas and abstractions; learns through a process of questioning, reasoning, and testing; and evaluates learning by standards of logic and the use of evidence.

■ *The Self-Expressive style learner* looks for images implied in learning; uses feelings and emotions to construct new ideas and products; and judges the learning process according to its originality, aesthetics, and capacity to surprise or delight.

■ *The Interpersonal style learner,*[1] like the Mastery learner, focuses on concrete, palpable information; prefers to learn socially; and judges learning in terms of its potential use in helping others.

Learning styles are not fixed throughout life, but develop as a person learns and grows. Our approximate breakdown of the percentages of people with strengths in each style is as follows: Mastery, 35 percent; Understanding, 18 percent; Self-Expressive, 12 percent; and Interpersonal, 35 percent (Silver and Strong 1997).

Most learning-style advocates would agree that all individuals develop and practice a mixture of styles as they live and learn. Most people's styles flex and adapt to various contexts, though to differing degrees. In fact, most people seek a sense of wholeness by practicing all four styles to some degree. Educators should help students discover their unique profiles, as well as a balance of styles.

Strengths and Limitations of a Learning-Style Model

The following are some *strengths* of learning-style models:

■ They tend to focus on how different individuals process information across many content areas.

■ They recognize the role of cognitive and affective processes in learning and, therefore, can significantly deepen our insights into issues related to motivation.

■ They tend to emphasize thought as a vital component of learning, thereby avoiding reliance on basic and lower-

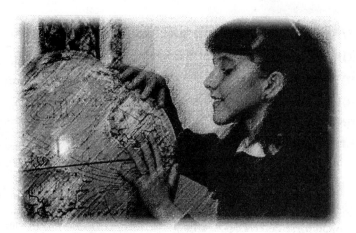

Multiple intelligence theory is concerned with differences in the *process* of learning, whereas learning-styles theory centers on the *content* and *products* of learning.

level learning activities.

Learning-styles models have a couple of limitations. First, they may fail to recognize how styles vary in different content areas and disciplines.

Second, these models are sometimes less sensitive than they should be to the effects of context on learning. Emerging

from a tradition that viewed style as relatively permanent, many learning-style advocates advised altering learning environments to match or challenge a learner's style. Either way, learning-style models have largely left unanswered the question of how context and purpose affect learning.

Multiple Intelligence Theory

Fourteen years after the publication of *Frames of Mind* (Gardner 1983), the clarity and comprehensiveness of Howard Gardner's design continue to dazzle the educational community. Who could have expected that a reconsideration of the word *intelligence* would profoundly affect the way we see ourselves and our students?

Gardner describes seven intelligences: linguistic, logical-mathematical, spatial, musical, bodily-kinesthetic, interpersonal, and intrapersonal.[2] The distinctions among these intelligences are supported by studies in child development, cognitive skills under conditions of brain damage, psychometrics, changes in cognition across history and within different cultures, and psychological transfer and generalization.

Thus, Gardner's model is backed by a rich research base that combines physiology, anthropology, and personal and cultural history. This theoretical depth is sadly lacking in most learning-style models. Moreover, Gardner's seven intelligences are not abstract concepts, but are recognizable through common life experiences. We all intuitively understand the difference between musical and linguistic, or spatial and mathematical intelligences, for example. We all show different levels of aptitude in various content areas. In all cases, we know that no individual is universally intelligent; certain fields of knowledge engage or elude everyone. Gardner has taken this intuitive knowledge of human experience and shown us in a lucid, persuasive, and well-researched manner how it is true.

Yet, there are two gaps in multiple intelligence theory that limit its application to learning. First, the theory has grown out of cognitive science—a discipline that has not yet asked itself why we have a field called cognitive science, but not one called affective science. Learning-style theory, on the other hand, has deep roots in psychoanalysis. Learning-style theorists, therefore, give psychological *affect* and individual personality central roles in understanding differences in learning.

Multiple intelligence theory looks where style does not: It focuses on the content of learning and its relation to the disciplines. Such a focus, however, means that it does not deal with the individualized process of learning. This is the second limitation of multiple intelligence theory, and it becomes clear if we consider variations within a particular intelligence.

Are conductors, performers,

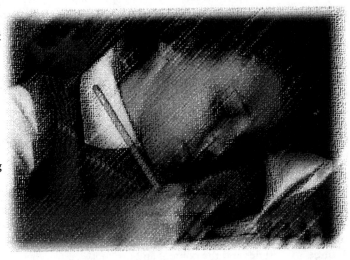

> Learning styles are not fixed throughout life, but develop as a person learns and grows.

composers, and musical critics all using the same musical intelligence? What of the differing linguistic intelligences of a master of free verse like William Carlos Williams and a giant of literary criticism like Harold Bloom? How similar are the bodily-kinesthetic intelligences of dancers Martha Graham and Gene Kelly or football players Emmitt Smith and golfer Tiger Woods? How can we explain the difference in the spatial intelligences of Picasso and Monet—both masters of modern art?

Most of us would likely agree that different types of intelligence are at work in these individuals. Perhaps one day, Gardner's work on the "jagged profile" of combined intelligences or, perhaps, his insistence on the importance of context will produce a new understanding of intelligence. But at the moment, Gardner's work does not provide adequate guidelines for dealing with these distinctions. Most of us, however, already have a way of explaining individual differences between Monet and Picasso, Martha Graham and Gene Kelly, or between different students in our classrooms: We refer to these individuals as having distinct *styles*.

Of course, as Gardner would insist, radically different histories and contexts go a long way in explaining distinctions between Monet and Picasso, for example. But how are teachers to respond to this explanation? As all teachers know, we must ultimately consider differences at the individual level. Learning styles, with their emphasis on differences in individual thought and feeling, are the tools we need to describe and teach to these differences.

Best of all, learning styles' emphasis on the individual learning process and

> We all intuitively understand the difference between musical and linguistic, or spatial and mathematical intelligences.

Gardner's content-oriented model of multiple intelligences are surprisingly complementary. Without multiple intelligence theory, style is rather abstract, and it generally undervalues context. Without learning styles, multiple intelligence theory proves unable to describe different processes of thought and feeling. Each theory responds to the weaknesses of the other; together, they form an integrated picture of intelligence and difference.

Integrating Learning Styles and Multiple Intelligences

In integrating these major theories of knowledge, we moved through three steps. First, we attempted to describe, for each of Gardner's intelligences, a set of four learning processes or abilities, one for each of the four learning styles. For linguistic intelligence, for example, the *Mastery* style represents the ability to use language to describe events and sequence activities; the *Interpersonal* style, the ability to use language to build trust and rapport; the *Understanding* style, the ability to develop logical arguments and use rhetoric; and the *Self-expressive* style, the ability to use metaphoric and expressive language.

Next, we listed samples of vocations that people are likely to choose, given particular intelligence and learning-style profiles. Working in this way, we devised a model that linked the process-centered approach of learning styles and the content and product-driven multiple intelligence theory.

Figure 2 shows how you might construct a classroom display of information about intelligences, styles, and possible vocations. Consider kinesthetic intelligence and the difference between a Tiger Woods and a Gene Kelly: People who excel in this intelligence, with an *Understanding* style, might be professional athletes (like Tiger Woods), dance critics, or sports analysts; people with a *Self-expressive* style might be sculptors, choreographers, dancers (like Gene Kelly), actors, mimes, or puppeteers.

The following outline shows how we categorized abilities and sample vocations for the seven intelligences, by learning style:

Linguistic

Mastery: The ability to use language to describe events and sequence activities (*journalist, technical writer, administrator, contractor*)

Interpersonal: The ability to use language to build trust and rapport (*salesperson, counselor, clergyperson, therapist*)

Understanding: The ability to develop logical arguments and use rhetoric (*lawyer, professor, orator, philosopher*)

Self-expressive: The ability to use metaphoric and expressive language (*playwright, poet, advertising copywriter, novelist*)

Logical-Mathematical:

Mastery: The ability to use numbers to compute, describe, and document (*accountant, bookkeeper, statistician*)

Interpersonal: The ability to apply mathematics in personal and daily life (*tradesperson, homemaker*)

Understanding: The ability to use mathematical concepts to make conjectures, establish proofs, and apply mathematics and data to construct arguments (*logician, computer programmer, scientist, quantitative problem solver*)

Self-expressive: The ability to be sensitive to the patterns, symmetry, logic, and aesthetics of mathematics and to solve problems in design and modeling (*composer, engineer, inventor, designer, qualitative problem solver*)

Spatial

Mastery: The ability to perceive and represent the visual-spatial world accu-

---

FIGURE 1

Sample "Kinesthetic" Vocations by Style

Mastery	Interpersonal
The ability to use the body and tools to take effective action or to construct or repair *Mechanic, Trainer, Contractor, Craftsperson, Tool and Dye Maker*	The ability to use the body to build rapport, to console or persuade, and to support others *Coach, Counselor, Salesperson, Trainer*

Kinesthetic

Understanding	Self-Expressive
The ability to plan strategically or to critique the actions of the body *Physical Educator, Sports Analyst, Professional Athlete, Dance Critic*	The ability to appreciate the aesthetics of the body and to use those values to create new forms of expression *Sculptor, Choreographer, Actor, Dancer, Mime, Puppeteer*

rately (*illustrator, artist, guide, photographer*)

Interpersonal: The ability to arrange color, line, shape, form, and space to meet the needs of others (*interior decorator, painter, clothing designer, weaver, builder*)

Understanding: The ability to interpret and graphically represent visual or spatial ideas (*architect, iconographer, computer graphics designer, art critic*)

Self-expressive: The ability to transform visual or spatial ideas into imaginative and expressive creations (*artist, inventor, model builder, cinematographer*)

Bodily-Kinesthetic

Mastery: The ability to use the body and tools to take effective action or to construct or repair (*mechanic, trainer, contractor, craftsperson, tool and dye maker*)

Interpersonal: The ability to use the body to build rapport, to console and persuade, and to support others (*coach, counselor, salesperson, trainer*)

Understanding: The ability to plan strategically or to critique the actions of the body (*physical educator, sports analyst, professional athlete, dance critic*)

Self-expressive: The ability to appreciate the aesthetics of the body and to use those values to create new forms of expression (*sculptor, choreographer, actor, dancer, mime, puppeteer*)

Musical

Mastery: The ability to understand and develop musical technique (*technician, music teacher, instrument maker*)

Interpersonal: The ability to respond emotionally to music and to work together to use music to meet the needs of others (*choral, band, and orchestral performer or conductor; public relations director in music*)

Understanding: The ability to interpret musical forms and ideas (*music critic, aficionado, music collector*)

Self-expressive: The ability to create imaginative and expressive perfor-

mances and compositions (*composer, conductor, individual/small-group performer*)

Interpersonal

Mastery: The ability to organize people and to communicate clearly what needs to be done (*administrator, manager, politician*)

Interpersonal: The ability to use empathy to help others and to solve problems (*social worker, doctor, nurse,*

F I G U R E 2

Student Choice: Assessment Products by Intelligence and Style

LINGUISTIC
Mastery
- Write an article
- Put together a magazine
- Develop a plan
- Develop a newscast
- Describe a complex procedure/object

Interpersonal
- Write a letter
- Make a pitch
- Conduct an interview
- Counsel a fictional character or a friend

Understanding
- Make a case
- Make/defend a decision
- Advance a theory
- Interpret a text
- Explain an artifact

Self-Expressive
- Write a play
- Develop a plan to direct
- Spin a tale
- Develop an advertising campaign

therapist, teacher)

Understanding: The ability to discriminate and interpret among different kinds of interpersonal clues (*sociologist, psychologist, psychotherapist, professor of psychology or sociology*)

Self-expressive: The ability to influence and inspire others to work toward a common goal (*consultant, charismatic leader, politician, evangelist*)

Intrapersonal

Mastery: The ability to assess one's own strengths, weaknesses, talents, and interests and use them to set goals (*planner, small business owner*)

Interpersonal: The ability to use understanding of oneself to be of service to others (*counselor, social worker*)

Understanding: The ability to form and develop concepts and theories based on an examination of oneself (*psychologist*)

Self-expressive: The ability to reflect on one's inner moods, intuitions, and temperament and to use them to create or express a personal vision (*artist, religious leader, writer*)

As the final step in constructing the intelligence-learning style menus, we collected descriptions of products that a person with strengths in each intelligence and style might create. For example, in the linguistic intelligence domain, a person with the *Mastery* style might write an article, put a magazine together, develop a newscast, or describe a complex procedure. By contrast, a person with a *Self-expressive* style might write a play, spin a tale, or develop an advertising campaign (see fig. 2). In the kinesthetic intelligence domain, a person with an *Understanding* style might choreograph a concept or teach a physical education concept; a person with a *Self-expressive* style might create a diorama or act out emotional states or concepts. A class display of such lists might accompany charts like the sample shown in Figure 2.

How to Use the Integrated Intelligence Menus

Several years ago, Grant Wiggins reminded us that we can't teach everything. It is also quite obvious that we can't use every teaching method nor every form of assessment. Here are some ways to use the Integrated Intelligence Menus—particularly for performance assessment—without trying to do everything at once.

1. Use the menus as a compass. Keep a running record of the styles and intelligences you use regularly and of those you avoid. When a particular form of assessment doesn't work, offer the student another choice from another part of the menu.

2. Focus on one intelligence at a time. Offer your students a choice in one of the four styles, or urge them to do two assessments: one from a style they like and one from a style they would normally avoid.

3. Build on student interest. When students conduct research, either individually or in groups, show them the menus and allow them to choose the product or approach that appeals to them. They should choose the best product for communicating their understanding of the topic or text. Students thus discover not only the meaning of quality, but also something about the nature of their own interests, concerns, styles, and intelligences.

In developing assessments, teachers must devise their own standards and expectations. But we can judge the model itself by two powerful standards:

■ Does it help us develop every student's capacity to learn what we believe all students need to know?

■ Does it help each student discover and develop his or her unique abilities and interests?

In conjunction, both multiple intelligences and learning styles can work together to form a powerful and integrated model of human intelligence and learning—a model that respects and celebrates diversity and provides us with the tools to meet high standards. ■

[1]The term *interpersonal style* overlaps with Gardner's *interpersonal intelligence.* In Gardner's model, interpersonal intelligence is a category related to the content and products of knowledge. In our learning-style model, the interpersonal style refers to a way of processing knowledge.

[2]Gardner has recently introduced an eighth intelligence—*naturalist.* Although our integrated intelligence menus can easily accommodate this new category, we have chosen to work only with the classic seven intelligences.

References
Briggs, K.C., and I.B. Myers. (1977). *Myers-Briggs Type Indicator.* Palo Alto, Calif.: Consulting Psychologists Press.
Butler, K. (1984). *Learning and Teaching Style in Theory and Practice.* Columbia, Conn.: The Learner's Dimension.
Gardner, H. (1983). *Frames of Mind: The Theory of Multiple Intelligences.* New York: Basic Books.
Gardner, H. (1993). *Multiple Intelligences: The Theory in Practice.* New York: Basic Books.
Gregorc, A. (1985). *Inside Styles: Beyond the Basics.* Maynard, Mass.: Gabriel Systems, Inc.
Jung, C. (1927). *The Theory of Psychological Type.* Princeton, N.J.: Princeton University Press.
McCarthy, B. (1982). *The 4Mat System.* Arlington Heights, Ill.: Excel Publishing Co.
Silver, H.F., and J.R. Hanson. (1995). *Learning Styles and Strategies.* Woodbridge, N.J.: The Thoughtful Education Press.
Silver, H.F., and R.W. Strong. (1997). *Monographs for Learning Style Models and Profiles.* (Unpublished research).

Harvey Silver is President, **Richard Strong** is Vice President, and **Matthew Perini** is Director of Publishing at Silver Strong & Associates, Inc., Aspen Corporate Park, 1480 Route 9 North, Woodbridge, NJ 07095 (e-mail: silver_strong @msn.com).

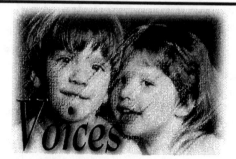

*L*ock-step, assembly-line learning violates a critical discovery about the human brain: each brain is not only unique, but is also growing on a very different timetable.

— *Eric Jensen,*
Super Teaching

Published by Turning Point for Teachers, Del Mar, CA: 1995 (p. 11)

Questions and Answers About Struggling Learners

In my conferences and customized trainings, I meet teachers who ask numerous questions about struggling learners. Often called "gray-area children," "tweeners," and "crackers," these students are in danger of falling between the cracks if they don't receive the modifications and adaptations they need in the classroom.

Here are answers to the twenty questions teachers ask most often about these children — who they are, what characteristics they have, and how we can meet their needs.

1. What is a struggling learner?

A struggling learner is a student who has difficulty keeping up with classmates of the same age in a developmentally appropriate learning environment.

The struggling learner does not qualify for special education services, or in many cases for remedial or other school services. Whereas the learning disabled child has peaks and valleys in knowledge and skill levels, often the struggling learner's strengths and needs can be described as "flat." Struggling learners often:

- have difficulty organizing themselves and their work environment.
- do not take oral directions the first time given.
- are overwhelmed by work tasks and need work chunked for them.
- have weak social and emotional skills.

These children can easily fall between the cracks of the educational system unless we provide them with the assistance they need.

2. Why are classroom teachers faced with an increasing number of struggling learners?

Today's classrooms reflect society. In this country we are dealing with young mothers, in both urban and rural areas, with inadequate prenatal care — which often results in premature, low birthweight babies. We have young parents who used alcohol and drugs during pregnancy. We have children being placed in inadequate child care facilities, or who are being cared for by teen mothers as young as fourteen. Additionally, many children are being raised in single-parent homes, or in homes where both parents may work several jobs, leaving little time for the children.

These children suffer on two fronts: their environment is lacking in the support and stimulation that allows them to learn some of the basic knowledge they need in order to succeed in school; and the energy required to survive in poverty, in stressful, sometimes dysfunctional home environments, robs children of the focus and concentration they need in the classroom.

Of course, not all struggling learners come from poverty or neglect, or from stressful homes. Many children are struggling in school because their natural learning patterns do not fit the learning structure of the classroom.

3. Will a summer school program cure these children?

Summer school programs can certainly help maintain a continuum for these children, so that they can progress at their own rate, retain knowledge from the previous year, and avoid losing ground over the summer. If a child is lagging only slightly behind his class, he may enter school in the fall more on a par with the other children.

However, a summer program can't accelerate the child's normal learning process, and if a child is a year behind the rest of his class, he is certainly not going to catch up to the other students in two or three months'

Excerpted from *More I Can Learn! Strategies and Activities for Gray-Area Children* (K-4), by Gretchen Goodman. Peterborough, NH: Crystal Springs Books, 1998.

time. The child who does catch up in September may start to lag behind again as the year progresses, because he is operating within his *normal learning pace*.

It is important to recognize that struggling learners *do not need to be cured*. Rather, they need material presented to them in a variety of ways, and in small chunks; and they need to be able to work in ways that show what they know while adapting to their special circumstances.

4. Is retention a viable option for the struggling learner?

Retention is appropriate for some children under some circumstances, but is usually *not* a good option for the struggling learner. Retention works best for children who are bright, but developmentally young; the extra year allows them to be placed in a classroom of students who are at the same age developmentally, and to catch up to grade level during the extra year.

Struggling learners, on the other hand, are working at their natural capacity. They will not rise to the top of their class with an extra year, but will continue to struggle as their classmates move on, because there is a disparity in their skill level and ability to learn compared with their "regular" classmates. All the extra time in the world will not change that.

A teacher who is faced with the decision of retaining a student should seek the guidance of a professional support team; this is not a decision that should be made independently. The team should evaluate the child and determine, among other things, whether the child is truly a slow learner or just developmentally young.

In ideal circumstances, the support team should include the teacher about to receive the struggling student. Once the team determines that the child is a slow learner, it can discuss as a group interventions and adaptations that will help the student succeed in the new grade.

5. Why not just put these students into special classes?

Very often these children don't meet the guidelines set up by school districts for special education services. Need for these services is determined by a combination of standardized assessment tools, such as IQ tests, and evaluation of a child's classroom performance. Many gray-area children are working within their ability range, which falls outside of the mandated criteria for special education or learning disabled status.

Learning-disabled children may have an IQ of 131 in verbal ability but an overall performance score of 91; this discrepancy between ability and classroom achievement could qualify them for support services. Struggling learners, on the other hand, may test at a straight across-the-board IQ of 80 to 89, and be performing at that level in the classroom—which could preclude their getting special services.

6. How can I ever teach to all the different ability levels within my classroom?

Many of the teaching strategies that work so well in today's classrooms are of special benefit to struggling learners — and to the teacher who has to attend to the diverse needs of his or her students. These methods help optimize the learning and teaching environment in a diverse classroom:
*   Use flexible grouping; have children work in whole group, small groups, with partners, and individually as needed. Team-teaching arrangements, wise use of aides, and "push in" arrangements in which special education personnel and other specialists come into the classroom and work with the classroom teacher, are great ways of optimizing flexible grouping strategies.
*   Use thematic learning, building lessons around key topics and ideas. This serves to integrate the curriculum and to heighten the children's interest levels.
*   Include topics chosen by students in the curriculum; allow students to choose *how* some topics will be studied.
*   Create a peer tutoring program within the classroom, so students can help each other learn.
*   Create a cross-age tutoring program to give younger students role models and to give older students the opportunity to *be* role models.
*   Utilize senior citizen volunteers as teacher aides or as special guests to present interesting topics to children. Some school districts have created programs for senior citizens who receive a tax break in exchange for volunteering in the schools.
*   Use cooperative learning strategies.

It's interesting to note that many of the instructional strategies which benefit struggling learners involve inter-personal relationships, either with other students or with a caring adult. Probably the single most important factor in motivating struggling learners is support and acceptance from the people in their lives.

7. Are there adaptations I can make in my teaching without changing a lot of the materials?

Yes, there are many things you can do:
- Begin by teaching in a variety of modalities. Most teachers have been taught in a combination auditory and visual style, listening to a college professor lecture in front of a large class while the professor writes information on a blackboard. We tend to carry that method of teaching into our classrooms. Unfortunately, struggling learners seldom learn well in a strictly auditory or visual manner, but need other methods, including tactile/kinesthetic experiences and a lot of interpersonal activities.
- Break the students' work into small, bite-size pieces. Instead of assigning a whole chapter on Monday to be completed by Friday, assign the student six to eight pages a night.
- Have a study buddy assigned to every student. The struggling learner can share study notes and call her study buddy with homework questions.
- Have materials and lessons taped for students. This will allow struggling readers to keep up with the class in terms of content. The student can also use the tapes to help follow along with written material.
- Give students plenty of breaks throughout the day. A break could be something as simple as walking to the office for supplies, feeding a class pet, or collecting papers.

8. Are these adaptations only used for the gray-area child?

Absolutely not! It is amazing how many teachers contact me after workshops and inservices to share the successes they've had with *all* children using some of the *I Can Learn* activities and adaptations. What makes a struggling learner's life simpler can often help ease learning for children not considered struggling. These adaptations can become a natural part of the teacher's bag of tricks in dealing with all students on a daily basis.

9. How can I help gray-area learners organize themselves and their materials?

It would be wonderful if parents taught young children the basics of organization: where to keep their toys and clothes, how to clean up after themselves, etc. Unfortunately, most children come to school without these skills. School is usually the first time the child is expected to be organized, so you have your work cut out for you. Here are some tips which are helpful for all students, but particularly for the struggling learner:
- Have a laminated "To Do" list on the child's desk. This will help the child organize his time.
- Have the child list the day's activities, then check off each item as it is completed.
- Have the student keep materials in the same location each day — a cubby, mailbox, chair pack, or desk.
- Teach the student to make a desk map to help organize the materials inside.
- Color-code book covers by subject, and have matching color-coded notebooks for the student —red for math, blue for writing, for instance.
- Use a parent letter or assignment book to keep parents informed of upcoming events and requirements. If necessary, ask the parent to sign the assignment book each night (after checking to see that the assignment has been completed) and return the book to the school with the student the following day.
- At the end of each week, send home a summary sheet tallying work completed, test or paper scores, and class participation.

10. What do I tell other students who say, "It's not fair that Johnny gets to do it a special way"?

It is our role as classroom teachers to communicate to students that we all have our strengths and needs in life. Some of us can do cursive writing, others excel with printing. Some students can play baseball, others hockey. Most importantly, we need to get across the idea that "fair" doesn't mean that everyone gets the same things in life; it means that everyone gets what he or she needs in order to succeed in life.

At the same time, try to avoid having struggling learners get too much special treatment. When one student uses a fun adaptation such as Post-It note writing, let other students try it too. If a student gets to do an oral book report rather than a written one, provide that option for other students as well, at least some of the time. Once in a while, give a test and allow all students to circle the ten questions they want to answer on the test.

Most importantly, we need to model behavior for students by presenting ourselves as individuals who struggle and ask for help in some areas, and excel in others.

11. How can we build self-esteem in the struggling learner?

When a child is struggling in school — when he can't grasp the material, when she sees herself falling behind her classmates, when parental anxiety (and sometimes pressure) rises at home — the struggling learner's self-esteem plummets. Building it up again is paramount.

The key is to discover and recognize the students' strengths outside the academic area:

- Struggling learners tend to be very empathetic with other learners, and often make outstanding helpers who eagerly assist the teacher with a variety of activities. Appoint them as wheelchair drivers and peer tutors to special-needs students. Let them assist in lower elementary grades and tutor younger students. Give them the opportunity to read to kinder-garteners or tape-record books for other classes.
- These children often relate very strongly to class pets. Make sure they have an opportunity to care for these animals.
- Pay attention to the lives these children have outside the classroom. If Mark hit a softball and made a home run at recess, mention it in class.
- Encourage children to bring in hobbies and discuss them during a sharing time. If they know how to do something involved with their hobby, ask them to teach the rest of the class.
- Have all the children in the class make an "I Can" collage, helping them focus on activities with which they can succeed. Let the children in the classroom suggest skills and abilities to each other. ("Mark, you sure can hit a ball!")

12. Should I grade these students differently than other students in my room?

If a school district continues to grade and evaluate student progress with a standardized letter report card, classroom teachers need to document all modifications made for a struggling learner in order to assist next year's teacher. It is also important to document the adaptations and modifications made for a student for his parents, and to keep the parents well informed about the child's progress and the use of specific modifications. For instance:

- Has the teacher read all the tests to the child?
- Has the reading material been taped for the child?
- Have directions given orally to the class also been written for the child?
- Has the material been retaught in a variety of ways?

Many school districts attach a modification sheet to the child's report card to inform both the parents and next year's teacher of the modifications.

Schools who have begun to use anecdotal records, authentic assessment, and portfolios to evaluate students are likely to get a more accurate view of what their struggling learners can do.

Struggling learners may need *some* modifications in *some* areas, rather than across the curriculum. For instance, a child can compute mathematics problems, but can't do as many in the same amount of time as the average learner. Another student may find an oral book report easier to do than a written one. In both instances, the modifications show mastery of the subjects and skills that need to be measured.

When the amount of needed modifications for a particular child exceeds the amount of learning taking place, it may be necessary to provide the child with more individually designed instruction in the form of special education.

13. How should I handle test taking with my struggling learners?

Test taking needs to be modified for struggling learners, just as notetaking and projects are adapted. Here are some adaptations that can be used as needed:

- For students with reading difficulties, read the tests to them.
- Provide a study guide to help students study before the test.
- Give untimed tests to students who work more slowly than their classmates.
- Give tests in small chunks. Alternatively, tell children to work on the test for twenty minutes; they will be scored only on what they complete.
- Have children try the whole test, then circle the ten questions on which they want to be scored.
- Allow children to choose ten out of twenty spelling words when they are first assigned. The children under-stand that they can study these ten words, and will only be tested on these words.
- Alternatively, the students can take the entire test, but will only be scored on these ten words.
- Give students an open-book test or notebook test, where they can use their class work for assistance.
- Try giving struggling learners the first letter of each answer as a clue.
- Allow these students to use word banks or answer keys during tests.

14. How can I help parents better understand and support their child?

All parents want their children to succeed; when it becomes evident that a child is having difficulty in school, parents experience tremendous anxiety. It's important for the school to provide as much information as they can, as well as a lot of support, for these parents as they work with the school to help their child.

A child experiencing problems academically may have been informally evaluated by a classroom teacher, or the evaluation may have gone beyond that to some type of formalized assessment tools or even special education screening.

Whatever form the evaluation takes, parents need to be given a complete, accurate understanding of the results, and the steps the school plans to take to address the child's learning difficulties. Parents need to be told: "Here's what we think the difficulty is; here's what we plan to do about it; here's what we hope to accomplish."

It's important to explain to parents the curriculum, the classroom structure, and instructional strategies utilized on a day-to-day basis in their child's classroom. Parents may not understand concepts like invented spelling, thematic teaching, and cooperative learning, and may blame these unfamiliar strategies for their child's lack of success. Here are other ways to include parents:

- Make periodic phone calls to parents to let them know of their child's successes in the classroom.
- Show parents work samples from both typical learners and struggling learners, so they can understand the difference in work products and expectations between these two groups of children. Work samples can also provide a goal and some type of guide as their child works on particular skills.
- Invite parents to the classroom frequently, not just for report card conferences. Let them see how your classroom functions, and what the expectations for your class are in terms of learning and behavior.
- Give parents of struggling learners the opportunity to participate in student workshops and book groups; this will give them a chance to work with a variety of students and gain some perspective on their own child's learning patterns.
- Have a school fun night for families. This allows parents to see their children in school having a good time and interacting in a way that doesn't involve academics. (Sometimes, when a child is having trouble in school, the school takes on an ominous presence for the entire family. Periodic, non-academic activities help to dispel this.)
- Videotape your classroom so that parents who can't break away from a job can see how the class functions on a daily basis, and how their own child functions within the class. (This is a valuable strategy for all parents; their children may act very differently when parents are in the classroom than they would ordinarily act.)
- Communicate with parents through communication logs, diaries, journals, and newsletters.
- Most importantly, encourage parents to attend all team meetings called to discuss modifications and supports implemented for their child in the classroom.

Be aware that many parents with struggling learners have been through numerous bouts of testing and evaluation of their children, sometimes with conflicting results, and many learning strategies may have been tried unsuccessfully. Parents will often come to you exhausted, confused, and frustrated at their inability to find answers for their child. You need to treat them with patience, respect, and kindness, and assure them that you're going to hang in there with them and their child.

15. Are there ways for parents to help these students at home?

There are many ways parents can help their children at home:

- Struggling learners often need to have material repeated at home, and need the chance to rehearse material. Teachers can help with this by providing parents with rehearsal calendars that tell the parents what subjects need to be reviewed. This gives the child the opportunity to acquire some basic knowledge about a subject before facing it in class.
- Parents must be included in all team meetings where interventions are being designed for the student.
- Send parents taped versions of books and oral classroom lectures so that they can review the material with the child.

If parent support is lacking in the home, it is the school's responsibility to provide the child with someone at school who can rehearse and review classroom material with the child. This person can be a paid teacher's aide, a high school volunteer, a PTO volunteer, or a mentor teacher from another classroom willing to volunteer time to help this student.

16. What happens when a child moves? I have worked so hard to develop adaptations for children, and I'm afraid the new teacher won't.

It's hard for us to accept that, when a child moves, we lose the ability to provide the help that we know the child needs. Concern over the capabilities of the child's next teacher is natural. We need to provide all the adaptations and modifications the child needs as long as she is in our care, and accept the fact that, once she is gone, there is not much we can do.

One thing we *can* do is document all the adaptations and modifications we have provided for the child, and include all specific adaptation and modification sheets we have used. Also send along a copy of any behavior management plan developed for the child. Make sure you let the new school's administration know that you will be willing to communicate personally with the new teacher and specialists in order to give them an understanding of how to help the child.My principal expects all students to be "on level" at the end of the school year. How can I inform her of the improbability of this happening?

17. My principal expects all students to be "on level" at the end of the school year. How can I inform her of the improbability of this happening?

First of all, you need to ask for a definition of "on level." Does this mean that all children exiting from a single-year first grade will be reading materials designated for "end-of-year" first grade? This is not only unlikely, it is virtually impossible.

If your principal believes it is possible, you have a problem. You need to share information with the principal on your own periodic assessments of the students, showing where the students were academically at the beginning of the year compared where they are at the end of the year. Being able to show the students' progress throughout the year will help, and will (one hopes) give the principal an inkling of the normal variations in academic development among students.

Of course, this means you have to have your own assessment act together. Make sure you have plenty of work samples contained in your student portfolios that accurately show your students' progression in skills. In terms of your struggling learners, you will be able to show growth on a continuum, even though it may not be at a specific grade level. You can also periodically audio- and videotape children working and reading in the classroom to show growth.

Invite your principal into your classroom to participate in book sharing with the students; have her observe the students as they work in learning centers, and as you apply a variety of adaptations throughout the classroom. Give your principal the opportunity to interact on a personal level with your struggling students so that she can gain an understanding of how these children function.

18. What kind of training do I need to motivate and teach struggling learners?

Unfortunately, there is no one easy answer in terms of teaching struggling learners. Teachers need to take a patient, trial-and-error approach to discover what works with each student.

However, training in certain instructional strategies and educational concepts will give the classroom teacher valuable tools in dealing with these students. Teachers should consider training to enable them to do the following:

- Combine literature-based reading and writing instruction with more structured methods. Struggling learners *need* structure, but do not react well to isolated drills. Integrating structured lessons in phonics and other decoding skills with exciting children's literature will provide both the structure and the motivation these learners need.
- Teachers need to understand how to adapt instruction for children who learn differently. For instance, when learning the concept of addition, some students will be able to add the numbers mentally without use of manipulatives, some may place objects next to the numbers and count them, and others will regroup the numbers. The teacher needs to be able to teach these different approaches as appropriate for a particular student.
- Develop adaptations and modifications in classroom instruction and assignments appropriate to the students' needs.
- Create student-centered classrooms in which instruction is geared toward the students' ability levels and needs, rather than providing a ready-made curriculum and fitting the students into the curriculum. Develop a method by which students can have input into the curriculum and the classroom's rules of conduct.
- Create learning centers as part of the classroom environment.
- Develop cooperative learning opportunities.
- Develop an assessment program using portfolios and work samples.

- Adjust the pace and presentation of subject matter according to the varying needs of the children in the class.
- Develop collaborative teaching and planning strategies to provide support for each other as teachers.
- Apply constructivist learning and brain-based learning concepts to instruction, emphasizing learning as a process rather than a product.
- Design lessons to begin with concrete activities and then move to abstract concepts.

19. How can I get support for myself within the school setting?

Some years ago, a teacher's only option in getting support was to refer the struggling learner to a child study team, which essentially meant the team would *test the child*.

There is a better way. Instead of sending the child down the hall to be tested, many schools are setting up strong building-based assistance teams which provide instructional support for the *teacher*. Teachers meet periodically with their peers in their own school to brainstorm suitable instructional adaptations for students. This has the advantage of being able to tap into ideas that other teachers have discovered in working with similar problems, and can have the side benefit of an increased comfort level when it becomes time to send a child on to his or her next teacher. Imagine being able to pass this child along to a teacher who has sat next to you for the past year in an assistance team meeting and helped you work out your instructional strategies for this child!

Having a strong, assistance-based team also provides a sense of community for teachers, a message of "We're all in this together," rather than "You're on your own." This sense of community can also be very reassuring to parents and their children.

20. Where can I go for help?

The days of teaching in isolation are over. No one person can handle the complex problems of today's learners without assistance. Luckily, there are many places to go for help and support:
- Connect with special education teachers and guidance personnel in your school; they have a wealth of information and resources to share.
- Consider team teaching, if possible. Often a competent teammate can provide solutions for problems that may elude you.
- Take advantage of schoolwide assistance teams to help you with problem solving. If none is available, talk to your administration about starting one.
- Connect with a knowledgeable teacher for peer coaching. If you are in a position to mentor someone else, do so.
- Read books and periodicals created for teachers.
- Take advantage of staff development resources; these are available through training organizations such as The Society for Developmental Education.*
- Do an ERIC search. ERIC has a wealth of information on specific educational topics, and is accessible via letter, phone, or the Internet:

> ERIC (Educational Resources Information Center)
> 5207 University of Oregon
> Eugene OR 97403-5207
> 1-800-LET-ERIC
> http://www.ed.gov/pubs/pubdb.html

*The Society For Developmental Education
Ten Sharon Road
PO Box 577
Peterborough, NH 03458
1-800-924-9621

How To Use This Booklet

For many of us, computers are exciting, but puzzling. Our children know far more about computers than we do! How do we bridge the gap between what our children know and what we know to be able to assist them with their school work and help them get ready for the information age of the next century? After all, being able to use technology is rapidly becoming a requirement for being an informed citizen and a productive worker.

Whether your children are experienced computer users or just getting started, they need your involvement, your experience, and your judgment. This booklet is designed to provide you with basic information about how to use the computer to find information and communicate with others. It tells you what you need to get started on the Internet—a vast network of computers that connects people and information all over the world—and points you to some of the many interesting, helpful, and fun resources available online for parents and children.

You'll find that the vocabulary of computers is taken from sources familiar to us. Computer language is borrowed from travel: *superhighway, engine, cruising, surfing, navigating;* from restaurants: *menu, server;* and from the environment: *Web, mouse, windows, site.* Computer vocabulary can also be descriptive of the movement or sound made to do something on the computer: to "click" or "drag" the mouse, for example. Other words come from words used for medieval manuscripts: *icon, scroll, cursor.* In the following sections, you'll find several key computer terms in italics. They are defined in the glossary at the end of this booklet.

You can see there is a great deal of variety in the thinking behind computers. Since the computer world is constantly growing and changing, there is some variety among different systems and software, as well. As you begin using the computer, you may notice some differences between instructions given in this booklet and the system you use. Feel free to experiment and explore.

You might want to use this booklet as a tutorial to help you learn. You can use the sites suggested in various sections to try out the computer. Remember, if you have questions, your children may know the answers. Don't hesitate to ask them. That's how we encourage our children to learn. You will find that your children, local librarians, friends, teachers, and others familiar with computers will be able to help.

Have a pleasant and safe journey down the information superhighway!

What Is the Information Superhighway?

When we talk about getting online, we mean being connected to the *Internet*—a giant network of computers that connects people and information all over the world. The Internet has a lot in common with other forms of communication:

World Wide Web

- Like the U.S. Postal Service, the Internet allows anyone who knows your Internet address to send you a letter. (It's called electronic mail, or *e-mail* for short).

- Like the telephone, the Internet allows you to "chat" with other people by participating in online discussion groups.

Excerpted from "Parents Guide to the Internet." Published by the U.S. Department of Education, Office of Educational Research and Improvement, Media and Information Services. Washington, D.C., 1997.

- Like the library, the Internet contains information on almost any topic you can imagine in many formats, including books, articles, videos, and music recordings.

- Like the newspaper, the Internet can give you new information every day, including world news, business, sports, travel, entertainment, and ads.

In addition to words, one part of the Internet—the *World Wide Web* (often shortened to WWW or the Web)—is especially interesting to people because it includes pictures and sounds.

A Short History Lesson

The Internet began in the 1960s as a U.S. Department of Defense communication network. Soon after, university researchers and professors began to use it to communicate with others in their fields. Internet use really took off in the early 1990s with the arrival of the Web, which made it easier to find and view information online. Today, millions of people throughout the world are connected to the Internet. No one—no country, organization, or company—is in charge of the Internet; it's growing and being changed by its users every day.

Benefits of Getting on the Information Superhighway

A computer that is connected to the Internet allows you to turn your home, community center, local library, or school into a place of unlimited information and communication. The Internet can help your family:

- **Find educational resources**, including up-to-the minute news, copies of important documents and photos, and collections of research information on topics ranging from weather conditions to population statistics.

- **Get help with homework** through online encyclopedias and other reference materials and access to experts.

- **Increase reading skills** by providing access to interesting materials and suggestions for additional reading.

- **Improve technology and information skills** necessary to find and use information, solve problems, communicate with others, and meet a growing demand for these skills in the workplace.

- **Connect with places around the world** to exchange mail with electronic pen pals and learn about other cultures and traditions.

- **Locate parenting information** and swap ideas with other families.

- **Learn and have fun together** by sharing interesting and enjoyable experiences.

In the next few sections, we'll discuss what you need to start using the Internet.

Starting the Engine

It's not necessary to buy a computer to begin exploring the Internet. You may be able to get started using free facilities in your community. Try:

- **A public institution** such as a library or community center. Some public housing complexes also have free computer centers with online access for their residents.

- **Your children's school** or a community college or university, if you're taking a class.

- **Your employer**, who may encourage you to learn new online skills by using company computer equipment for a limited amount of time each day.

- **Your local shopping mall**, which may have a room with computers for use by those visiting the mall.

Some communities sponsor *freenets* to give all their members free access to a wealth of information. To see if there is a freenet in your area, have someone with Web access go to http://www.lights.com/freenet/.

Understanding the Basics

To take advantage of online offerings, you need to use a computer set up with certain *hardware* (equipment) and *software* (instruction programs for the computer) as well as online access. Internet essentials include:

- **A computer** with a monitor (screen), a keyboard for typing text and numbers onto the screen, and a *mouse*, (a small hand-controlled device for pointing and clicking to select choices on the screen). You may also want a printer, which will allow you to get paper copies of what you see on a screen.

- **A modem** (either inside your computer or as a separate piece of equipment outside) to allow your computer to communicate with other computers through the phone line. Communications software works with the *modem* to give the computer instructions for connecting to the online world.

- **A connection to the Internet** through either an *Internet Service Provider (ISP)* or an *online service*. An ISP simply offers connection to the Internet, while an online service provides additional services (See below "Internet Service Provider or Online Service: Which is Right for My Family?").

- **Software for using the Internet** (may already be provided on the computer or through the Internet connection). To move around on the Web, you'll need *Web browser* software such as Netscape Navigator or Communicator or NCSA Mosaic. You'll also need software such as Eudora or cc:mail for sending and receiving electronic mail.

Internet Service Provider or Online Service: Which Is Right for My Family?

An *Internet Service Provider* (ISP) provides you with the software you need to get on the Internet. ISPs include local and regional companies, nationwide providers such as UUNet and Netcom, and telecommunications companies such as AT&T and MCI. If your family is ready to explore the Internet independently, an ISP can be a wise choice. Ask a friend with Web access to download and print for you a list of ISPs for your area using the Web address http://www.thelist.com.

Online services such as America Online and Prodigy offer members partial or full Internet access along with a number of additional resources, such as travel planning, financial management services, children's areas, and *chat rooms* in which several individuals participate in a group discussion about a selected topic at the same time. Although many of the resources available through online services can also be found on the Internet, online services organize them attractively and make them easy for you and your children to access with the click of a mouse. Within their own resource areas, online services can also exercise more control over what their members see and do by blocking access to certain sites and monitoring communication, particularly in children's areas.

Before you choose, you should consider:

- **Cost.** Will you pay a monthly fee for unlimited usage or are charges based on the actual time online? Will you pay the price of a local call or a long-distance call each time you go online?

- **Assistance.** If you have trouble with your connection, what kind of telephone help (sometimes called technical support) is available?

- **Contract.** Some ISPs and online services offer free trial periods or allow you to get a refund for the unused part of a service contract. This can be helpful as you experiment to find the best arrangement for your family.

Be aware that while you're online, the modem will be using your phone. You won't be able to make or receive any telephone calls until you disconnect from the Internet or unless you have a separate phone line for your modem.

Buying the Set Up You Need

If you're thinking about buying a computer set up to go on the Internet, keep these considerations in mind:

Talk with your family and decide how the computer will be used. Will you be using the computer mostly for typing (word processing) school assignments, sending e-mail, and browsing the Web? Do you plan to purchase additional software and games that will require a *CD-ROM* drive? Do you need sound and video capabilities for games and some World Wide Web sites, or can you do without these functions for a while?

Do your homework. You can get guidance about buying a computer from many sources:

- Consumer guides, computer magazines, and books available at the library.
- Family members, friends, coworkers, and computer experts at your child's school or your workplace.
- Workshops or classes sponsored by community colleges, libraries, and computer stores.
- Computer user groups.

Become familiar with computer features so you can decide what makes sense for your family. A computer's capabilities depend on:

- the size of its memory, measured in megabytes (MG) of RAM (random access memory),
- the speed of its processor, measured in megahertz (MHz),
- the size of its hard drive, measured in mega bytes or gigabytes (GB), and
- the speed of its modem, measured in kilobits per second (Kbps).

The greater these capabilities, the more quickly you'll be able to move around the Internet, look at Web sites, save, and print files—the more expensive you'll find the set up.

Decide whether to invest in new or used equipment. When you buy a new computer, you'll generally receive everything you need to go online immediately. You'll probably be advised to buy the biggest hard drive, the most memory, and the fastest processor and modem that you can afford, so your computer has enough capacity to work well now and in the future. You'll spend somewhere between $1,200 and several thousand dollars.

For several hundred dollars, in contrast, you may be able to buy an older model used computer and a printer, and add a modem and communications software. This set up may be all your family needs to write letters and school reports, use e-mail, and browse the Web. Of course there will be tradeoffs in terms of speed and performance, and you may run a higher risk of equipment breakdown. Some stores specialize in refurbishing used equipment, or inspecting it and replacing worn parts. If you take this route, find out what parts are new before you buy and ask whether you can get a warranty. Also, with any used set up, make sure that any software that is included is licensed, rather than an illegal copy.

Add upgrades over time. You can buy additions you want or need later and install the upgrades yourself as you learn more about working with computers. Before you buy software, ask someone you know with Web access to check a site like **Tucows** http://www.tucows.com or **Stroud** http://www.stroud.com to learn what free and low-cost programs are available through the Internet.

Navigating the Journey

On any trip, you need a map with guideposts to navigate well. This section offers some basics to help you begin to explore the World Wide Web and communicate with others on the Internet.

Surfing the Net or Cruising the Superhighway

When you go on the Internet, you may have a specific destination in mind, or you may wish to browse through the Web, the way you would browse through a library or a catalog, looking for topics or things that interest you. This browsing is often called surfing the Net or cruising the Superhighway. There are several ways to get around on the Web.

- **Using Web addresses.** To get to a special destination, such as one of the sites described in Sites Along the Way on p. 11, you'll type in an *internet address* in the space provided on the Web browser. Web addresses, sometimes called uniform resource locators (*URL*), begin with http://, which stands for *hypertext transfer protocol.* After you type in the Web address, it may take awhile for the site's *home page* to appear on the screen, especially if it includes many pictures. Once it does, you'll probably see several choices you can click your mouse on to take you further into the site. (If you type in an address incorrectly, or too many people are trying to use a site at once, you'll get an error message on your computer screen. Just try again).

- **Following links.** Many sites include *hypertext links* to other sites with related content. When you click on one of these highlighted areas, your computer will connect to another Web site without your having to know or type its address.

- **Using search engines.** *Search engines* are programs that you can select from your Web browser to enable you to search the Internet by keywords or topics. If you or your child are interested in finding out more about Jackie Robinson, for example, you can click on a search engine, enter his name, then pull up several Web sites for further exploration.

Using the Internet To Do a School Project

Assignment: Write a 2–3 page essay on the life of Jackie Robinson. Include facts about his life, his greatest accomplishments, and why you believe he deserves a place in history.

Here's how you can find the information to do this project:

- Sign onto the Internet; once connected, *click* the mouse on the search key.

- From the *menu*, select a *search engine* based on your topic. (Here we have selected AltaVista).

- At the subject box, type in Jackie Robinson and *click* on the search key.

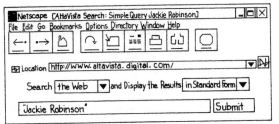

- Review search results: "Found 1 *category* and 19 *site* matches for Jackie Robinson."

- Select one or all site matches (all sites are underlined). Each *site* has additional *sites* for more information.

- Print or *download* all the information you need for the essay.

- Use this information to write the report.

Examples of search engines include:

Infoseek
http://www.infoseek.com

Webcrawler
http://webcrawler.com

Yahoo
http://www.yahoo.com

Yahooligans (for children)
http://www.yahooligans.com

You can find these search engines and many more at the All-in-One site http://www.albany.net/allinone/ or your Web browser's *home page.* If a search on one doesn't produce good results, try another.

- **Using bookmarks.** As you look through the Internet, you'll probably find sites you'll want to revisit. If so, you can create a *bookmark* by saving the address on your computer, usually with just a click of the mouse. The help feature on your Web browser can give you specific instructions. When you want to return to the site, you'll just click its address on your list.

Saving Information from the Internet

In your travels on the Internet, you'll probably come across information you want to keep. You can either make a paper or "hard" copy directly from the Web, or you can *download* a copy of the information onto your own computer.

- **Printing a copy.** While you're looking at the information you wish to print, you can click on the print command or *icon*, and the printer connected to the computer will print a copy for you. Using the mouse, you can also highlight the information you would like to print and click on the print command or icon. Text usually prints quickly, but graphics can take a long time. If you don't need the images, you may wish to check your online help feature to see how to remove them before printing.

311

- **Downloading a copy.** If you'd like to be able to use the information you've found on the Internet on your own computer (perhaps to include it in a report or send it by e-mail to someone else), you can use your mouse to click on a command or icon to download it. Be careful, though. When you travel online, you can bring back *viruses*, or programs that can destroy your personal files and software. For protection, it's important to buy—and regularly update—an anti-virus program. For added safety, download files and e-mail messages to a disk and do a virus check before copying the information to the hard drive inside your computer.

Electronic Communication

The most popular online activity is communicating with individuals and groups through e-mail, listserv, and Usenet newsgroups.

- **E-mail.** You and your children may want to send notes to friends and family. To send an e-mail message, you'll need the e-mail address of the person to whom you are sending a message. E-mail addresses often start with a version of the person's name and continue with the "at" sign (@), the Internet service provider's name (usually abbreviated), a period (called "dot"), and a three-letter extension. Extensions include *com* for businesses, *edu* for educational institutions, *gov* or *mil* for the federal government, *org* for nonprofit organizations, and *net* for networks. Make sure that when you type an address, you key it exactly as it is given to you—copy the capitalization, spacing, and punctuation. Some examples of e-mail addresses are:
  jdoe@ed.gov
  cbass@school.edu
  sgreene@nonprofit.org

> **Important:** It's a good safety precaution to make up names and never use your real name in order to make it difficult for strangers to contact you and other family members by phone or in person.

- **Listservs.** You can use e-mail to participate in discussion groups focused on topics that interest you. When you put your name on a *listserv*, you can read all the messages sent to members of the group, and you, too, can send messages to the entire group. Each group has an administrator who sets the rules for how the group will operate. If the listserv is moderated, the administrator will also keep the discussion on track and make sure participants treat each other courteously, or follow *Netiquette*. A list of listservs and the e-mail addresses for subscribing to them is available from http://www.list.com/.

- **Usenet newsgroups.** Usenet is a system of thousands of special interest groups that allows people to post messages for anyone else to read. Readers can respond by posting a general message or sending an e-mail to the author of an earlier message. Unlike listservs, *usenet newsgroups* do not require people to subscribe; however, newsgroups must be registered with Usenet. You can probably find newsgroups through your Internet Service Provider. Most ISPs let you search for newsgroups that interest you by using keywords. Try "parenting," for example. Because Usenet newsgroup messages can take up a lot of space, ISPs aren't able to carry all newsgroups. If you know of a newsgroup that you can't find through your ISP, ask to see whether it can be added.

Caution: Most newsgroups are not moderated; no one keeps the discussion focused on the topic or exercises control over inappropriate behavior. Some topics are not suitable for children.

Children with Special Needs

Children with special needs can often benefit from the use of assistive technology to support communication, self-expression and positive social interaction. Parents and teachers tell stories of children who overcome obstacles and achieve success online—the child with a writing disability who wins second place in a nationwide writing contest or the teenager with a learning disability who becomes an electronic pen pal with a scientist across the country who shares his fascination with fossils

Technology is available to help people with special needs. If your child has a mobility or sensory impairment, for example, you may decide to replace the mouse with another device for giving the computer commands. A joystick, for instance, can be controlled with the entire hand. Other devices require only a single finger for control. Magnifying the screen can help individuals with low vision, while voice synthesis technology can read screen information to those who are blind.

The ERIC Clearinghouse on Disabilities and Gifted Education operated by the Council for Exceptional Children offers information about disabilities and accommodations. Call 1–800–328–0272 or TTY 703–264–9449, send e-mail to ericec@cec.sped.org, or visit the Web site http://www.cec.sped.org/ericec.htm.

Other Web sites are also helpful. For example, Winners on Wheels is a team-oriented youth program that uses learning and fun to promote self-esteem and independence in children with disabilities http://www.wowusa.com/. Visit http://www.isc.rit.edu/~easi/ which provides information on adaptive computer technology for individuals with disabilities. Starbright, another site, applies the latest advancement in technology to positively affect the lives of disabled children http://www.starbright.org.

Tips for Safe Traveling

Like most parents, you probably have rules for how your children should deal with strangers, which TV shows, movies, and videos they're allowed to watch, what stores they're allowed to enter, and where and how far from home they're allowed to travel. It's important to make similar rules for your children's Internet use and to be aware of their online activities.

You'll also want to make sure that surfing the Net doesn't take the place of homework, social activities, or other important interests. You might even set an alarm clock or timer if you or your child tend to lose track of time. This section offers tips for ensuring that your children have safe, productive, and enjoyable experiences on the Internet.

Interacting with Others on the Internet

Just as we tell our children to be wary of strangers they meet, we need to tell them to be wary of strangers on the Internet. Most people behave reasonably and decently online, but some are rude, mean, or even criminal. Teach your children that they should:

- **Never** give out personal information (including their name, home address, phone number, age, race, family income, school name or location, or friends' names) or use a credit card online without your permission.

- **Never** share their password, even with friends.

- **Never** arrange a face-to-face meeting with someone they meet online unless you approve of the meeting and go with them to a public place.

- **Never** respond to messages that make them feel confused or uncomfortable. They should ignore the sender, end the communication, and tell you or another trusted adult right away.

- **Never** use bad language or send mean messages online.

Also, make sure your children know that people they meet online are not always who they say they are and that online information is not necessarily private.

Limiting Children to Appropriate Content on the Internet

Even without trying, your children can come across materials on the Internet that are obscene, pornographic, violent, hate filled, racist, or offensive in other ways. One type of material—child pornography—is illegal. You should report it to the Center for Missing and Exploited Children by calling 1–800–THE LOST (843–5678) or going to http://www.missingkids.org/.

While other offensive material is not illegal, there are steps you can take to keep it away from your children and out of your home.

- Make sure your children understand what you consider appropriate for them. What kinds of sites are they welcome to visit? What areas are off limits? How much time can they spend, and when? How much money, if any, can they spend? Set out clear, reasonable rules and consequences for breaking them.

- Make online exploration a family activity. Put the computer in the living room or family room. This arrangement involves everyone and helps you monitor what your children are doing.

- Pay attention to games your older child might download or copy. Some are violent or contain sexual content.

- Look into software or online services that filter out offensive materials and sites. Options include stand alone software that can be installed on your computer, and devices that label or filter content directly on the web. In addition, many Internet Service Providers and commercial online services offer site blocking, restrictions on incoming e-mail, and children's accounts that access specific services. Often, these controls are available at no additional cost. Be aware, however, children are often smart enough to get around these restrictions. Nothing can replace your supervision and involvement.

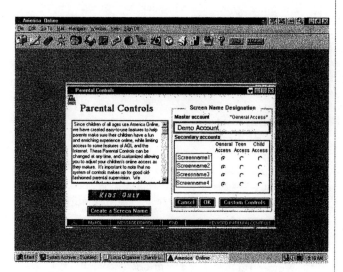

- Find out what the Internet use policy is at your local library.

- Ask about the Internet use policy at your child's school.

Encouraging Information Literacy

Show your children how to use and evaluate information they find on the Internet. Not all online information is reliable. Some individuals and organizations are very careful about the accuracy of the information they post, but others are not. Some even mislead on purpose. Remind your children not to copy online information and claim it's their own or copy software unless it is clearly labeled as free.

Help children understand the nature of commercial information, advertising, and marketing, including who created it and why it exists. Encourage them to think about why something is provided and appears in a specific way. Steer your children to noncommercial sites and other places that don't sell products specifically to children. It is important to be aware of the potential risks involved in going online, but it is also important to keep them in perspective. Common sense and clear guidelines are the place to start.

Supporting School Use of Technology

You can encourage your children's online activities at home and at school. Talk with your children, school staff, and other parents about what online experiences are already part of classroom activities and what is being planned. Get involved by:

- Helping schools get technology, including used equipment from government agencies or businesses. For information on computer recycling, visit http://www.microweb.com/pepsite/Recycle/recycle_index.html and the Computer Recycling Project at http://www.voicenet.com/~cranmer/recycling.html.

- Helping your school and community participate in **NetDay**, a grassroots volunteer effort to wire schools so their computers are networked and have Internet access http://www.netday.org/.

- Sharing your expertise by volunteering in the classroom or organizing training for teachers and other parents.

- Asking your local PTA to set up a "family night" on computers, technology, and the Internet.

- Helping schools develop "rules of the road" that are discussed with students before they go online.

- Joining the school's technology planning group.

Special Opportunity for Schools

In May 1997, the Federal Communications Commission (FCC) approved a rule (known as the E-rate) giving schools 20 to 90 percent discounts in access charges to the Internet and telecommunications services, including wiring school buildings for the Internet. (The amount of the discount depends on how many low-income students a school serves and whether it is located in a rural, suburban, or urban area). Starting in January 1998, more than $2 billion a year will be available for the discounts (see http://www.fcc.gov/learnnet/ and http://www.ed.gov/Technology/ for more information).

To apply for a discount, a school must have a technology plan that explains how the school will integrate technology into the curriculum. The plan must also address hardware, software, training, and maintenance issues. As a parent, you can play an active role in helping your school develop a technology plan.

NOTES

(ALMOST) THE *Only Site* YOU'LL EVER NEED

BY JIM MOULTON

*P*resenter Jim Moulton has created the ultimate in linked sites for educators; this site is composed entirely of links to other sites! To access all the sites on the following pages, type in the URL: **http://www.col.k12.me.us/teachers/sites.html** (Don't type in the information in the parentheses; this is a description of the site and not part of the address.)

Check in often; Jim revises this site on a regular basis.

Web Sites Designed Primarily for Teachers
http://www.capecod.net/schrockguide (*Kathy Schrock's Guide*)
http://topcat.bridgew.edu/~kschrock/#classwork (*Kathy's Class Projects*)
http://www.ceismc.gatech.edu/busyt/ (*The Busy Teacher*)
http://www.bellsouth.net/dp/educ/ (*Bellsouth's Education Gateway*)
http://www.edbriefs.com (*News from the education world and more*)
http://falcon.jmu.edu/~ramseyil/ (*Internet School Library/Media Center*)
http://www.pacificnet.net/~mandel/ (*Lesson Plan & Ideas Sharing Place*)
http://www.brainstation.com/ (*Brainstation; Tutorials and Resources*)
http://www.classroom.net/resource/CitingNetResources.html (*Citations*)
http://www.enc.org/nf_index.htm (*Eisenhower National Clearinghouse*)
http://tristate.pgh.net/~pinch13/ (*B.J. Pinchbeck's Homework Helper*)
http://www.col.k12.me.us/lon/lonlinks (*Longfellow Links, By Grade Level*)
http://www.gsn.org/teach/ (*Global School Net*)

http://topcat.bridgew.edu/~kschrock/spring98/ryan/grantweb.htm (*Grants*)
http://www.hmco.com/hmco/school/School.html (*Education Place*)
http://web66.coled.umn.edu/schools.html (*Web 66; Schools Online*)
http://www.expage.com (*Make your own 'Links Page'*)
http://www.motted.hawaii.edu/et_tools/surveymaker.html (*Survey Maker*)
http://www.schoolnotes.com (*Free Teacher Web Pages*)
http://www.classroom.net/ (*Classroom Connect*)
http://www.schoolnet.ca/ (*Canada's Schoolnet*)

Curriculum Materials
http://www.acs.ucalgary.ca/~dkbrown/ (*Children's Literature*)
http://www.scvol.com/States/ (*50 States & Capitals*)
http://forum.swarthmore.edu/ (*The Math Forum*)
http://www.sciencenetlinks.com (*Science NetLinks*)
http://www.clearinghouse.net/ (*A list of Hot Lists*)
http://www.miningco.com (*The Mining Co; Great Sites*)
http://www.nmmnh-abq.mus.nm.us/nmmnh/online.html (*Science Museums*)
http://www.ipl.org/ (*Internet Public Library*)
http://groundhog.sprl.umich.edu/curriculum/ (*Weather Curriculum*)
http://covis.atmos.uiuc.edu/covis/visualizer/ (*The Weather Visualizer*)
http://www.scicentral.com (*SciCentral; Great Science Resources*)
http://www.siec.k12.in.us/~west/sites/art.htm (*Art and Music Sites*)
http://www.girltech.com/index_home.html (*Club Girl Tech*)
http://www.discovery.com/news/earthalert/earthalert.html (*Earth Alert*)

http://www.surfnetkids.com (*Curriculum Materials by Topic*)
http://www.mapquest.com (*MapQuest, home of the interactive atlas*)
http://www.city.net (*Information about 5,000+ cities worldwide*)
http://www.kn.pacbell.com/wired/bluewebn/ (*PacBell's Blue Web'n*)
http://www.askanexpert.com/askanexpert (*Ask an Expert*)
http://pages.prodigy.com/kidsmoney/ (*Kids' Money*)
http://infoserver.etl.vt.edu/~/PE.Central/ (*Physical Education Central*)
http://www.odci.gov/cia/publications/nsolo/wfb-all.htm (*CIA Factbook*)
http://www.oit.itd.umich.edu/projects/ADW/ (*The Animal Diversity Web*)
http://www.writeenvironment.com/linksto.html (*Online Writing Resources*)
http://157.182.12.132/omdp yearbook/YearBook.htm (*Full Projects!!*)
http://lcweb2.loc.gov/ammem (*Library of Congress; The American Memory*)
http://www.si.edu (*Smithsonian Institution*)
http://www.nasa.gov (*NASA*)

Organizations
http://www.ed.gov/ (*U.S. Department of Education*)
http://www.nsta.org/ (*National Science Teachers Association*)
http://www.ncte.org/ (*National Council of Teachers of English*)
http://www.nea.org/ (*National Education Association*)
http://www.aft.org//index.htm (*American Federation of Teachers*)
http://www.pta.org/ (*National Parent Teachers Association*)
http://www.ascd.org (*Association for Supervision and Curriculum Dev.*)
http://www.socdeved.com/ (*Society for Developmental Education*)

http://nces.ed.gov (*National Center for Educational Statistics*

Tutorials
http://www.techlinx.org/inttut.htm (*Internet Tutorials*)

Publications & Media
http://www.techlearning.com (*Technology & Learning*)
http://www.edweek.com (*Education Week*)
http://www.edweek.com/tm/tm.htm (*Teacher Magazine*)
http://www.teachingk-8.com/ (*Teaching K-8*)
http://place.scholastic.com/instructor/home.htm (*Instructor Magazine*)
http://www.newslink.org/news.htm (*Complete List of Online Publications*)

http://www.pbs.org (*Public Broadcasting*)
http://www.cnn.com/ (*CNN*)
http://www.usatoday.com/ (*USA Today*)

Parents' Resources
http://www.ed.gov/PFIE/index.html (*Partnership for Family Involvement*)
http://kidshealth.org/parent/ (*Parents' Health Resource*)
http://www.parentsoup.com/ (*Parenting Site*)
http://www.smartparent.com (*SmartParent Site - Internet Safety, etc.*)
http://www.iamyourchild.org (*I Am Your Child*)

Search Engines
http://www.altavista.digital.com (*Altavista*)
http://www.yahoo.com (*Yahoo*)
http://www.infoseek.com (*Infoseek*)
http://www.webcrawler.com (*Webcrawler*)
http://www.lycos.com (*Lycos*)
http://www.dogpile.com (*Dogpile*)
http://www.four11.com/ (*Find people online*)
http://www.liszt.com/ (*Searchable list of Internet Listservs*)
http://www.dejanews.com (*To search newsgroups*)
http://www.searchenginewatch.com (*Search Engine Watch*)

Jim Moulton may be contacted at: jmoulton@horton.col.k12.me.us

Child Advocacy Organizations

Children's Defense Fund
25 E. St. NW, Washington, DC 20001
   If you are interested in finding out information about the Children's Sabbath program, please write to the above address c/o The Religious Affairs Division, National Observance of Children's Sabbaths.

Learning Disabilities / Inclusion

A.D.D. Warehouse
300 Northwest 70th Ave. Suite 102
Plantation, FL 33317
1-800-233-9273
FAX: (954) 792-8545
Internet: www.addwarehouse.com
   Books, tapes, videos on ADD, hyperactivity, and related disorders, including learning disabilities and Tourette's syndrome.

Paul H. Brookes Publishing Co. (catalog available)
P.O. Box 10624
Baltimore, MD 21285-0624
1-800-638-3775
FAX: (410) 337-8539
e-mail: custserv@pbrookes.com
Website: http://www.pbrookes.com

Centre for Integrated Education and Community
24 Thome Crescent
Toronto, Ontario M6H 2S5

CH.A.D.D. (Children with Attention Deficit Disorder)
499 NW 70th Ave., Suite 101
Plantation, FL 33317
(954) 587-3700

The Council for Exceptional Children
1920 Association Drive
Reston, VA 20191-1589
Toll-free: 1-888-CEC-SPED
(703) 620-3660
   (publishes *Exceptional Children, Teaching Exceptional Children* and *CEC Today*.)

Down Syndrome News
National Down Syndrome Congress
1605 Chantilly Dr., Suite 250
Atlanta, GA 30324
1-800-232-6372

Exceptional Children's Assistance Center
PO Box 16
Davidson, NC 28036
(704) 892-1321
1-800-962-6817 (NC only)
FAX: (704) 892-5028

The Exchange
The Learning Disabilities Network
72 Sharp St., Suite A-2
Hingham, MA 02043
(781) 340-5605 • FAX: (781) 340-5603
e-mail: LDNTWK@aol.com

Impact
Publications Office
Institute on Community Integration
University of Minnesota
109 Pattee Hall, 150 Pillsbury Dr. S.E.
Minneapolis, MN 55455
(612) 624-4512

Inclusion Press International
24 Thome Crescent
Toronto, Ontario M6H 2S5
(416) 658-5363 • FAX: (416) 658-5067
e-mail: Compuserve: 74640, 1124
Web Page: http: //inclusion.com

Learning Disabilities Association
4156 Library Rd.
Pittsburgh, PA 15234
(412) 341-1515 • FAX: (412) 344-0224

MPACT (Missouri Parents Act)
8631 Delmar, Suite 300
St. Louis, MO 63124
1-800-995-3160

Parents Active for Vision Education (P.A.V.E.)
National Headquarters
9620 Chesapeake Drive, Suite 105
San Diego, CA 92123
Phone: (619) 467-9620
1-800-PAVE-988
Fax: (619) 467-9624
   This organization believes that undetected vision disorders often contribute to learning problems in school.

PEAK (Parent Center, Inc.)
6055 Lehman Dr., Suite 101
Colorado Springs, CO 80918
(719) 531-9400 • FAX: (719) 531-9452
e-mail: info@peakparent.org
   Inclusion resources, practical tools for educating ALL students in general education classrooms

Whole Language Hotline

The Center for the Expansion of Language and Thinking (CELT) operates a crisis hotline to support teachers and administrators who come under attack for their child-centered practices. For further information, contact:
   The Center for Establishing Dialogue in Teaching and Learning (CED)
   325 E. Southern Ave., Suite 107-108, Tempe, AZ 85282
   1-602-894-1333 • FAX 602-894-9547

Paperback Book Clubs

Troll Book Club
2 Lethbridge Plaza
Mahwah, NJ 07430
1-800-541-1097

Publications

Children's Literature

Book Links: Connecting Books, Libraries and Classrooms
American Library Association
50 Huron St.
Chicago, IL 60611

The Bulletin of the Center for Children's Books
University of Illinois Press
1325 S. Oak St.
Champaign, IL 61820

CBC Features
Children's Book Council
568 Broadway, Suite 404
New York, NY 10012

Children's Literature and Reading
(special interest group of the
International Reading Association)
Membership: Dr. Miriam A. Marecek
10 Marchant Rd.
Winchester, MA 01890

The Horn Book Magazine
11 Beacon St., Suite 1000
Boston, MA 02108
The Horn Book also publishes *The Horn Book Guide to Children's and Young Adult Books*, a semi-annual publication reviewing nearly 4000 hardcover trade books each year.

Journal of Children's Literature
Children's Literature Assembly
Membership Chair: Dr. Linda M. Pavonetti, Ed.D.
c/o Department of Reading
and Language Arts
Rochester, MI 48309-4494
(248) 608-8852
e-mail: <pavonett@oakland.edu>

The Kobrin Letter
732 Greer Rd.
Palo Alto, CA 94303
    This free newsletter reviews nonfiction books.

The New Advocate
Christopher-Gordon Publishers, Inc.
1502 Providence Highway, Suite 12
Norwood, MA 02062

Reading Is Fundamental (RIF)
600 Maryland Ave. S.W., Suite 600
Washington, D.C. 20024-2569
(202) 287-3220
http://www.si.edu/rif
    For information on starting a RIF program or for parent brochures.

The WEB (Wonderfully Exciting Books)
The Ohio State University
Room 200 Ramseyer Hall
29 West Woodruff
Columbus, OH 43210

Early Childhood / Developmental Education

Childhood Education
Journal of the Association for Childhood
    Education International
Suite 215
17904 Georgia Ave.
Olney, MD 20832

Early Childhood News
Peter Li, Inc.
330 Progress Road
Dayton, OH 45449
(513) 847-5900

Early Childhood Today
Scholastic, Inc.
555 Broadway
New York, NY 10012

Young Children
National Association for the Education of Young Children
    (NAEYC)
1509 16th St. NW
Washington, DC 20036-1426
1-800-424-2460
FAX: (202) 328-1846
e-mail: naeyc@naeyc.org
website: http://www.naeyc.org

General Education — Classroom Focus

Creative Classroom
Children's Television Workshop
Subscriptions: PO Box 7691
                Red Oak, IA 51519-0691

Instructor Magazine
Scholastic, Inc.
555 Broadway
New York, NY 10012

Learning
1607 Battleground Avenue
Greensboro, NC 27408

The Private Eye Newsletter
7710 31st Avenue NW
Seattle, WA 98117
(206) 784-8813
Fax: (206) 781-2172
e-mail: ruef@halcyon.com
website: http://www.the-private-eye.com/ruef/

Teaching K-8
40 Richards Ave.
Norwalk, CT 06854

General Education — Issues/Research/Technology Focus

The American School Board Journal and
    Electronics School
National School Boards Association
1680 Duke St.
Alexandria, VA 22314

Democracy and Education
The Institute for Democracy in Education
College of Education
313 McCracken Hall, Ohio University
Athens, OH 45701-2979
(614) 593-4531 • FAX: (614) 593-0177

Education Week
Editorial: 6935 Arlington Rd., Suite 100
                  Bethesda, MD 20814
Subscriptions: P.O. Box 2083
                  Marion, OH 43305

Educational Leadership
Journal of the Association for Supervision and
    Curriculum Development (ASCD)
1250 N. Pitt St.
Alexandria, VA 22314-1403
1-800-933-2723

FairTest
The National Center for Fair & Open Testing
342 Broadway
Cambridge, MA 02139
   FairTest has serious issues with standardized tests as administered and used in today's schools and offers alternative options, including performance assessments.

Phi Delta Kappan
Eighth and Union
P.O. Box 789
Bloomington, IN 47402
Journal of Phi Delta Kappa International
The professional fraternity in education

Principal
National Association of Elementary School Principals
   (NAESP)
1615 Duke St.
Alexandria, VA 22314-3483

The Responsive Classroom: A Newsletter for Teachers
Northeast Foundation for Children
71 Montague City Rd.
Greenfield, MA 01301
1-800-360-6332

The School Administrator
American Association of School Administrators
1801 North Moore St.
Arlington, VA 22209

Teaching Voices
The Massachusetts Field Center for Teaching & Learning
University of Massachusetts
100 Morrissey Blvd.
Boston, MA 02125
(617) 287-7660
FAX: (617) 287-7664

TIP (Theory into Practice)
Subscription Dept.
Ohio State University
174 Arps Hall
1945 N. High St.
Columbus, OH 43210-1172

Language

Language Arts
National Council of Teachers of English
1111 W. Kenyon Rd.
Urbana, IL 61801-1096

Literacy
The International Institute of Literacy Learning
Box 1414
Commerce, TX 75429

Primary Voices K-6
National Council of Teachers of English
1111 W. Kenyon Rd.
Urbana, IL 61801-1096

The Reading Teacher
International Reading Association
P.O. Box 8139
Newark, DE 19714-8139
(IRA also publishes Journal of Adolescent and Adult Literacy, Reading Today, Reading Research Quarterly; Lectura y Vida — a Spanish language journal.)

Math and Science

Science and Children
National Science Teachers Association
1840 Wilson Blvd.
Arlington, VA 22201-3000

Teaching Children Mathematics
National Council of Teachers of Mathematics
1906 Association Dr.
Reston, VA 20191-1593
(703) 620-9840
Website: http://www.nctm.org
Other journals include: Mathematics Teaching in the Middle School; Mathematics Teacher; Journal for Research in Mathematics Education.

Whole Language

The Whole Idea
The Wright Group
19201 120th Ave. NE
Bothell, WA 98011
(425) 486-8011 • FAX: (425) 486-7704

Whole Language Network
Teaching K-8
40 Richards Ave.
Norwalk, CT 06854

The Whole Language Teachers Association Newsletter
P.O. Box 216
Southboro, MA 01772

WLSIG Newsletter
Talking Points
Whole Language Umbrella

For membership inquiries:	National Council of Teachers of English 1111 W. Kenyon Road Urbana, IL 61801 1-800-369-6283 (217) 328-3870 • FAX: (217) 328-9645
President:	Kittye Copeland
Newsjournal:	Shirley Crenshaw and Dorothy King

Sources of Multiage Materials

Crystal Springs Books
Ten Sharon Road
PO Box 500
Peterborough, NH 03458
1-800-321-0401
FAX: 1-800-337-9929

Creative Teaching Press, Inc.
P.O. Box 6017
Cypress, CA 90630-0017
1-800-444-4287

Richard C. Owen Publishers, Inc.
P.O. Box 585
Katonah, NY 10536
1-800-336-5588

Interact (Simulation Units)
1825 Gillespie Way, #101
El Cajon, CA 92020-1095
1-800-359-0961 • FAX: 1-800-700-5093
Website: www.interact-simulations.com
   Produce multiage, cross-curriculum, interactive simulations.

Big Book Publishers

Sundance Publishing
P.O. Box 1326
Littleton, MA 01460
1-800-343-8204

The Wright Group
19201 12th Ave. NE
Bothell, WA 98011
1-800-523-2371

Publishers & Distributors of Math Books & Products

Creative Publications
5623 W. 115th Street
Alsip, IL 60803
1-800-624-0822

Crystal Springs Books
Ten Sharon Road, PO Box 500
Peterborough, NH 03458
1-800-321-0401

Cuisenaire
PO Box 5026
White Plains, NY 10602-5026
1-800-237-0338

Dale Seymour Publications
PO Box 10888
Palo Alto, CA 94303-0879
1-800-872-1100

Dandy Lion Publications
3563-L Sueldo
San Luis Obispo, CA 93401
1-800-776-8032

Delta Education
PO Box 3000
Nashua, NH 03061-9912
1-800-442-5444

Educational Electronics (Calculator Dist.)
70 Finnell Drive
Weymouth Landing, MA 02188
1-800-526-9060

The Math Shop
Quantexx
PO Box 694
Canfield, OH 44406
1-800-798-MATH

National Council of Teachers of Mathematics
PO Box 25405
Richmond, VA 23260-5405
1-800-235-7566

Scholastic, Inc.
2931 E. McCarty Street
Jefferson City, MO 65101
1-800-325-6149

Materials

Big Book Materials
Sticky pockets — Demco Library Supplies and Equipment, 1-800-356-1200
Velour paper — Dick Blick Art Supply, 1-800-345-3042
Grommets — Hardware stores
Alphabet & number stickers — Childcraft Education Corp., 1-800-631-5652
"Scribbles" Glitter Writers — Arts and crafts stores or Duncan Hobby, (209) 291-2515

Binding Machines and Spiral Binding
General Binding Corporation
One GBC Plaza, Northbrook, IL 60062
(847) 723-4000
Scholastic, Inc. — 1-800-724-6527

Book Racks/Easels
Fixturecraft Corp.
443 East Westfield Ave.
P.O. Box 292, Roselle Park, NJ 07204-0292
1-800-275-1145

Chart Paper/Sentence Strips
School Specialty – New England Division
P.O. Box 3004, Agawam, MA 01101-8004
1-800-628-8608

J.L.Hammett Company
P.O. Box 859057, Braintree, MA 02185-9057
1-800-333-4600

Computer Programs
Print Shop
Broderbund
500 Redwood Blvd.
P.O. Box 6121, Novato, CA 94948-6121
1-800-521-6263

SuperPrint
Scholastic
P.O. Box 7502, Jefferson City, MO 65102
1-800-724-6527

Educational Records Center
Catalog for Songs
3233 Burnt Mill Drive, Suite 100
Wilmington, NC 28403-2655
1-800-438-1637

Highlight Tape
Available from Crystal Springs Books • 1-800-321-0401

Kinesiology
Brain Gym®
Developmental activities to help children learn more effectively
Educational Kinesiology Foundation
P.O. Box 3396, Ventura, CA 93006-3396
1-800-356-2109

Manatee Adoption ($10.00/year)
Save the Manatee Club
500 N. Maitland Ave., Suite 210
Maitland, FL 32751
(407) 539-0990

Metal Shower Curtain Rings
Department Stores

Plastic Rings/Bird Bands
Farm Feed Stores

Ribbons and Awards
Hodges Badge Company, Inc. • 1-800-556-2440

Sea Monkey Eggs
Sea Monkeys
Transcience Corporation
P.O. Box 809, Bryans Road, MD 20616

Stencil Machines
The Ellison LetterMachine
Ellison Educational Equipment, Inc.
P.O. Box 8209, Newport Beach, CA 92658-8209
1-800-253-2238

Touch phonics Reading Systems
Manipulative Phonics System
4900 Birch Street, Newport Beach, CA 92660
(714) 975-1141 • FAX (714) 975-1056
1-800-92-TOUCH (928-6824)
http://www.touchphonics.com

Whale Adoption
Whale Adoption Project
International Wildlife Coalition
634 N. Falmouth Highway, P.O. Box 388
N. Falmouth, MA 02556-0388

Wikki Stix
Available from Crystal Springs Books • 1-800-321-0401

Children's Magazines

Publication / Subscription Address	Interest Area/Age Group
AppleSeeds 30 Grove Street Peterborough, NH 03458 website: http://cobblestonepub.com	Social Studies/Reading 7-9
Big Book Magazine Scholastic, Inc. P.O. Box 10805 Des Moines, IA 50380-0813 1-800-788-7017	General Interest 4-7
Boys' Life Boy Scouts of America 1325 Walnut Hill Lane P.O. Box 152079 Irving, TX 75015-2079	General Interest 7-18
California Cobblestone 30 Grove Street Peterborough, NH 03458 website: http://cobblestonepub.com	California History 8-14
Classical Calliope 30 Grove Street Peterborough, NH 03458 website: http://cobblestonepub.com	World History 9-16
Cobblestone 30 Grove Street Peterborough, NH 03458 website: http://cobblestonepub.com	American History 8-14
* *Creative Kids* P.O. Box 8813 Waco, TX 76714-8813 1-800-998-2208 FAX: 1-800-240-0333 e-mail: Creative-Kids@prufrock.com	Student Art/Writing 8-14
* *Cricket* P.O. Box 7433 Red Oak, IA 51591-4433 Submissions: 315 5th St., P.O. Box 300 Peru, IL 61354	Literature/Art 9-14
Faces 30 Grove Street Peterborough, NH 03458 website: http://cobblestonepub.com	World Cultures 8-14
FootSteps 30 Grove Street Peterborough, NH 03458 website: http://cobblestonepub.com	African-American Heritage 8-14
* *Highlights for Children* P.O. Box 269 Columbus, OH 43216-0269 (614) 486-0631 FAX: (614) 487-2700 Street Address: 2300 W. Fifth Ave. Columbus, OH 43215 Submissions: 803 Church St. Honesdale, PA 18431	General Interest 2-12
KIDS Discover P.O. Box 54209 Boulder, CO 80321-4209	Science/General Interest 5-12

Publication / Subscription Address	Interest Area/Age Group
Kids City *Contact Kids* Submissions: Children's Television Workshop One Lincoln Plaza New York, NY 10023	Entertainment/Education
Ladybug Red Oak, IA 51591	Literature 2-6
* *Merlyn's Pen* Fiction, Essays, and Poems by America's Teens P.O. Box 1058 East Greenwich, RI 02818	Student Writing 12-16
* *Odyssey* 30 Grove Street Peterborough, NH 03458 http://cobblestonepub.com	Space Exploration/ Astronomy 8-14
Plays 120 Boylston St. Boston, MA 02116-4615	Drama 6-18
Ranger Rick National Wildlife Federation 8925 Leesburg Pike Vienna, VA 22180-0001	Science/Wildlife Nature, Environment 7-12
* *School Mates* 186 Route 9W New Windsor, NY 12553	Chess for Beginners 7 and up
Scienceland 501 Fifth Ave. Suite 2108 New York, NY 10017-6107	Science 5-11
Sesame Street Magazine P.O. Box 52000 Boulder, CO 80321-2000	General Interest 2-6
Sports Illustrated for Kids P.O. Box 830609 Birmingham, AL 35283-0609	Sports 8-13
Stone Soup The Magazine by Young Writers and Artists P.O. Box 83 Santa Cruz, CA 95063	Student Writing/Art 6-14
Storyworks Scholastic 555 Broadway New York, NY 10012-3999	Literature 8-11
3-2-1 Contact P.O. Box 51177 Boulder, CO 80321-1177	Science 8-14
Your Big Backyard National Wildlife Federation 8925 Leesburg Pike Vienna, VA 22184 Includes parents guide	Animals/Nature 3-6

*encourages children's submissions

Workshops and Conferences

The Society For Developmental Education
Ten Sharon Road, Box 577, Peterborough, NH 03458
1-800-924-9621 • e-mail: sde.csb@socdeved.com • Website at: http://www.socdeved.com

The Society For Developmental Education (SDE) presents workshops, conferences, and staff development inservices throughout the year and around the country for elementary educators on multiage, school readiness, inclusion education, multiple intelligences, character education, discipline, whole language, authentic assessment, math, science, and related topics. SDE sponsors a National Multiage and Looping Conference each July. For information on dates and location, please call 1-800-462-1478 or write to the address above.

Other Resources

ERIC

ERIC (Educational Resources Information Center) is a clearinghouse or central agency responsible for the collection, classification, and distribution of written information related to education. If you need help finding the best way to use ERIC, call ACCESS ERIC toll-free at 1-800-LET-ERIC. If you need specific information about multiage education, call Norma Howard at 1-800-822-9229.

A Value Search: Multiage or Nongraded Education is available for $7.50 and can be ordered from Publication Sales, ERIC Clearinghouse on Educational Management, 5207 University of Oregon, Eugene, OR 97403-5207. A handling charge of $4.00 is added to all billed orders.

National Association for Year-Round Education (NAYRE)
P.O. Box 711386, San Diego, CA 92171-1386
(618) 276-5296 • FAX: (619) 571-5754 • e-mail: info@nayre.org • website: www.nayre.org

The National Association for Year-Round Education (NAYRE) has its membership among schools who follow a year-round academic schedule; some members, for instance, have a nine-weeks-in-school, nine-week-vacation schedule, rather than giving students three months off during the summer. This type of year-round schedule provides academic continuity. NAYRE provides information on its programs and membership to interested parties.

Multiage Classroom Exchange
Teaching K-8
40 Richards Ave., Norwalk, CT 06854

The Multiage Classroom Exchange puts teachers in contact with others who are interested in swapping ideas, activities, and experiences relating to the multiage, progressive classroom. To join, send your name, address, age levels you teach, years of experience with multiage education, and a self-addressed, stamped envelope to the address listed. You'll receive a complete, up-to-date list of teachers who are interested in exchanging information.

Under Construction
Jane Meade-Roberts
202 Riker Terrace Way, Salinas, CA 93901
Phone (408) 455-1831 (to leave message) • FAX: (408) 424-2829

Under Construction's goal is to assist teachers, parents and administrators in gaining an understanding of how children and adults construct knowledge, and to support experienced teachers who are working to understand constructivist theory and its implications for teaching. (Constructivism is a scientific theory of learning, based on Piaget's theory of cognitive development, that explains how people come to build their own knowledge and understand the things and people in their own world.)

The organization feels that multiage classrooms are wonderfully suited for helping adults learn more about how children develop and construct knowledge. Many of the teachers and parents in the group are currently involved in multiage classrooms or are interested in developing their understanding of constructivism so that they may begin a multiage learning environment for children in their own school.

Under Construction is an umbrella for several groups working toward this end. The Constructivist Network of Monterey County, which meets monthly, is largely composed of university personnel and some school teachers. The network provides a speaker series for the community. A focus group includes teachers involved in coaching and classroom visitations. The organization is collaborating with the local adult school to provide classes for parents of children in multiage classrooms, and has just begun to work with a new local university, with the object of working with people in the community. An advisory board oversees the organization. The organization is funded by the Walter S. Johnson Foundation.

Bibliography
(compiled by SDE Presenters)

Attention Deficit Disorder (ADD) / Attention Deficit Hyperactivity Disorder (ADHD)

Barkley, Russell A. *ADHD in the Classroom (Video and Program Guide)*. New York: Guilford Publications, 1994.

Einstein, Carol. *Be Your Own Reading Specialist: A Guide For Teachers of Grades 1-3*. Rosemont, NJ: Modern Learning Press, 1997.

Hallowell, Edward M., and Ratey, John J. *Driven to Distraction*. New York: Touchstone, 1994.

Hartmann, Thom. *Attention Deficit Disorder: A Different Perception*. Penn Valley, CA, and Lancaster, PA: Underwood-Miller, 1993.

Ingersoll, Barbara, Ph.D. *Your Hyperactive Child: A Parent's Guide to Coping With Attention Deficit Disorder*. New York: Doubleday, 1988.

Moss, Deborah. *Shelley, the Hyperactive Turtle*. Rockville, MD: Woodbine House, 1989.

Moss, Robert A., and Dunlap, Helen Huff. *Why Johnny Can't Concentrate: Coping with Attention Deficit Problems*. New York: Bantam Books, 1990.

Parker, Harvey. *The ADD Hyperactivity Handbook for Schools*. Plantation, FL: Impact Publications, 1992.

———.*The ADD Hyperactivity Workbook for Parents, Teachers, and Kids*. Plantation, FL: Impact Publications, 1988.

———.*The ADAPT Accommodation Planbook for Teachers*. Plantation, FL: Impact Publications, 1992.

———.*The ADAPT Student Planbook*. Plantation, FL: Impact Publications, 1992.

Rief, Sandra. *How to Reach and Teach ADD/ADHD Children*. West Nyack, NY: The Center for Applied Research in Education, 1993.

Shapiro, Lawrence E. *Sometimes I Drive My Mom Crazy, But I Know She's Crazy About Me*. King of Prussia, PA: The Center for Applied Psychology, Inc., 1993.

Taylor, John F. *Helping Your Hyperactive/Attention Deficit Child*. Rocklin, CA: Prima Publishing, 1994.

Anti-Hurrying

Elkind, David, Ph.D. *All Grown Up & No Place To Go*. Reading, MA: Addison-Wesley, 1984.

———. *The Hurried Child*. Reading, MA: Addison-Wesley, 1981.

———. *Miseducation: Preschoolers at Risk*. New York: Alfred A. Knopf, 1987.

———. *Reinventing Childhood: Raising and Educating Children in a Changing World*. Rosemont, NJ: Modern Learning Press, 1998.

Gilmore, June E.. *The Rape of Childhood: No Time to Be a Kid*. Middletown, OH: J & J Publishing, 1990.

National Education Commission on Time and Learning. *Prisoners of Time*. Washington, DC: U.S. Government Printing Office, Superintendent of Documents, 1994.

Uphoff, James K.. *Real Facts From Real Schools: What You're Not Supposed to Know About School Readiness and Transition Programs*. Rosemont, NJ: Modern Learning Press, 1990, 1995.

Uphoff, James K.; Gilmore, June; and Huber, Rosemarie. *Summer Children: Ready (or Not) for School*. Middletown, OH: The Oxford Press, 1986.

Winn, Marie. *Children Without Childhood*. New York: Penguin Books, 1984.

Assessment

Batzle, Janine. *Portfolio Assessment and Evaluation: Developing and Using Portfolios in the K-6 Classroom*. Cypress, CA: Creative Teaching Press, 1992.

Bridges, Lois. *Assessment: Continuous Learning*. York, ME: Stenhouse Publishers, The Galef Institute, 1995.

Clay, Marie. *An Observation Survey of Early Literacy Achievement*. Portsmouth, NH: Heinemann, 1993.

———. *Sand* and *Stones: "Concepts About Print" Tests*. Portsmouth, NH: Heinemann, 1980.

Clemmons, J.; Laase, L.; Cooper, D.; Areglado, N.; and Dill, M. *Portfolios in the Classroom: A Teacher's Sourcebook*. New York: Scholastic Inc., 1993.

Fiderer, Adele. *35 Rubrics & Checklists to Assess Reading and Writing: Time-Saving Reproducible Forms for Meaningful Assessment*. New York: Scholastic Inc., 1998.

Goodman, Yetta, et al. *Reading Miscues Inventory: Alternative Procedures*. New York: Richard C. Owen Publishers, 1987.

Graves, Donald, and Sustein, Bonnie, eds. *Portfolio Portraits*. Portsmouth, NH: Heinemann, 1992.

Keshner, Judy. *The Kindergarten Teacher's Very Own Student Assessment and Observation Guide*. Rosemont, NJ: Modern Learning Press, 1996.

Lazear, David. *Multiple Intelligence Approaches to Assessment: Solving the Assessment Conundrum*. Palatine, IL: IRI/Skylight Publishing, Inc., 1994.

MacDonald, Sharon. *Portfolio and Its Use Book II: A Road Map for Assessment*. Little Rock, AR: Southern Early Childhood Association, 1996.

Parsons, Les. *Response Journals*. Portsmouth, NH: Heinemann, 1989.

Power, Brenda Miller. *Taking Note: Improving Your Observational Notetaking*. York, ME: Stenhouse, 1996.

Power, Brenda Miller, and Chandler, Kelly. *Well-Chosen Words: Narrative Assessments and Report Card Comments*. York, ME: Stenhouse Publishers, 1998.

Schipper, Beth, and Rossi, Joanne. *Portfolios in the Classroom: Tools for Learning and Instruction*. York, ME: Stenhouse Publishers, 1997.

Traill, Leanna. *Highlight My Strengths*. Reed Publications, 1993.

Vail, Priscilla L. *A Language Yardstick: Understanding and Assessment*. Rosemont, NJ: Modern Learning Press, 1998.

Audio/Video

Ames, Louise Bates. *Part I: Ready Or Not: Here I Come!* and *Part II: An Evaluation of the Whole Child*, video. Modern Learning Press, 1983.

Anderson, Robert, and Pavan, Barbara. *The Nongraded School*. Bloomington, IN: Phi Delta Kappa. An interview with the authors of *Nongradedness: Helping It to Happen*. Video, 30 minutes.

Feldman, Jean. *Fresh Ideas for Active Teaching*. Video. Crystal Springs Books, 1997.

Forsten, Char, and Grant, Jim. *The Looping Video*. Video. Crystal Springs Books, 1998.

Fountas, Irene C., and Pinnell, Gay Su. *The Essentials of Guided Reading*. Audiotape. Heinemann, 1997.

Gesell Institute of Human Development. *Ready or Not Here I Come*. Video/16mm film. Modern Learning Press, 1984.

Goodman, Gretchen. *Classroom Strategies for "Gray-Area" Children*. Video. Crystal Springs Books, 1995.

Grant, Jim. *Avoid the Pitfalls of Implementing Multiage Classrooms*. Video. Crystal Springs Books, 1995.

———. *Do You Know Where Your Child Is?* Video. Modern Learning Press, 1985.

———. *Grade Replacement*. Audiotape. Modern Learning Press, 1988.

———. *Making Informed Decisions About Retention*. Video. Crystal Springs Books, 1997.

———. *Worth Repeating*. Video. Modern Learning Press, 1988.

Pavelka, Pat. *Creating and Managing Effective Centers & Themes*. Video. Crystal Springs Books, 1997.

Thompson, Ellen. *A Day in a Multiage Classroom*. Video. Crystal Springs Books, 1994.

———. *The Nuts and Bolts of Multiage Classrooms*. Video, 90 minutes. Crystal Springs Books, 1994.

Behavior / Discipline

Bailey, Dr. Becky. *There's Gotta Be a Better Way: Discipline That Works!* Oviedo, FL: Loving Guidance, 1997.

Braman, O. Randall. *The Oppositional Child*. Charlotte, NC: Kidsrights, 1997.

Burke, Kay. *What to Do with the Kid Who ... Developing Cooperation, Self-Discipline and Responsibility in the Classroom*. Palatine, IL: IRI/Skylight Publishing, 1992.

Charles, C.M. *Building Classroom Discipline*. New York: Longman, 1992.

Coletta, Anthony. *What's Best for Kids: A Guide to Developmentally Appropriate Practices for Teachers & Parents of Children Ages 4-8*. Rosemont, NJ: Modern Learning Press, 1991.

Curwin, Richard L., and Mendler, Allen N. *Discipline with Dignity*. Alexandria, VA: Association for Supervision and Curriculum Development, 1993.

Feldman, Jean. *Transition Time: Let's Do Something Different!* Beltsville, MD: Gryphon House, 1995.

Fox, Lynn. *Let's Get Together*. Rolling Hills, CA: Jalmar Press, 1993.

Kohn, Alfie. *Punished by Rewards: The Trouble with Gold Stars, Incentive Plans, A's, Praise, and Other Bribes*. Boston: Houghton Mifflin, 1993.

Kreidler, William. *Conflict Resolution Through Children's Literature*. New York: Scholastic Inc., 1994.

———. *Creative Conflict Resolution: Strategies for Keeping Peace in the Classroom*. Rocklin, CA: Prima Publishing, 1993.

Nelson, Jane; Lott, Lynn; and Glenn, Stephen. *Positive Discipline in the Classroom.*. Rocklin, CA: Prima Publishing, 1993.

Payne, Ruby K, Ph.D. *Poverty: A Framework for Understanding and Working With Students and Adults from Poverty*. Baytown, TX: RFT Publishing, 1995.

Vail, Priscilla. *Emotion: The On-Off Switch for Learning*. Rosemont, NJ: Modern Learning Press, 1994.

Wright, Esther. *Good Morning, Class — I Love You!* Rolling Hills, CA: Jalmar Press, 1988.

———. *Loving Discipline A to Z*. San Francisco: Teaching From the Heart, 1994.

Curriculum — Overview

Avi. *Poppy*. New York: Avon Books, A Division of The Hearst Corporation, 1995.

Bredekamp, Sue, and Rosegrant, Teresa, eds. *Reaching Potentials: Appropriate Curriculum and Assessment for Young Children*, Vol. 1. Washington, DC: NAEYC, 1992.

Charney, Ruth Sidney. *Habits of Goodness: Case Studies in the Social Curriculum.* Greenfield, MA: Northeast Foundation for Children, 1997.

Chertok, Bobbi; Hirshfeld, Goody; and Rosh, Marilyn. *Teaching American History with Art Masterpieces.* New York: Scholastic Inc., 1998.

Coates, Grace Davila, and Stenmark, Jean Kerr. *Family Math for Young Children: Comparing.* Berkeley, CA: Lawrence Hall of Science, University of California at Berkeley, 1997.

Cummings, Carol, Ph.D. *Managing a Diverse Classroom: Practical Ideas for Thematic Units, Reading and Writing, Learning Centers, and Assessments.* Edmonds, WA: Teaching, Inc., 1995.

Daniels, Harvey, and Bizar, Marilyn. *Methods that Matter: Six Structures for Best Practice Classrooms.* York, ME: Stenhouse Publishers, 1998.

Dodge, Diane Trister; Jablon, Judy R.; and Bickart, Toni S. *Constructing Curriculum for the Primary Grades.* Washington, DC: Teaching Strategies, Inc., 1992.

Edinger, Monica and Fins, Stephanie. *Far Away and Long Ago: Young Historians in the Classroom.* York, ME: Stenhouse Publishers, 1998.

Fisher, Bobbi. *Inside the Classroom: Teaching Kindergarten and First Grade.* Portsmouth, NH: Heinemann, 1996.

Fogarty, Robin. *The Mindful School: How to Integrate the Curricula.* Palatine, IL: IRI/Skylight Publishing, 1991.

Hall, G.E., and Loucks, S. F. "Program Definition and Adaptation: Implications for Inservice." Journal of Research and Development in Education (1981) 14, 2:46-58.

Hildum, Kristin K. *Write to Publish: Teaching Writing Skills through Classroom Magazine Publishing* (Grades 4-8). Cypress, CA: Creative Teaching Press, 1996.

Hohmann, C. *Mathematics: High Scope K-3 Curriculum Guide* (illustrated field test edition). Ypsilanti, MI: High Scope Press, 1991.

Jensen, Eric. *Brain Compatible Strategies.* Del Mar, CA: Turning Point Publishing, 1997.

———. *Over 1,000 Easy-to-Use & Practical Strategie!* Del Mar, CA: Turning Point Publishing, 1995.

Julio, Susan. *Great Map Mysteries: 18 Stories and Maps to Build Geography and Map Skills* (Grades 3-6). New York: Scholastic Inc., 1997.

Katz, Bobbi. *American History Poems.* New York: Scholastic Inc., 1998.

Lee, Martin, and Miller, Marcia. *Real-Life Math Investigations: 20 Activities that Help Students Apply Mathematical Thinking to Real-Life Situations.* New York: Scholastic Inc., 1997.

Maehr, J. *Language and Literacy: High Scope K-3 Curriculum Guide* (illustrated field test edition). Ypsilanti, MI: High Scope Press, 1991.

MacDonald, Sharon. *Everyday Discoveries: Amazingly Easy Science and Math Using Stuff You Already Have.* Beltsville, MD: Gryphon House, 1998.

Moore, Helen H. *A Poem A Day: 180 Thematic Poems and Activities That Teach and Delight All Year Long* (Grades K-3). New York: Scholastic Inc., 1997.

Murdock, Maureen. *Spinning Inward: Using Guided Imagery With Children for Learning, Creativity & Relaxation.* Boston: Shambhala Publications, 1987.

National Association of Elementary School Principals. *Standards for Quality Elementary and Middle Schools: Kindergarten through Eighth Grade.* Alexandria, VA: NAESP, 1990.

Olien, Rebecca. *Exploring Plants.* New York: Scholastic Inc., 1997.

Richardson, Kathy. *Developing Number Concepts Using Unifix Cubes.* Menlo Park, CA: Addison-Wesley, 1984.

Rowan, Thomas E., and Morrow, Lorna J. *Implementing the K-8 Curriculum and Evaluation Standards: Readings from the "Arithmetic Teacher."* Reston, VA: National Council of Teachers of Mathematics, 1993.

Silver, Donald M. and Wynne, Patricia J. *Amazing Earth Model Book: Easy-to-Make Hands-on Models That Teach* (Grades 3-6). New York: Scholastic Inc., 1997.

Stenmark, Jean Kerr; Thompson, Virginia; and Cossey, Ruth. *Family Math.* Berkeley, CA: Lawrence Hall of Science, 1986.

Stone, Sandra J. *Playing: A Kid's Curriculum* (Ages 2-6). Glenview, IL: ScottForesman, GoodYearBooks, 1993.

Curriculum — Integrated Activities

Bauer, Karen, and Drew, Rosa. *Alternatives to Worksheets.* Cypress, CA: Creative Teaching Press, 1992.

Brainard, Audrey, and Wrubel, Denise H. *Literature-Based Science Activities: An Integrated Approach.* New York: Scholastic, 1993.

Cherkerzian, Diane. *The Complete Lesson Plan Book.* Peterborough, NH: Crystal Springs Books, 1993.

Feldman, Jean R. *Wonderful Rooms Where Children Can Bloom!* Peterborough, NH: Crystal Springs Books, 1997.

Hiatt, Catherine; Wolven, Doug; Botka, Gwen; and Richmond, Jennifer. *More Alternatives to Worksheets.* Cypress, CA: Creative Teaching Press, 1994.

Kohl, MaryAnn, and Potter, Jean. *ScienceArts: Discovering Science Through Art Experiences.* Bellingham, WA: Bright Ring Publishing, 1993.

Ruef, Kerry. *The Private Eye. Looking/Thinking by Analogy: A Guide to Developing the Interdisciplinary Mind.* Seattle: The Private Eye Project, 1992.

Short, Kathy G.; Schroeder, Jean; Laird, Julie; Kauffman, Gloria; Ferguson, Margaret J.; Crawford, Kathleen Marie. *Learning Together Through Inquiry: From Columbus to Integrated Curriculum.* York, ME: Stenhouse Publishers, 1996.

Steffey, Stephanie, and Hood, Wendy J., eds. *If This Is Social Studies, Why Isn't It Boring?* York, ME: Stenhouse Publishers, 1994.

Developmental Education / Readiness

Ames, Louise Bates. *What Do They Mean I'm Difficult?* Rosemont, NJ: Modern Learning Press, 1986.

Ames, Louise Bates; Baker, Sidney; and Ilg, Frances L. *Child Behavior (Specific Advice on Problems of Child Behavior).* New York: Barnes & Noble Books, 1981.

Ames, Louise Bates, et al. *The Gesell Institute's Child from One to Six.* New York: Harper & Row, 1946.

Boyer, Ernest. *The Basic School: A Community for Learning.* Ewing, NJ: The Foundation for the Advancement of Teaching, 1991.

Brazelton, T. Berry. *To Listen to a Child: Understanding the Normal Problems of Growing Up.* Reading, MA: Addison-Wesley, 1986.

———. *Touchpoints: The Essential Reference. Your Child's Emotional and Behavioral Development.* Reading, MA: Addison-Wesley, 1994.

———. *Working and Caring.* Reading, MA: Addison-Wesley, 1985.

Bredekamp, Sue, ed. *Developmentally Appropriate Practice in Early Childhood Programs Serving Children From Birth Through Age 8,* expanded edition. Washington, DC: National Association for the Education of Young Children, 1987.

Charney, Ruth Sidney. *Teaching Children to Care: Management in the Responsive Classroom.* Greenfield, MA: Northeast Foundation for Children, 1991.

Elovson, Allanna. *The Kindergarten Survival Book.* Santa Monica, CA: Parent Ed Resources, 1991.

Grant, Jim. *Childhood Should Be a Precious Time.* (poem anthology) Rosemont, NJ: Modern Learning Press, 1989.

Grant, Jim, and Johnson, Bob. "First Grade Readiness Checklist." Peterborough, NH: Crystal Springs Books, 1997.

———. "Kindergarten Checklist." Peterborough, NH: Crystal Springs Books, 1997.

———. "I Hate School!" Some Common Sense Answers for Educators & Parents Who Want to Know Why and What to Do About It. Rosemont, NJ: Programs for Education, 1994.

Grant, Jim, and Azen, Margot. *Every Parent's Owner's Manuals.* (Three-, Four-, Five-, Six-, Seven-Year- Old). Rosemont, NJ: Programs for Education.

Healy, Jane M. *Endangered Minds: Why Children Don't Think and What We Can Do About It.* New York: Simon and Schuster, 1990.

———. *Your Child's Growing Mind: A Guide to Learning and Brain Development From Birth to Adolescence.* New York: Doubleday, 1987.

Karnofsky, Florence, and Weiss, Trudy. *How to Prepare Your Child for Kindergarten.* Carthage, IL: Fearon Teacher Aids, 1993.

Lamb, Beth, and Logsdon, Phyllis. *Positively Kindergarten: A Classroom-proven, Theme-based Developmental Guide for the Kindergarten Teacher.* Rosemont, NJ: Modern Learning Press, 1991.

Mallory, Bruce, and New, Rebecca, eds. *Diversity and Developmentally Appropriate Practices: Challenges for Early Childhood Education.* New York: Teachers College Press, 1994.

Miller, Karen. *Ages and Stages: Developmental Descriptions and Activities Birth Through Eight Years*. Chelsea, MA: Telshare Publishing Co., 1985.

National Association of Elementary School Principals. *Early Childhood Education and the Elementary School Principal*. Alexandria, VA: NAESP, 1990.

National Association of State Boards of Education. *Right from the Start: The Report of the NASBE Task Force on Early Childhood Education*. Alexandria, VA: NASBE, 1988.

Singer, Dorothy, and Revenson, Tracy. *How a Child Thinks: A Piaget Primer*. Independence, MO: International University Press, 1978.

Wood, Chip. *Yardsticks: Children in the Classroom Ages 4-14*. Greenfield, MA: Northeast Foundation for Children, 1997.

Grade Replacement

Ames, Louise Bates. *What Am I Doing in This Grade?* Rosemont, NJ: Modern Learning Press, 1985.

———. *Is Your Child in the Wrong Grade?* Rosemont, NJ: Modern Learning Press, 1978.

Ames, Louise Bates; Gillespie, Clyde; and Streff, John W. *Stop School Failure*. Rosemont, NJ: Modern Learning Press, 1972.

Grant, Jim. *Retention and Its Prevention: Making Informed Decisions About Individual Children*. Rosemont, NJ: Modern Learning Press, 1997.

Grant, Jim, and Richardson, Irv. *The Retention/Promotion Checklist (K-8)*. Peterborough, NH: Crystal Springs Books, 1998.

Hobby, Janice Hale. *Staying Back*. Gainesville, FL: Triad, 1990.

Moore, Sheila, and Frost, Roon. *The Little Boy Book*. New York: Clarkson N. Potter, 1986.

Inclusion / Differently Abled / Learning Disabilities

Dunn, Kathryn B., and Dunn, Allison B. *Trouble with School: A Family Story about Learning Disabilities*. Rockville, MD: Woodbine House, 1993.

Goodman, Gretchen. *I Can Learn! Strategies and Activities for Gray-Area Children*. Peterborough, NH: Crystal Springs Books, 1995.

———. *More I Can Learn!* Peterborough, NH: Crystal Springs Books, 1998.

———. *Inclusive Classrooms from A to Z: A Handbook for Educators*. Columbus, OH: Teachers' Publishing Group, 1994.

Irlen, Helen. *Reading by the Colors: Overcoming Dyslexia and Other Reading Disabilities Through the Irlen Method*. Garden City Park, NY: Avery Publishing Group Inc., 1991.

Lang, Greg, and Berberich, Chris. *All Children are Special: Creating an Inclusive Classroom*. York, ME: Stenhouse Publishers, 1995.

Phinney, Margaret. *Reading with the Troubled Reader*. Portsmouth, NH: Heinemann, 1989.

Rhodes, Lynn, and Dudley-Marling, Curtis. *Readers and Writers with a Difference: A Holistic Approach to Teaching Learning Disabled and Remedial Students*. Portsmouth: Heinemann, 1988.

Society For Developmental Education. *Creating Inclusive Classrooms: Education for All Children*. Peterborough, NH, 1994.

Vail, Priscilla. *About Dyslexia*. Rosemont, NJ: Programs for Education, 1990.

———. *Smart Kids with School Problems*. New York: E.P. Dutton, 1987.

The Internet (See pages 313-314 for internet resources)

Issues in Education

Barrs, Myra, and Pidgeon, Sue, eds. *Gender and Reading in Elementary Classrooms*. York, ME: Stenhouse Publishers, 1994.

Carbo, Marie. *What Every Principal Should Know About Teaching Reading: How to Raise Test Scores and Nurture and Love of Reading*. Syosset, NY: National Learning Styles Institute, 1997.

Cummings, Carol, Ph.D. *Managing a Diverse Classroom: Practical Ideas for Thematic Units, Reading and Writing, Learning Centers, and Assessments*. Edmonds, WA: Teaching, Inc., 1995.

DuVall, Rick. *Building Character & Community in the Classroom*. Cypress, CA: Creative Teaching Press, 1997.

Goodman, Kenneth S., ed. *In Defense of Good Teaching: What Teachers Need to Know About the "Reading Wars."* York, ME: Stenhouse Publishers, 1998.

Jensen, Eric. *Brain-Based Learning*. Del Mar, CA: Turning Point Publishing, 1996.

Ledell, Marjorie, and Arnsparger, Arleen. *How to Deal with Community Criticism of School Change*. Alexandria, VA: Association for Supervision and Curriculum Development, 1993.

Rasell, Edith, and Rothstein, Richard, eds. *School Choice: Examining the Evidence*. Washington, DC: Economic Policy Institute, 1993.

Wortman, Robert, and Matlin, Myna. *Leadership in Whole Language: The Principal's Role*. York, ME: Stenhouse Publishers, 1995.

Wortman, Robert. *Administrators Supporting School Change*. York, ME: Stenhouse Publishers, The Galef Institute, 1995.

Language Arts

Atwell, Nancie. *Coming to Know: Writing to Learn in the Middle Grades*. Portsmouth, NH: Heinemann, 1990.

———. *In the Middle: Writing, Reading, and Learning with Adolescents*. Portsmouth, NH: Heinemann, 1987.

———. *Side by Side: Essays on Teaching to Learn*. Portsmouth, NH: Heinemann, 1991.

———. *Workshop 1: Writing and Literature*. Portsmouth, NH: Heinemann, 1989.

———. *Workshop 2: Beyond the Basal*. Portsmouth, NH: Heinemann, 1989.

———. *Workshop 3: The Politics of Process*. Portsmouth, NH: Heinemann, 1991.

Bean, Wendy, and Bouffler, Chrys. *Read, Write, Spell*. York, ME: Stenhouse Publishers, 1997.

Beeler, Terri. *I Can Read! I Can Write! Creating a Print-Rich Environment*. Cypress, CA: Creative Teaching Press, 1993.

Bromley, Karen. *Journaling: Engagements in Reading, Writing, and Thinking*. New York: Scholastic, 1993.

Buros, Jay. *Why Whole Language?* Rosemont, NJ: Programs for Education, 1991.

Calkins, Lucy M. *The Art of Teaching Writing*. Portsmouth, NH: Heinemann, 1986.

———. *Living Between the Lines*. Portsmouth, NH: Heinemann, 1990.

Carbo, Marie. *What Every Principal Should Know About Teaching Reading: How to Raise Test Scores and Nurture a Love of Reading*. Syosset, NY: National Learning Styles Institute, 1997.

Carey, Patsy; Holzschuher, Cynthia; and Kilpatrick, Susan. *Activities for Any Literature Unit* (Primary). Huntington Beach, CA: Teacher Created Materials, Inc., 1995.

Chambers, Aidan. *The Reading Environment: How Adults Help Children Enjoy Books*. York, ME: Stenhouse Publishers, 1996.

———. *Tell Me: Children, Reading and Talk*. York, ME: Stenhouse Publishers, 1996.

Clay, Marie. *Becoming Literate*. Portsmouth, NH: Heinemann, 1991.

———. *Observing Young Readers*. Portsmouth, NH: Heinemann, 1982.

———. *Reading Recovery: A Guidebook for Teachers in Training*. Portsmouth, NH: Heinemann, 1993.

Cloonan, Kathryn L. *Sing Me A Story, Read Me A Song* (Books I and II). Beverly Hills, FL: Rhythm & Reading Resources, 1991.

———. *Whole Language Holidays*. (Books I and II). Beverly Hills, FL: Rhythm & Reading Resources, 1992.

Cunningham, Patricia, and Allington, Richard. *Classrooms That Work: They Can All Read & Write*. New York: HarperCollins College Publishers, 1994.

Daniels, Harvey. *Literature Circles: Voice and Choice in the Student-Centered Classroom*. York, ME: Stenhouse Publishers, 1994.

Einstein, Carol. *Be Your Own Reading Specialist: A Guide for Teachers of Grades 1-3*. Rosemont, NJ: Modern Learning Press, 1997.

Eisele, Beverly. *Managing the Whole Language Classroom: A Complete Teaching Resource Guide for K-6 Teachers*. Cypress, CA: Creative Teaching Press, 1991.

Fisher, Bobbi. *Joyful Learning: A Whole Language Kindergarten*. Portsmouth, NH: Heinemann, 1991.

Fountas, Irene C., and Pinnell, Gay Su. *Guided Reading: Good First Teaching for All Children*. Portsmouth, NH: Heinemann, 1996.

Frank, Marjorie. *If You're Trying to Teach Kids How to Write, You've Gotta Have This Book*. Nashville, TN: Incentive Publications, 1979.

Graves, Donald. *Build a Literate Classroom*. Portsmouth, NH: Heinemann, 1991.

———. *A Researcher Learns to Write*. Portsmouth, NH: Heinemann, 1984.

———. *Discover Your Own Literacy*. Portsmouth, NH: Heinemann, 1990.

———. *Experiment with Fiction*. Portsmouth, NH: Heinemann, 1990.

———. *Investigate Nonfiction*. Portsmouth, NH: Heinemann, 1989.

———. *Writing: Teachers and Children at Work*. Portsmouth, NH: Heinemann, 1983.

Goodman, Kenneth S., ed. *In Defense of Good Teaching: What Teachers Need to Know About the "Reading Wars."* York, ME: Stenhouse Publishers, 1998.

Haack, Pam, and Merrilees, Cynthia. *Ten Ways to Become a Better Reader*. Cleveland, OH: Modern Curriculum Press, 1991.

———. *Write on Target*. Peterborough, NH: The Society For Developmental Education, 1991.

Harvey, Stephanie. *Nonfiction Matters: Reading, Writing, and Research in Grades 3-8*. York, ME: Stenhouse Publishers, 1998.

Hetzel, June. *Responding to Literature: Activities to Use with Any Literature Selection*. Cypress, CA: Creative Teaching Press, Inc., 1993.

Johnson, Linda Mele. *Teaching Beginning Reading*. Torrance, CA: Fearon Teacher Aids, A Division of Frank Schaffer Publications, Inc., 1997.

Krensky, Stephen. *Write Away! One Author's Favorite Activities That Help Ordinary Writers Become Extraordinary Writers* (Grades 3-6). New York: Scholastic Inc., 1998.

Lamme, Linda. *Highlights for Children: Growing Up Reading*. Reston, VA: Acropolis Books, 1984.

———. *Growing Up Writing*. Reston, VA: Acropolis Books, 1984.

Lapin, Gloria. *Sight Word Stories: Alternate Strategies for Emergent Readers*. Torrance, CA: Fearon Teacher Aids, 1997.

McCarthy, Tara. *Descriptive Writing*. New York: Scholastic Inc., 1998.

———. *Expository Writing*. New York: Scholastic Inc., 1998.

———. *Narrative Writing* (Grades 4-8). New York: Scholastic Inc., 1998.

———. *Persuasive Writing* (Grades 4-8). New York: Scholastic Inc., 1998.

McTeague, Frank. *Shared Reading in the Middle and High School Years*. Portsmouth, NH: Heinemann, 1992.

Opitz, Michael F. *Flexible Grouping in Reading: Practical Ways to Help All Students Become Better Readers*. New York: Scholastic Inc., 1998.

Pavelka, Patricia. *Making the Connection: Learning Skills Through Literature (K-2)*. Peterborough, NH: Crystal Springs Books, 1995.

———. *Making the Connection: Learning Skills Through Literature (3-6)*. Peterborough, NH: Crystal Springs Books, 1997.

Picciotto, Linda Pierce. *Managing an Integrated Language Arts Classroom*. Ontario: Scholastic, 1995.

Pigdon, Keith, and Woolley, Marilyn. *The Big Picture: Integrating Children's Learning*. Portsmouth, NH: Heinemann, 1993.

Rief, Linda. *Seeking Diversity: Language Arts With Adolescents*. Portsmouth, NH: Heinemann, 1988.

———. *Invitations: Changing as Teachers and Learners K-12*. Portsmouth, NH: Heinemann, 1991.

———. *Literacy at the Crossroads: Crucial Talk About Reading, Writing, and Other Teaching Dilemmas*. Portsmouth, NH: Heinemann, 1996.

Samway, Katherine Davies, and Whang, Gail. *Literature Circles in a Multicultural Classroom*. York, ME: Stenhouse Publishers, 1996.

Sampson, Michael. *Pathways to Literacy*. New York: Holt, Rinehart & Winston, 1991.

Schell, Leo. *How to Create an Independent Reading Program*. New York: Scholastic Inc., 1991.

———. *Building Literacy with Interactive Charts*. New York: Scholastic Inc., 1991.

Span, Mary Beth. *26 Interactive Alphabet Mini-Books: Easy-to-Make Reproducible Books That Promote Literacy*. New York: Scholastic Inc., 1997.

Stitt, Neil. *Take Any Book: Hundreds of Activities to Develop Basic Learning Skills Using Any Book*. Torrance, CA: Fearon Teacher Aids, A Division of Frank Schaffer Publications, Inc., 1998.

Tarlow, Ellen. *Teaching Story Elements with Favorite Books: Creative and Engaging Activities to Explore Character, Plot, Setting, and Themes That Work With ANY Book!* New York: Scholastic Inc., 1998.

Wollman-Bonilla, Julie. *Response Journals*. New York: Scholastic Inc., 1991.

Language Arts — Bilingual

Samway, Katharine Davies, and Whang, Gail. *Literature Study Circles in a Multicultural Classroom*. York, ME: Stenhouse Publishers, 1996.

Whitmore, Kathryn F., and Crowell, Caryl G. *Inventing a Classroom: Life in a Bilingual, Whole Language Learning Community*. York, ME: Stenhouse Publishers, 1994.

Language Arts — Spelling and Phonics

Cunningham, Patricia M. *Phonics They Use: Words For Reading and Writing*. 2nd edition. New York: HarperCollins College Publishers, 1995.

Cunningham, Patricia M., and Hall, Dorothy P. *Making Big Words: Multilevel, Hands-On Spelling and Phonics Activities (Grades 3-6)*. Torrance, CA: Good Apple, A Division of Frank Schaffer Publications, 1994.

———. *Making More Big Words: Multilevel, Hands-On Phonics and Spelling Activities*. Torrance, CA: Good Apple, A Division of Frank Schaffer Publications, 1997.

———. *Making Words: Multilevel, Hands-On, Developmentally Appropriate Spelling and Phonics Activities*. Torrance, CA: Good Apple, A Division of Frank Schaffer Publications, 1994.

———. *Making More Words: Multilevel, Hands-On Phonics and Spelling Activities (Grades 1-3)*. Torrance, CA: Good Apple, A Division of Frank Schaffer Publications, 1997.

Dorn, Linda J.; French, Cathy; and Jones, Tammy. *Apprenticeship in Literature: Transitions Across Reading and Writing*. York, ME: Stenhouse Publishers, 1998.

Erickson, Rhonda. *The Amazing Alphabet Puppets*. Cypress, CA: Creative Teaching Press, 1995.

Fitzpatrick, Jo. *Phonemic Awareness: Playing With Sounds to Strengthen Beginning Reading Skills*. Cypress, CA: Creative Teaching Press, 1997.

Fry, Edward, Ph.D. *How to Teach Reading (for Teachers, Parents, Tutors)*. Laguna Beach, CA: Laguna Beach Educational Books, 1995.

———. *1000 Instant Words*. Laguna Beach, CA: Laguna Beach Educational Books, 1994.

———. *Phonics Patterns: Onset and Rhyme Word Lists*. Laguna Beach Educational Books, 1994.

Gentry, J. Richard. *My Kid Can't Spell*. Portsmouth, NH: Heinemann, 1996.

———. *Spel . . . Is a Four-Letter Word*. New York: Scholastic, 1987.

Gentry, J. Richard, and Gillet, Jean Wallace. *Teaching Kids to Spell*. Portsmouth, NH: Heinemann, 1993.

Hong, Min, and Stafford, Patsy. *Spelling Strategies That Work: Practical Ways to Motivate Students to Become Successful Spellers*. New York: Scholastic Inc., 1997.

McCracken, Marlene J. and Robert A. *Spelling Through Phonics* (Second Edition). Winnipeg, Canada: Peguis Publishers, 1996.

Scholastic Guide to Balanced Reading: Making It Work for You (Grades 3-6). New York: Scholastic Inc., 1993.

Trisler, Alana, and Cardiel, Patrice. *My Word Book.* Rosemont, NJ: Modern Learning Press, 1994.

———.*Words I Use When I Write.* Rosemont, NJ: Modern Learning Press, 1989.

———.*More Words I Use When I Write.* Rosemont, NJ: Modern Learning Press, 1990.

Wagstaff, Janiel. *Phonics That Work! New Strategies for the Reading/Writing Classroom.* New York: Scholastic Inc., 1995.

Learning Centers

Cook, Carole. *Math Learning Centers for the Primary Grades.* West Nynack, NY: The Center for Applied Research, 1992.

Ingraham, Phoebe Bell. *Creating and Managing Learning Centers: A Thematic Approach.* Peterborough, NH: Crystal Springs Books, 1996.

Isabell, Rebecca. *The Complete Learning Center Book.* Beltsville, MD: Gryphon House, 1995.

MacDonald, Sharon. *Squish, Sort, Paint & Build: Over 200 Easy Learning Center Activities.* Beltsville, MD: Gryphon House, 1996.

Marx, Pamela. *Classroom Museums: Touchable Tables for Kids!* New York: Scholastic Inc., 1992.

Morrow, Lesley Mandel. *The Literacy Center: Contexts for Reading and Writing.* York, ME: Stenhouse, 1997.

Learning Strategies / Multiple Intelligences

Armstrong, Thomas. *Multiple Intelligences in the Classroom.* Alexandria, VA: Association for Supervision and Curriculum Development, 1994.

Campbell, Bruce. *The Multiple Intelligences Handbook: Lesson Plans and More . . . .* Stanwood, WA: Campbell & Associates, 1994.

Campbell, Linda; Campbell, Bruce; and Dickinson, Dee. *Teaching and Learning Through Multiple Intelligences.* Needham Heights, MA: Allyn & Bacon, 1991.

Carriero, Paul. *Tales of Thinking: Multiple Intelligences in the Classroom.* York, ME: Stenhouse Publishers, 1998.

Chapman, Carolyn. *If the Shoe Fits . . . How to Develop Multiple Intelligences in the Classroom.* Arlington Heights, IL: IRI/Skylight Training and Publishing, Inc., 1993.

Gardner, Howard. *Frames of Mind: The Theory of Multiple Intelligences.* New York: Basic Books, 1985.

———. *Multiple Intelligences: The Theory in Practice.* New York: Basic Books, 1990.

———. *The Unschooled Mind: How Children Think and How Schools Should Teach.* New York: Basic Books, 1990.

Grant, Janet Millar. *Shake, Rattle and Learn: Classroom-Tested Ideas That Use Movement for Active Learning.* York, ME: Stenhouse Publishers, 1995.

Lazear, David. *Multiple Intelligence Approaches to Assessment: Solving the Assessment Conundrum.* IRI/Skylight Publishing, Inc., 1994.

———. *Seven Pathways of Learning: Teaching Students and Parents About Multiple Intelligences.* Tucson, AZ: Zephyr Press, 1994.

———. *Seven Ways of Knowing: Teaching for Multiple Intelligences.* Palatine, IL: IRI/Skylight Publishing, Inc., 1991.

———. *Seven Ways of Teaching: The Artistry of Teaching With Multiple Intelligences.* Palatine, IL: IRI/Skylight Publishing, Inc. 1991.

New City School Faculty. *Celebrating Multiple Intelligences: Teaching for Success.* St. Louis, MO: The New City School, Inc., 1994.

Short, Kathy G.; Schroder, Jean; Laird, Julie; Kauffman, Gloria; Ferguson, Margaret J.; and Crawford, Kathleen Marie. *Learning Together Through Inquiry: From Columbus to Integrated Curriculum.* York, ME: Stenhouse, 1996.

Vail, Priscilla. *Gifted, Precocious, or Just Plain Smart.* Rosemont, NJ: Programs for Education, 1987.

Looping

Forsten, Char. *The Multiyear Lesson Plan Book.* Peterborough, NH: Crystal Springs Books, 1996.

Forsten, Char; Grant, Jim; Johnson, Bob; and Richardson, Irv. *Looping Q&A: 72 Practical Answers to Your Most Pressing Questions.* Peterborough, NH: Crystal Springs Books, 1997.

Grant, Jim; Johnson, Bob; and Richardson, Irv. *The Looping Handbook: Teachers and Students Progressing Together.* Peterborough, NH: Crystal Springs Books, 1996.

Hanson, Barbara. "Getting to Know You: Multiyear Teaching," *Educational Leadership,* November 1995.

Jacoby, Deborah. "Twice the Learning and Twice the Love." *Teaching K-8,* March 1994.

Million, June. "To Loop or Not to Loop? This is a Question for Many Schools." *NAESP Communicator.* Vol. 18, Number 6, February 1996.

Multiage Education

American Association of School Administrators. *The Nongraded Primary: Making Schools Fit Children,* Arlington, VA, 1992.

Anderson, Robert H., and Pavan, Barbara Nelson. *Nongradedness: Helping It to Happen.* Lancaster, PA: Technomic Press, 1992.

Bingham, Anne A.; Dorta, Peggy; McClasky, Molly; and O'Keefe, Justine. *Exploring the Multiage Classroom.* York, ME: Stenhouse Publishers, 1995.

Bridge, Connie A.; Reitsma, Beverly S.; and Winograd, Peter N. *Primary Thoughts: Implementing Kentucky's Primary Program.* Lexington, KY: Kentucky Department of Education, 1993.

Burruss, Bette, and Fairchild, Nawanna. *The Primary School: A Resource Guide for Parents.* Lexington, KY: The Prichard Committee for Academic Excellence and The Partnership for Kentucky School Reform, 1993. PO Box 1658, Lexington, KY 40592-1658, 800-928-2111.

Chase, Penelle, and Doan, Joan. *Full Circle: A New Look at Multiage Education.* Portsmouth, NH: Heinemann, 1994.

Davies, Anne; Politano, Colleen; and Gregory, Kathleen. *Together is Better.* Winnipeg, Canada: Peguis Publishers, 1993.

Fogarty, Robin, ed. *The Multiage Classroom: A Collection.* Palantine, IL: Skylight Publishing, 1993.

Gaustad, Joan. "Making the Transition From Graded to Nongraded Primary Education." *Oregon School Study Council Bulletin,* 35(8), 1992.

———."Nongraded Education: Mixed-Age, Integrated and Developmentally Appropriate Education for Primary Children." *Oregon School Study Council Bulletin,* 35(7), 1992.

———."Nongraded Education: Overcoming Obstacles to Implementing the Multiage Classroom." 38(3,4) *Oregon School Study Council Bulletin,* 1994.

Gayfer, Margaret, ed. *The Multi-grade Classroom: Myth and Reality.* Toronto: Canadian Education Association, 1991.

Goodlad, John I., and Anderson, Robert H. *The Nongraded Elementary School.* New York: Teachers College Press, 1987.

Grant, Jim, and Johnson, Bob. *A Common Sense Guide to Multiage Practices.* Columbus, OH: Teachers' Publishing Group, 1995.

Grant, Jim; Johnson, Bob; and Richardson, Irv. *Multiage Q&A: 101 Practical Answers to Your Most Pressing Questions.* Peterborough, NH: Crystal Springs Books, 1995.

———. *Our Best Advice: The Multiage Problem Solving Handbook.* Peterborough, NH: Crystal Springs Books, 1996.

Grant, Jim and Richardson, Irv, compilers. *Multiage Handbook: A Comprehensive Resource for Multiage Practices.* Peterborough, NH: Crystal Springs Books, 1996.

Gutierrez, Roberto, and Slavin, Robert E. *Achievement Effects of the Nongraded Elementary School: A Retrospective Review.* Baltimore, MD: Center for Research on Effective Schooling for Disadvantaged Students, 1992.

Hunter, Madeline. *How to Change to a Nongraded School.* Alexandria, VA: Association for Supervision and Curriculum Development, 1992.

Kasten, Wendy, and Clarke, Barbara. *The Multi-age Classroom.* Katonah, NY: Richard Owen, 1993.

Katz, Lilian G.; Evangelou, Demetra; and Hartman, Jeanette Allison. *The Case for Mixed-Age Grouping in Early Education.* Washington, DC: National Association for the Education of Young Children, 1990.

Maeda, Bev. *The Multi-Age Classroom*. Cypress, CA: Creative Teaching Press, 1994.

Miller, Bruce A. *Children at the Center: Implementing the Multiage Classroom*. Portland, OR: Northwest Regional Educational Laboratory, 1994.

———. *The Multigrade Classroom: A Resource Handbook for Small, Rural Schools*. Portland, OR: Northwest Regional Educational Laboratory, 1989.

———. *Training Guide for the Multigrade Classroom: A Resource for Small, Rural Schools*. Portland, OR: Northwest Regional Laboratory, 1990.

National Education Association. *Multiage Classrooms*. NEA Teacher to Teacher Books, 1995.

Ostrow, Jill. *A Room With a Different View: First Through Third Graders Build Community and Create Curriculum*. York, ME: Stenhouse Publishers, 1995.

Politano, Colleen, and Davies, Anne. *Multi-Age and More*. Winnipeg, Canada: Peguis Publishers, 1994.

Rathbone, Charles; Bingham, Anne; Dorta, Peggy; McClaskey, Molly; and O'Keefe, Justine. *Multiage Portraits: Teaching and Learning in Mixed-age Classrooms*. Peterborough, NH: Crystal Springs Books, 1993.

Stone, Sandra J. *Creating the Multiage Classroom*. Indianapolis, IN: ScottForesman, GoodYearBooks, 1996.

Virginia Education Association and Appalachia Educational Laboratory. *Teaching Combined Grade Classes: Real Problems and Promising Practices*. Charleston, WV: Appalachian Educational Laboratory, 1990.

Parent Involvement / Resources for Parents

Bluestein, Jane, and Collins, Lynn. *Parents in a Pressure Cooker*. Rosemont, NJ: Modern Learning Press, 1990.

Elkind, David, Ph.D. *Reinventing Childhood: Raising and Educating Children in a Changing World*. Rosemont, NJ: Modern Learning Press, Inc., 1998.

Elovson, Allanna. *The Kindergarten Survival Book*. Santa Monica, CA: Parent Ed Resources, 1991.

Grant, Jim, and Azen, Margot. *Every Parent's Owner's Manuals. (Three-, Four-, Five-, Six-, Seven-Year- Old)*. Rosemont, NJ. Programs for Education. 16 pages each manual.

Henderson, Anne T.; Marburger, Carl L.; and Ooms, Theodora. *Beyond the Bake Sale: An Educator's Guide to Working with Parents*. Columbia, MD: National Committee for Citizens in Education, 1990.

Karnofsky, Florence, and Weiss, Trudy. *How to Prepare Your Child for Kindergarten*. Carthage, IL: Fearon Teacher Aids, 1993.

Lansky, Vicki. *Divorce Book for Parents*. New York: New American Library, 1989.

Lazear, David. *Seven Pathways of Learning: Teaching Students and Parents About Multiple Intelligences*. Tucson, AZ: Zephyr Press, 1994.

Picciotto, Linda Pierce. *Student-Led Parent Conferences: How to Launch and Manage Conferences that Get Parents Involved and Improve Student Learning*. New York: Scholastic Inc., 1996.

Vopat, James. *The Parent Project: A Workshop Approach to Parent Involvement*. York, ME: Stenhouse Publishers, 1994.

Teachers and Teaching

Fujawa, Judy. *(Almost) Everything You Need to Know About Early Childhood Education*. Beltsville, MD: Gryphon House, Inc., 1998.

Norris, Dennis M. *Get a Grant: Yes You Can!* New York: Scholastic Inc., 1998.

Northern Nevada Writing Project Teacher-Researcher Group. *Team Teaching*. York, ME: Stenhouse, 1996.

Terry, Alice. *Every Teacher's Guide to Classroom Management*. Cypress, CA: Creative Teaching Press, 1997.

Woodfin, Linda. *Familiar Ground: Traditions That Build School Community*. Greenfield, MA: Northeast Foundation for Children, 1998.

Thematic Learning and Teaching

Borst, Donna, ed. *Quick and Easy Teacher Tips*. Torrance, CA: Good Apple, A Division of Frank Schaffer Publications, 1998.

Eagan, Robynne. *Celebrate 2000: Two Thousand Things to Think About, Learn and Do for the Year 2000*. Carthage, IL: Teaching & Learning Company, 1998.

Eagan, Robynne, and Schofield, Tracey Ann. *Weather Wise: Creative Activities About the Environment* (Grades 1-4). Carthage, IL: Teaching & Learning Company, 1997.

Flagg, Ann. *Apples, Pumpkins and Harvest: Ready-to-Go Activities, Games, Literature Selections, Poetry and Everything You Need for a Complete Theme Unit* (K-1). New York: Scholastic Inc., 1998.

———. *Weather: Ready-to-Go Activities, Games, Literature Selections, Poetry and Everything You Need for a Complete Theme Unit* (K-1). New York: Scholastic Inc., 1997.

Flemming, Maria. *Homes: Ready-to-Go Activities, Games, Literature Selections, Poetry and Everything You Need for a Complete Theme Unit* (K-1). New York: Scholastic Inc., 1997.

Herr, Judy, and Libby, Yvonne. *Creative Resources for the Early Childhood Classroom*. Albany, NY: Delmar, 1990.

Kurth, Mary J. *Kindergarten Themes*. Cypress, CA: Creative Teaching Press, 1998.

McCarthy, Tara. *150 Thematic Writing Activities*. New York: Scholastic Inc., 1993.

Schlosser, Kristin. *Thematic Units for Kindergarten*. New York: Scholastic Inc., 1994.

Silk, Courtney. *Colors: Ready-to-Go Activities, Games, Literature Selections, Poetry and Everything You Need for a Complete Theme Unit* (K-1). New York: Scholastic Inc., 1997.

Strube, Penny. *Theme Units for Kindergarten*. NY: Scholastic Inc., 1994.

Thompson, Gare. *Teaching Through Themes*. New York: Scholastic Inc., 1991.

West, Tracey. *5 Senses: Ready-to-Go Activities, Games, Literature Selections, Poetry and Everything You Need for a Complete Theme Unit* (K-1). New York: Scholastic Inc., 1997.

Tracking / Untracking

Daniels, Harvey, and Bizar, Marilyn. *Methods That Matter: Six Structures for Best Practice Classrooms*. York, ME: Stenhouse Publishers, 1998.

George, Paul. *How to Untrack Your School*. Alexandria, VA.: Association for Supervision and Curriculum Development, 1992.

Kohn, Alfie. *No Contest: The Case Against Competition*. Boston, MA: Houghton Mifflin, 1992.

Kozol, Jonathan. *Savage Inequalities: Children in America's Schools*. New York: Crown, 1991.

Oakes, Jeannie. *Keeping Track: How Schools Structure Equality*. New Haven: Yale University Press, 1985.

Tomlinson, Carol Ann. *How to Differentiate Instruction in Mixed-Ability Classrooms*. Alexandria, VA: Association for Supervision and Curriculum Development, 1995.

Wheelock, Anne. *Crossing the Tracks: How "Untracking" Can Save America's Schools*. New York: New Press, 1992.

Index

NOTES

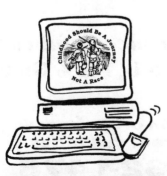
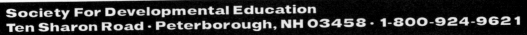

Mark your calendar now for the best multiage conference in the country!

The Society For
Developmental Education's

7th Annual
National Conference on
Multiage & Looping Practices

July 18-21, 1999 · Columbus, Ohio

Four days of comprehensive instruction focused on meeting your professional development needs

➢ Over 100 nationally renowned presenters and practitioners

➢ More than 200 sessions on teacher-requested topics

➢ Dozens of new ideas and 1,000+ pages of handouts

➢ Choice of basic, intermediate or advanced sessions

➢ Networking opportunities with fellow educators from around the country

This conference is designed to meet the needs of professionals working in multiage as well as single-grade classrooms:

✦ Multiage Classroom Teachers (K-6)

✦ Single-grade Classroom Teachers (K-6)

✦ Special Education Teachers

✦ Principals & Superintendents

✦ Title I Teachers & Directors

✦ Curriculum Coordinators

✦ Directors of Instruction

✦ Inservice/Staff Development Coordinators

✦ Early Childhood Specialists

✦ Instructional Aides & Support Staff

Recertification and Graduate Credit Options are available

Committed to helping you create successful classrooms and students — Your Satisfaction is 100% Guaranteed

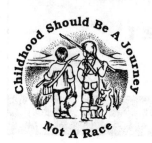

For more information or to reserve your space risk-free, call today

1-800-462-1478

The Society For Developmental Education
Ten Sharon Road, PO Box 577, Peterborough, NH 03458

Primary Grades Teachers — Join us in the summer of '99 for

The 2nd Annual National Conference for PreK-Grade 3 Educators

August 1-4, 1999 · Atlanta, Georgia

Dozens of hand-picked sessions on the critical issues facing primary teachers today, including:

- ➤ Guided Reading
- ➤ Writing
- ➤ Phonics
- ➤ Themes & Centers

- ➤ Struggling Learners
- ➤ Multiple Intelligence
- ➤ Assessment
- ➤ *And much more!*

Other Benefits of Attending:

- Comprehensive workshop handouts including *Into Teachers' Hands: Creating Classroom Success*, SDE's 11th annual sourcebook
- Nationally recognized trainers with teacher-tested ideas and strategies
- Pre-conference Institute with keynote presentation and luncheon
- Outstanding Book Fair and Exhibits

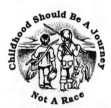

Call today for more information or to enroll risk-free!

1-800-462-1478

The Society For Developmental Education
Ten Sharon Road, PO Box 577, Peterborough, NH 03458

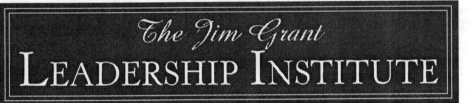

The Jim Grant
LEADERSHIP INSTITUTE

Enhancing Your Effectiveness as an Administrator, Educator and Leader

> Share this Institute information with your school administrator

A powerful three-day conference designed to focus on the most pressing issues facing you today as an educational leader. Guaranteed to learn practical solutions to your real-world problems.

- ■ World-class presenters
- ■ Timely topics
- ■ Recertification and graduate credit

- ■ Networking opportunities
- ■ One-on-one consultations available
- ■ Inservice training options

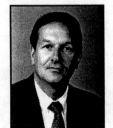

Join us in one of the following 4 locations in 1999:

- ☑ New Orleans - Winter
- ☑ New England - Summer

- ☑ San Antonio - Summer
- ☑ Washington, DC - Fall

For more information on the Jim Grant Leadership Institute call 1-800-462-1478

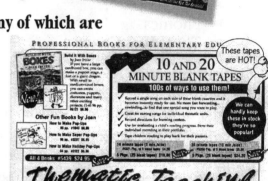
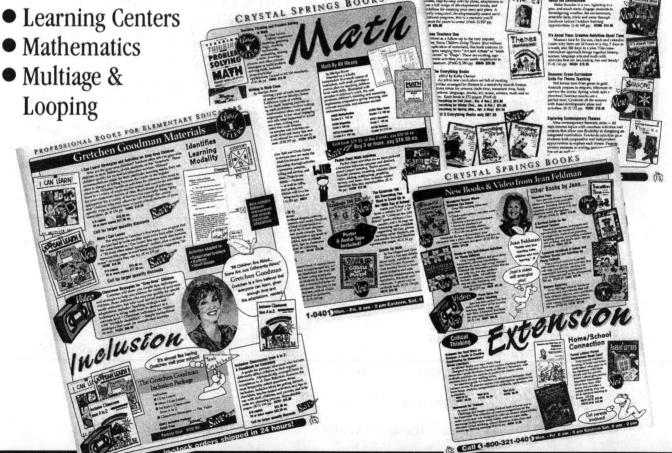